AF680234

CardioPREP

For DM/DNB Cardiology Aspirants (INICET SS/NEET SS)

Compiled by

Dr Asharam Panda

MBBS, MD Medicine(PGIMER Chandigarh),

DM Cardiology (AIIMS New Delhi)

notionpress
.com

INDIA • SINGAPORE • MALAYSIA

ISBN 979-8-90392-936-8

First Edition: 2026
Printed in India

Message for the Readers

- This book is a concise compilation of essential information specifically intended for INICET SS/ NEET SS examination, presented in a structured and reader-friendly manner. It is intended as an aid for the entrance examination and **not** as a substitute for standard textbooks.
- Many readers who have already gone through the recommended textbooks may use this for rapid revision. If you haven't yet covered the textbooks, don't be disheartened—these summaries aim to bring together almost all commonly tested topics in a clear and approachable manner.
- All summaries are prepared from the latest editions of standard textbooks and current guidelines. Topics have been selected based on their relevance and frequency in entrance examinations. However, given the continuously evolving nature of medical evidence and guidelines, minor discrepancies may be unavoidable.
- The MCQs are inspired by previous years' INI-CET SS and NEET SS questions, with several questions framed to reflect the expected difficulty level of these examinations.
- We sincerely welcome feedback, suggestions, and error corrections, and are always happy to provide academic support.
- Communicate at cardioprep2026@gmail.com and get updated summary of landmark trials.

Dr Asharam Panda

cardioprep2026@gmail.com

Acknowledgement

I sincerely thank my mentors for guiding my academic journey with their wisdom and encouragement. I am equally grateful to my patients and students, who continue to be my greatest teachers, constantly shaping my understanding and growth.

While many have contributed to this effort, the true strength behind this book is my family. I am deeply grateful to my parents and my wife, *Dr Priyanka*, for their unwavering support, patience, and understanding at every step of this journey. And to my baby *Aavisa*, whose innocent smiles have been my greatest source of joy, strength, and constant motivation throughout.

Special contribution

I extend my heartfelt thanks to Dr Kritesh, Dr Manna, Dr Vijay, Dr Seshkaran, Dr Viswajit, and Dr Vishal for their valuable support in preparing this manuscript and for their constant encouragement and moral support throughout the process.

Contents

MCQ Level I

1. In which of the following conditions should VSD not be closed?
   A. VSD with irreversible severe PAH
   B. H/o infective endocarditis
   C. infant with heart failure
   D. Qp: Qs>2
2. Underlying mechanism of arrhythmogenesis in Long QT syndrome?
   A. EAD
   B. DAD
   C. Enhanced automaticity
   D. Prolonged action potential duration
3. Which is a common cause of ostial LMCA stenosis?
   A. Aortoarteritis
   B. Syphilis
   C. Familial hypercholesterolemia
   D. All of the above
4. Which is not an example of idiopathic VT?
   A. Fascicular VT
   B. RVOT VT
   C. Brugada syndrome
   D. Papillary muscle VT
5. False about outflow tract (RVOT) VT?
   A. Vagal manoeuvre and adenosine may terminate
   B. Positive in inferior leads
   C. Suppressed during exercise
   D. Amenable for ablation
6. Bidirectional VT – false is?
   A. Digitalis toxicity predisposes
   B. Frontal axis changes from (-60 to -90 degrees) to (+120 to +130 degrees)
   C. Alternate RBBB and LBBB
   D. CPVT is a cause

7. Exercise precipitates VT in?
   A. RVOT VT
   B. LQTS
   C. CPVT
   D. All of the above
8. Idiopathic ventricular tachycardia includes?
   A. RVOT VT
   B. Annular VT
   C. Papillary muscle VT
   D. All of the above
9. Not a cause of acquired long QT?
   A. Hypokalemia
   B. Quinidine
   C. Digoxin toxicity
   D. MVP
10. Which is not a QT-opathy?
    A. Idiopathic VF
    B. Triadon knockout syndrome
    C. Timothy syndrome
    D. Ankyrin-B syndrome
11. M-FACT risk stratification score for?
    A. LQTS
    B. SQTS
    C. Brugada syndrome
    D. Early repolarization
12. Indication of ICD therapy in LQTS are all except?
    A. Recurrent syncope despite beta blocker
    B. SCD survivor on beta blocker therapy
    C. All SCD survivor without beta blocker therapy
    D. Very high QT interval (>550)

13. False statement regarding digoxin?

    A. It can be used safely in acute coronary syndrome

    B. Hypokalemia worsens arrhythmic side effects

    C. DIG trial showed no mortality benefit in heart failure patients

    D. Half-life is 36-48 hrs

14. Digoxin toxicity: all are true except

    A. Nausea and vomiting

    B. Bradycardia and AV block

    C. Non-paroxysmal atrial tachycardia

    D. Increased AV conduction

15. True statement regarding management of digoxin toxicity?

    A. Phenytoin and lidocaine are useful for tachyarrhythmia

    B. Cardioversion usually safe

    C. Magnesium sulfate usually safe to suppress tachycardia

    D. Dig-Fab immunotherapy not very useful

16. Most characteristic arrhythmic complication of digoxin toxicity?

    A. Non -paroxysmal atrial tachycardia with AV block

    B. Bidirectional VT

    C. Complete AV block

    D. Frequent VPC

17. Which isn't a new revision in the modified Jones criteria 2015

    A. Subclinical carditis

    B. Different CRP cut-off for low and high-risk populations

    C. Monoarthritis as a major criterion

    D. Definition of fever

18. False statement regarding acute rheumatic carditis?

    A. The commonest manifestation of ARF

    B. Higher chances of RHD with severe carditis

    C. Pericarditis common

    D. Surgery is indicated in refractory heart failure

19. Which of the following echocardiographic features is not included in the manifestation of subclinical carditis as per the modified Jones criteria?

    A. Early diastolic jet in pathologic AR

    B. Pansystolic jet in pathologic MR

    C. Colour jet visible in at least 2 views

    D. High velocity colour jet

20. Most specific manifestation of Acute Rheumatic Fever?

    A. Erythema marginatum

    B. Carditis

    C. Polyarthritis

    D. S.C nodules

21. Major focus of the revised Jones criteria (2015) for the diagnosis of Acute Rheumatic Fever?

    A. Subclinical carditis by ECHO Doppler

    B. Low-grade fever

    C. Geographic variation of the prevalence of RHD

    D. Monoarthritis as a major criterion

22. What is the common cause of diastolic dysfunction?

    A. Hyperthermia

    B. CAD

    C. VHD

    D. All of the above

23. Which of the following drugs has shown mortality benefit in Heart failure with preserved EF(HFpEF)?

    A. Metoprolol

    B. Spironolactone

    C. Hydralazine

    D. None

24. MPI (Myocardial performance index) false is?

    A. (IVCT+IVRT)/ET

    B. Reflect both systolic and diastolic function

    C. More than 0.5 is considered abnormal

    D. Systolic dysfunction decreases MPI

25. The first coronary angiogram was done in human by?
    A. Monitz
    B. Forssman
    C. Mason sones
    D. Andreas gruentzig
26. All of the following cardiac structures have a dual blood supply, except?
    A. Interventricular septum
    B. Left posterior fascicle
    C. Anterolateral papillary muscle
    D. Left anterior fascicle
27. Causes of bidirectional VT, all except?
    A. Digoxin toxicity
    B. CPVT
    C. Aconite poisoning
    D. Flecainide toxicity
28. False statement regarding Tetralogy of Fallot (TOF) physiology?
    A. RV pressure is systemic
    B. VSD is usually non-restrictive
    C. Left axis deviation is common
    D. PS usually severe
29. Side effects seen with SGLT2 inhibitors, all except?
    A. Ketoacidosis
    B. Hypoglycemia
    C. UTI
    D. Bone fracture
30. Which drug class has shown mortality benefit in both HFrEF & HFpEF?
    A. SGLT2 inhibitors
    B. ACE inhibitors
    C. Beta blocker
    D. Hydralazine nitrate

31. High-intensity statin reduces serum LDL level by?

    A. 20%

    B. 50%

    C. 95%

    D. 90%

32. Device closure is useful in?

    A. OS-ASD

    B. OP-ASD

    C. SV-ASD

    D. CS-ASD

33. Commonly described pathogenesis of acute coronary syndrome, all except?

    A. Plaque disruption

    B. Plaque erosion

    C. Calcified nodules

    D. Plaque hematoma

34. What is the most common cause of sudden cardiac death (SCD)?

    A. CAD

    B. LQTS

    C. HOCM

    D. Idiopathic

35. Which of the following risk factors has the highest attributable risk for cardiovascular disease (CVD)?

    A. Hypertension

    B. Diabetes mellitus

    C. Smoking

    D. Elevated LDL

36. The resting membrane potential (RMP) of cardiac myocytes is determined by?

    A. K+

    B. Na+

    C. Ca2+

    D. Cl-

37. What is the best modality to assess the depth of coronary calcium?

   A. Angiography

   B. IVUS

   C. OCT

   D. Angioscopy

38. Wrongly matched antidote?

   A. Apixaban- Idarucizumab

   B. Digoxin-Digibind Ab

   C. Dabigatran-Idarucizumab

   D. Flecainide- sodium bicarbonate

39. Cyanosis with a structurally normal heart, all except?

   A. PAVM

   B. Extracardiac TAPVC

   C. V/Q mismatch

   D. Methemoglobinemia

40. Congenital complete heart block (CHB) is commonly associated with all except?

   A. AVSD

   B. TOF

   C. Single ventricle

   D. Maternal autoimmune disease

41. False statement regarding Eisenmenger syndrome?

   A. Starts early in life

   B. Rare in ASD

   C. C/I for surgical closure of VSD

   D. Device closure can be done with PDA

42. Pregnancy is usually well tolerated in?

   A. Severe MR

   B. Severe PAH

   C. Severe MS

   D. Marfanoid with Aortic aneurysm

43. Are all causes of continuous murmur except?

    A. VSD with AR

    B. RSOV

    C. BT shunt

    D. Coronary AV fistula

44. ECG abnormality in Ebstein anomaly?

    A. Himalayan P wave

    B. Pre-excitation

    C. RBBB

    D. All of the above

45. The following are common causes of neonatal LV dysfunction, except?

    A. Critical aortic stenosis

    B. Coarctation of the aorta

    C. ALCAPA (anomalous origin of the left coronary artery from the pulmonary artery)

    D. Birth asphyxia

46. ARNI compared to ACE inhibitors is false?

    A. More hypotension

    B. More renal dysfunction

    C. More hyperkalemia

    D. More mortality benefit

47. Which of the following drug has atrial fibrillation as an adverse effect?

    A. Ivabradine

    B. Flecainide

    C. Ibutilide

    D. Amiodarone

48. What is false about the Bicuspid aortic valve (BAV)?

    A. AS is more common than AR

    B. Most common CHD

    C. RCC-NCC fusion common

    D. Aortopathy associated

49. Which antianginal is useful in diabetes with a HbA1c-lowering effect?
    A. Ranolazine
    B. Ivabradine
    C. Trimetazidine
    D. Nicorandil
50. Which is a metabolic antianginal?
    A. Ivabradine
    B. Trimetazidine
    C. Nicorandil
    D. Statins
51. Cyanosis is seen in all except?
    A. Gerbode defect
    B. Pulmonary AVF
    C. Eisenmenger syndrome
    D. TAPVC
52. Which of the following drug is most preferred in resistant HTN?
    A. Spironolactone
    B. Prazosin
    C. Clonidine
    D. ARNI
53. Systolic area index is useful in distinguishing –
    A. PAH
    B. Chronic constrictive pericarditis
    C. Diastolic heart failure
    D. RV dysfunction
54. False about CCTGA-
    A. May be associated with congenital CHB
    B. May be associated with VSD -PS
    C. RV faces systemic circulation
    D. LV fails early

55. The resting membrane potential of a myocardial cell is-

    A. -80 to -90

    B. +80 t0 +90

    C. -60 to -70

    D. -20 to -30

56. The correct statement while choosing a bioprosthetic Vs a mechanical heart valve is-

    A. Bioprosthetic degeneration is higher in the aortic than mitral position

    B. Higher rate of degeneration in younger patients

    C. Life-long anticoagulation with a bioprosthetic valve

    D. A bioprosthetic valve is preferred in younger individuals

57. An adolescent with a large VSD and exertional cyanosis. Which is a false statement regarding the treatment of this condition

    A. VSD closure should be advised

    B. Anticoagulation usually avoided

    C. Pulmonary vasodilators may be useful

    D. Survival is better than idiopathic PAH

58. Which condition doesn't warrant antibiotic prophylaxis before a bacteremic dental procedure?

    A. Small PDA

    B. Post Fontan palliation

    C. History of IE

    D. Mechanical heart valve

59. School-going girl with restrictive perimembranous VSD. What is the correct advice for management?

    A. Antibiotic prophylaxis before a dental procedure

    B. Close follow-up with echocardiography

    C. Both A and B

    D. Prophylactic closure

60. Which of the valve needs focused monitoring following TOF repair

    A. Pulmonary

    B. Aortic

    C. Mitral

    D. Tricuspid

61. Most common reoperation/intervention following corrective surgery for TOF

    A. Pulmonary valve intervention

    B. Residual vsd

    C. Pulmonary valvotomy

    D. Aortic valve intervention

62. Which is not a common association of a bicuspid aortic valve (BAV)?

    A. Coarctation of the aorta

    B. Aortopathy

    C. Coronary anomaly

    D. Parachute mitral valve

63. Which is a complication of isolated corrected TGA(CCTGA)

    A. AV block

    B. Heart failure

    C. Cyanosis

    D. Both A and B

64. The Ross procedure is useful in

    A. Aortic stenosis in young patients

    B. Pulmonary stenosis

    C. Pulmonary stenosis

    D. Tricuspid atresia

65. Treppe phenomena involve

    A. Increased contractility with increased heart rate

    B. Increased contractility with increased afterload

    C. Increased contractility with increased preload

    D. Decreased contractility with increased heart rate

66. Pansystolic murmur is seen in all except

    A. Traumatic TR

    B. VSD

    C. Rheumatic MR

    D. High-pressure TR

67. All are diabetogenic except

    A. Atenolol

    B. Chlorthalidone

    C. Statin

    D. Ranolazine

68. Which is not seen during exercise

    A. Increased cardiac output

    B. Increased mean blood pressure

    C. Increased total peripheral resistance

    D. Increase in systolic blood pressure

69. Which non-invasive modality has the least diagnostic value for detecting CAD in patients with stable ischemic heart disease

    A. Stress ECG

    B. SPECT MPI

    C. Stress echocardiography

    D. CT coronary angiography

70. Cyanosis is seen commonly in all except

    A. Truncus arteriosus

    B. AV canal defect

    C. Single ventricle

    D. Common atrium

71. The most common cause of sudden cardiac death

    A. CAD

    B. HOCM

    C. Coronary anomalies

    D. Channelopathies

72. Parenteral adenosine is not used in

    A. FFR measurement

    B. IFR measurement

    C. Stress MPI

    D. Termination of SVT

73. The lowest oxygen saturation (SpO2) is seen in

A. Coronary sinus

B. SVC

C. IVC

D. Renal vein

74. Chest X-ray after permanent pacemaker implantation. What should be the next line of management?

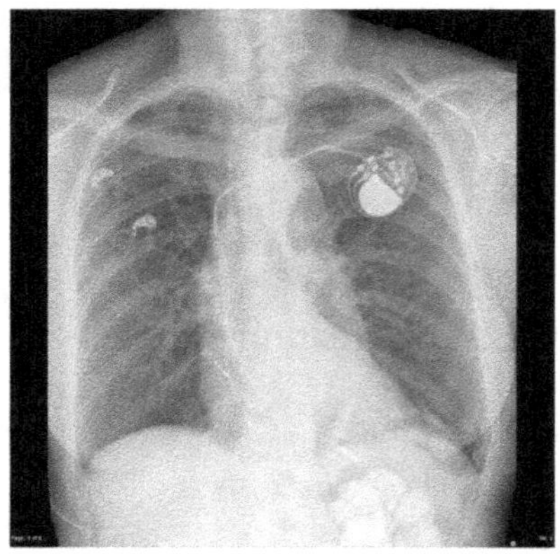

A. Urgent angiography

B. Echocardiography

C. High flow Oxygen

D. Lead revision

75. Ventricular arrhythmia depicted in the ECG is seen in all of the following conditions except-

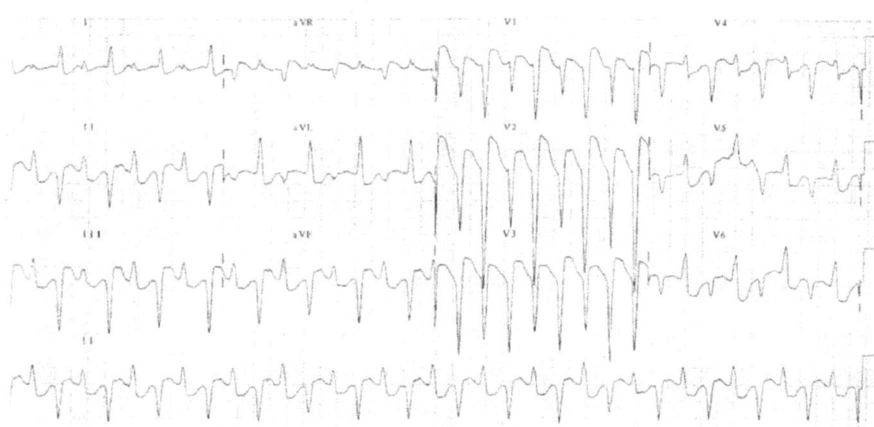

A. Aconite poisoning

B. CPVT

C. Digitalis toxicity

D. LQT3

76. Which is not a management strategy of chronic thromboembolic PAH(CTEPH)

    A. Pulmonary endarterectomy

    B. Riociguat

    C. Pulmonary balloon angioplasty

    D. Pulmonary sympathetic denervation

77. Disparity in pulse between the right and left upper limbs is seen in all except

    A. Takayasu

    B. Supravalvular AS

    C. Aortic dissection

    D. Kyphoscoliosis

78. Which is not an example of drug interaction?

    A. Digoxin and verapamil

    B. Pravastatin and ketoconazole

    C. Sildenafil and NTG

    D. Amiodarone and digoxin

79. Extra heart sound heard after S2 can't be-

    A. Ejection click

    B. Opening snap

    C. Pericardial knock

    D. S3

80. Renal artery stenosis is commonly seen in –

    A. Neurofibromatosis

    B. William syndrome

    C. Turner syndrome

    D. Marfan syndrome

81. Not a minor criterion in the modified Jones criteria for acute rheumatic fever-

    A. Polyarthralgia

    B. Monoarthritis

    C. ESR> 60

    D. Fever > 38 degrees

82. Cardiomyopathy caused by a mutation of the Desmosomal protein
    A. ARVC
    B. EMF
    C. RCMP
    D. Non-sarcomeric HCM
83. The most common congenital heart disease at birth
    A. ASD
    B. VSD
    C. TOF
    D. TGA
84. Which drug is usually withheld before coronary angioplasty
    A. Metformin
    B. Ramipril
    C. Statin
    D. Metoprolol
85. ACE inhibitor of choice in hepatic failure
    A. Lisinopril
    B. Ramipril
    C. Enalapril
    D. Perindopril
86. All are seen normally in old age, except
    A. Narrow pulse pressure
    B. S3
    C. Stiff aorta
    D. High diastolic blood pressure
87. Drugs which doesn't affect the bypass tract in WPW syndrome
    A. Verapamil
    B. Flecainide
    C. Amiodarone
    D. Quinidine

88. Poor prognostic factor during exercise stress test, all except

A. Hypotension

B. Persistent ST depression 5min post exercise

C. ST elevation

D. Failure to attain the target BP

89. Rotational atherectomy is useful in

A. Calcified lesion

B. Bifurcation

C. Ostial LM stenosis

D. Thrombotic lesion

90. Cancer with the highest propensity to metastasise to the heart

A. Ca breast

B. Melanoma

C. Osteosarcoma

D. Thyroid tumor

91. 34-year-old female with progressive pedal oedema and ascites. The most likely diagnosis is-

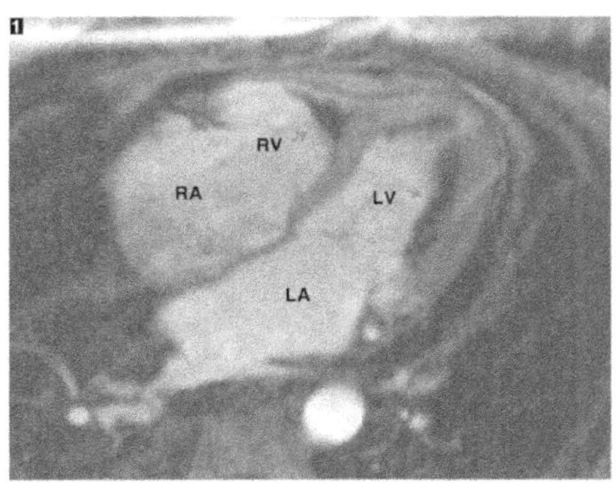

A. Endomyocardial fibrosis (EMF)

B. Apical HCM

C. Ebstein anomaly

D. Cardiac amyloidosis

92. A 72-year-old male with rest angina for 2 hours presents to casualty with the following ECG. Most likely site of coronary occlusion is

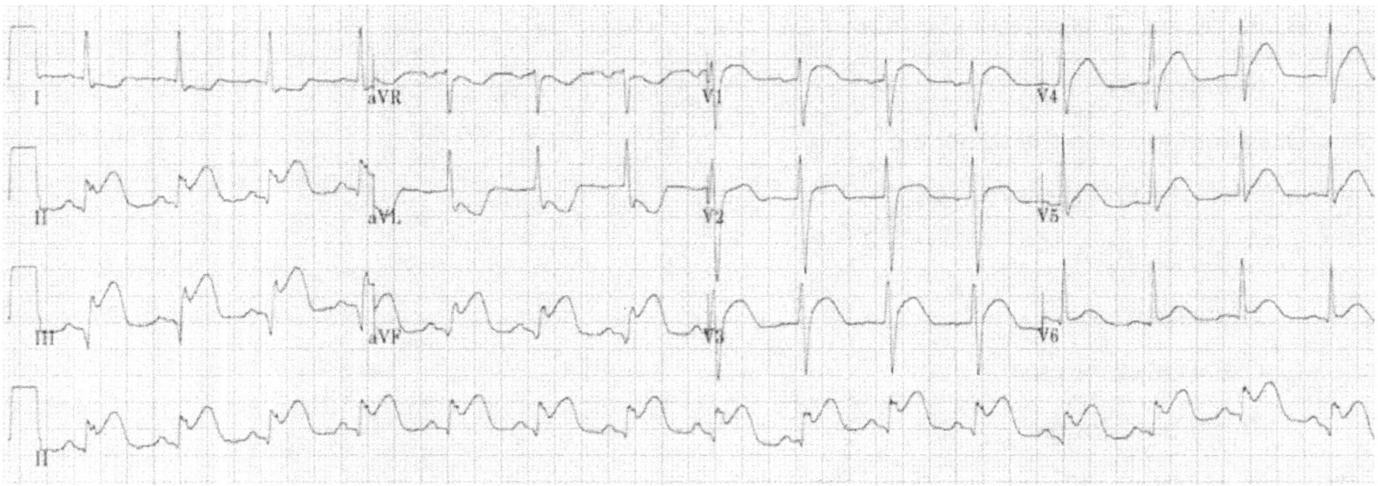

A. Proximal RCA

B. Proximal LCX

C. LAD

D. Distal LCX

93. The most common arrhythmia in infancy and childhood is

A. AVNRT

B. AVRT

C. CHB

D. Torsades

94. Drug of choice for recurrent pericarditis

A. NSAID

B. Corticosteroid

C. Methotrexate

D. Colchicine

95. Straightened left heart border in CXR, all except-

A. CCTGA

B. Severe MS

C. Absent pericardium

D. Tricuspid atresia

96. Balloon atrial septostomy (BAS)- most commonly done in

A. D-TGA

B. Ebstein

C. Tricuspid atresia

D. TOF

97. Which is not a feature of RVH

A. Rsr with r >0.5mv

B. qR pattern in V1

C. p pulmonale

D. RAD

98. Which of the following drug is not useful in CPVT

A. Amiodarone

B. Carvedilol

C. Flecainide

D. Verapamil

99. Listeria endocarditis is common with which condition

A. Iv drug abuser

B. Dental procedure

C. Ureteric stent implantation

D. Prosthetic heart valve

100. Wrong match in cardiac embryology

A. Rt 6th arch- PDA

B. Pulmonary vein- smooth part of the left atrium

C. Right horn of the sinus venosus

D. Vein of Marshall- left SVC

101. PCI in a patient with stable CAD is done mainly for

A. Reduce sudden death

B. Reduce MI

C. Angina relief

D. Prevent LV dysfunction

102. Which is not a marker of effective CPR
    A. ET CO_2 above 20 mmHg
    B. Compression depth at least 2 inches
    C. Rate 100-120 compressions per minute
    D. Compression ventilation ratio 15:2
103. The most specific indicator of successful CPR is
    A. Warm peripheries
    B. Palpable carotid pulse
    C. Sinus rhythm
    D. ET $CO_2 > 20$ mmHg
104. Massive cardiomegaly in CXR is seen in all except
    A. Aortic regurgitation
    B. Tricuspid regurgitation
    C. Ebstein
    D. Tamponade
105. A 2-year-old child with heart failure and cyanosis with the following chest X-ray. Mark the structure

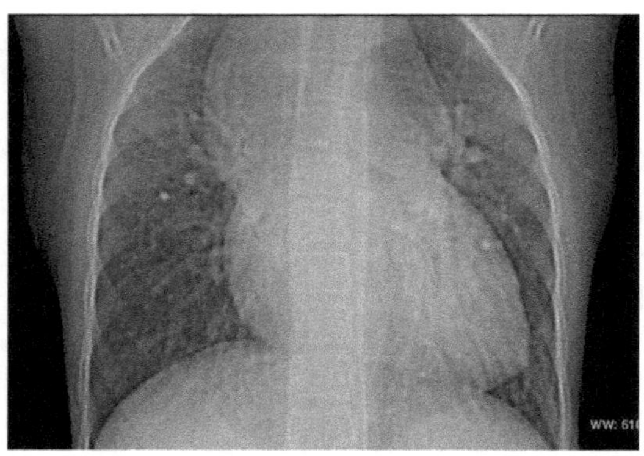

    A. Vertical vein of TAPVC
    B. SVC
    C. Pulmonary vein
    D. Pulmonary artery
106. Continuous murmur is seen in all except
    A. Mammary suffle
    B. Peripheral PS
    C. CoA
    D. VSD with AR

107. Syncope in a patient with Long QT syndrome with SCN5A mutation is usually precipitated by

A. Sleep

B. Exercise

C. Door bell

D. Peripartum

108. Signs of severe mitral stenosis are all except

A. Loud murmur

B. Narrow S2-OS gap

C. Loud P2

D. Long duration of the diastolic murmur

109. Single second heart sound (S2) in Eisenmenger seen in

A. ASD

B. VSD

C. PDA

D. AVSD

110. The most potent vasoconstrictor is

A. Endothelin

B. Adenosine

C. Ach

D. Bradykinin

111. Arrhythmia not responsive to DC cardioversion

A. Fascicular VT

B. Atrial fibrillation

C. Ectopic atrial tachycardia

D. Scar VT

112. Idaricuzumab is an antidote for

A. UFH

B. Clopidogrel

C. Dabigatran

D. Apixaban

113. The wrong match with regards to X-ray sign in congenital heart disease is-

    A. Figure 8- supracardiac TAPVC

    B. Egg on side- TGA

    C. Figure 3- Coarctation of the aorta

    D. Hilar water fall sign- pulmonary atresia

114. All are associated with fever and constitutional symptoms except

    A. Takayasu arteritis

    B. LA myxoma

    C. Carcinoid heart disease

    D. Rhabdomyoma

115. What is the structure marked in the echocardiographic short-axis view

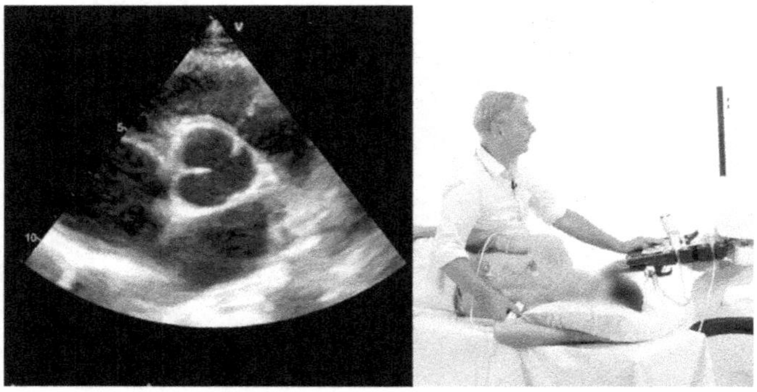

    A. Aortic valve

    B. RSOV

    C. Pulmonary valve

    D. Vegetation

116. Which of the following ECG features doesn't differentiate VT from SVT

    A. QRS duration

    B. AV dissociation

    C. Fusion beat

    D. Concordance in chest leads

117. Which of the following genetic abnormalities is not seen in homozygous familial hypercholesterolemia

    A. LDL receptor mutation

    B. Gain of function of the PCSK9 gene

    C. Apo B100 mutation

    D. Gain-of-function mutation of the LDL receptor

118. Which is not a treatment option for ATTR amyloidosis

   A. Tafamidis

   B. Patisiran

   C. Mipomersan

   D. Inotersan

119. Which of the following lipid-lowering agent is a suitable alternative to statin-induced myopathy

   A. Bempedoic acid

   B. Fibrate

   C. Omega-3 fatty acid

   D. Ezetimibe

120. Most potent statin

   A. Pitavastatin

   B. Fluvastatin

   C. Rosuvastatin

   D. Atorvastatin

121. Intranasal calcium channel blocker for PSVT

   A. Etripamil

   B. Rosapamil

   C. Diltiazem noso

   D. Verapamil

122. AICD is usually not advised in which condition

   A. VT with prior MI

   B. Fascicular VT

   C. Family h/o SCD

   D. Significant LGE burden in cardiac MRI

123. Which of the following drug increases the risk of atrial fibrillation

   A. Nicorandil

   B. Teimetazidine

   C. Ivabradine

   D. Ranolazine

124. Carney complex comprises all except

A. Cardiac myxoma

B. Skin lentigines

C. Rhabdomyoma

D. Hyperadrenalism

125. Which valvular lesion is common in homozygous familial hypercholesterolemia

A. Aortic regurgitation

B. Mitral stenosis

C. Aortic stenosis

D. Tricuspid stenosis

126. A 36-year-old male presented with one episode of syncope. There is a family history of sudden cardiac death. ECG recorded at admission is as below. Most likely diagnosis is

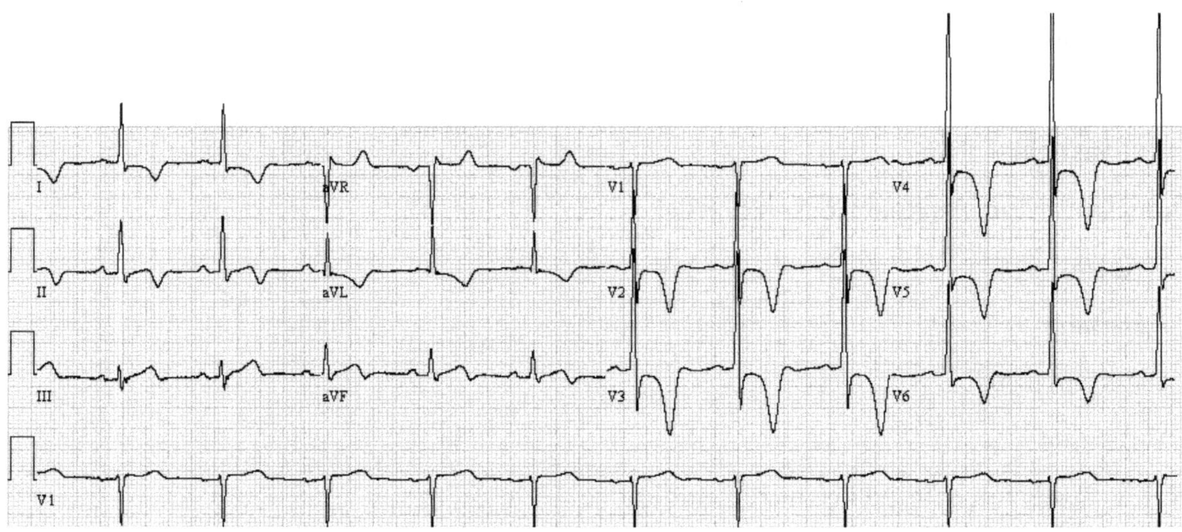

A. Apical HCM

B. LQT3

C. Brugada

D. ARVC

127. A patient with intermittent rest angina comes to the casualty with the following ECG, most likely has

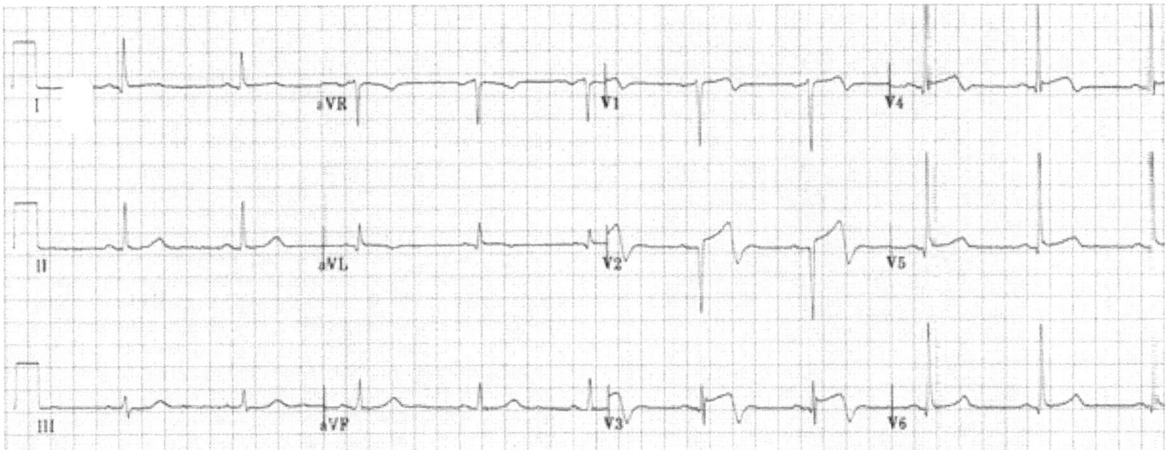

A. Critical LAD stenosis

B. Ventricular aneurysm

C. Prinzmetal angina

D. Brugada syndrome

128. The best management plan for the above-mentioned patient is

A. Emergency coronary angiography and revascularisation

B. Nitrate

C. Medical management

D. CT coronary angiography

129. CXR after permanent pacemaker implantation shows this. What is the next line of management?

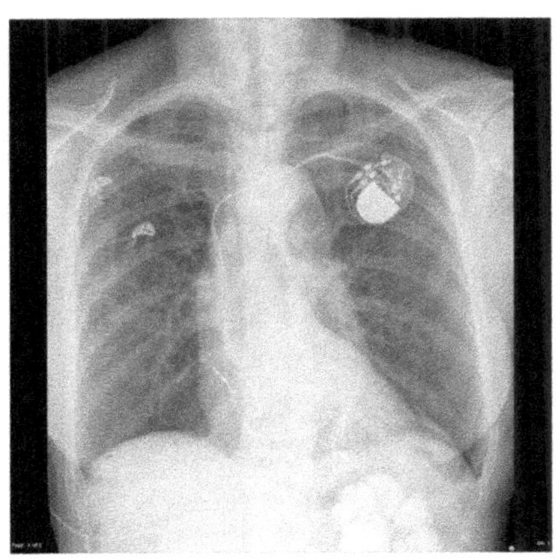

A. ICTD insertion

B. Reimplantation of the lead

C. Reimplantation of pacemaker

D. Reimplantation in the opposite side

130. The best management strategy for the following arrhythmia is

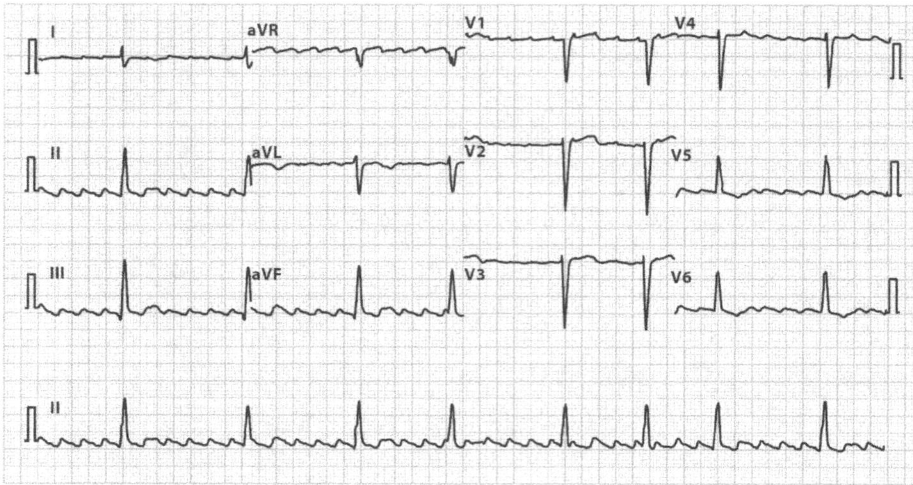

A. Catheter ablation

B. Beta blocker

C. Calcium channel blocker

D. DC cardioversion

131. Wrongly matched arrhythmia and its mechanism

A. Torsades - DAD

B. RVOT VT- DAD

C. Scar VT- reentry

D. EAT- Enhanced automaticity

132. Which of the following drugs doesn't target the PCSK9 pathway of LDL metabolism

A. Evolocumab

B. Alirocumab

C. Incliseran

D. Tafamidis

133. True statement regarding PCSK9, all except

A. Gain-of-function mutation leads to familial hypercholesterolemia

B. Decrease LDL clearance

C. Inhibitors given orally

D. Degrades LDL receptor

134. Wrong statement regarding fibrates
   A. Increases hepatic fatty acid uptake
   B. Reverse cholesterol transport
   C. First line for management of increased TG level
   D. Increase lipoprotein lipase activity
135. S. bovis endocarditis associated with
   A. Respiratory tract infection
   B. Dental infection
   C. Genitourinary infection
   D. Colon carcinoma
136. Which is not advised during routine management of TOF
   A. Fluid restriction
   B. Beta blocker
   C. Iron supplementation
   D. Avoid heavy exertion
137. A mismatched combination is
   A. Right atrium- right horn of sinus venosus
   B. Left atrium- pulmonary vein
   C. PDA- 6th arch
   D. Left SVC- left horn of sinus venosus
138. The wrong match is
   A. Noonan- HCM
   B. Alagille- peripheral PS
   C. NF1- renal artery stenosis
   D. Marfan- aortic stenosis
139. In a patient with mitral stenosis, the LA pressure is not elevated in
   A. Tachycardia
   B. Anaemia
   C. Pregnancy
   D. ASD

140. Continuous murmur seen in all except
    A. Mitral stenosis with ASD
    B. TOF with absent pulmonary valve
    C. TAPVC
    D. Peripheral PS
141. Eisenmangerization involves all except
    A. Increase in PA pressure
    B. Decrease PVRI
    C. Bidirectional shunt
    D. Cyanosis
142. All are true about HFpEF, except
    A. LV hypertrophy
    B. Decrease in LA size
    C. Near normal ejection fraction
    D. Increase in LVEDP
143. Which is not common in massive pulmonary embolism
    A. Hemoptysis
    B. Hypotension
    C. Dilated RV
    D. Syncope
144. Antiarrhythmic drug of choice in a patient with atrial fibrillation in the presence of CAD
    A. Flecainide
    B. Amiodarone
    C. Quinidine
    D. Procainamide
145. All are true regarding congenital CHB except
    A. Infrahisian pathology
    B. Associated with maternal autoantibody
    C. Most patients require a pacemaker
    D. Narrow QRS escape rhythm

146. Mitral annular calcification is commonly associated with

   A. Mitral regurgitation

   B. Mitral stenosis

   C. Supramitral stenosis

   D. LVOT obstruction

147. Most useful parameter before heart transplant assessment

   A. NYHA class

   B. Ejection fraction

   C. Peak oxygen consumption(VO2 max)

   D. HLA

148. Which is not considered an indication for mitral valve surgery in primary mitral regurgitation

   A. LV end systolic dimension > 40mm

   B. LVEF < 60 %

   C. Symptomatic severe MR

   D. Calcified valve

149. The most important predictor of mortality after MI is

   A. Ejection fraction (EF)

   B. QT dispersion

   C. Frequent VPC

   D. Heart rate variability

150. The following condition is not caused by

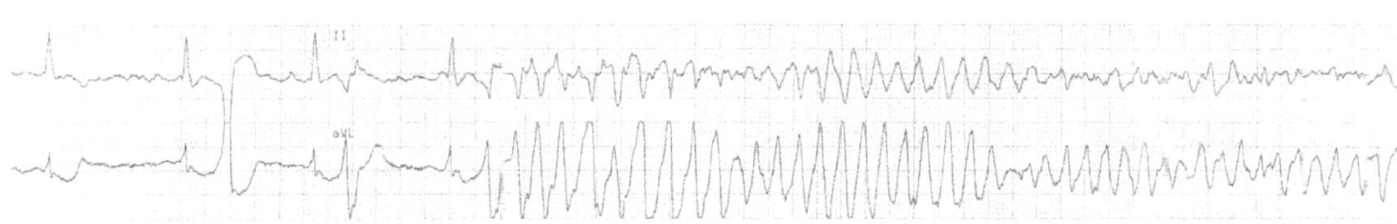

   A. TCA overdose

   B. Hypokalemia

   C. Gain-of-function mutation KCNQ1

   D. Quinidine overdose

151. Antiarrhythmic drug of choice in a patient with paroxysmal AF and dilated cardiomyopathy

A. Amiodarone

B. Dronedarone

C. Sotalol

D. Disopyramide

152. 25-year-old female with progressive dyspnoea, limb claudication with following aortic angiogram. Most likely diagnosis is

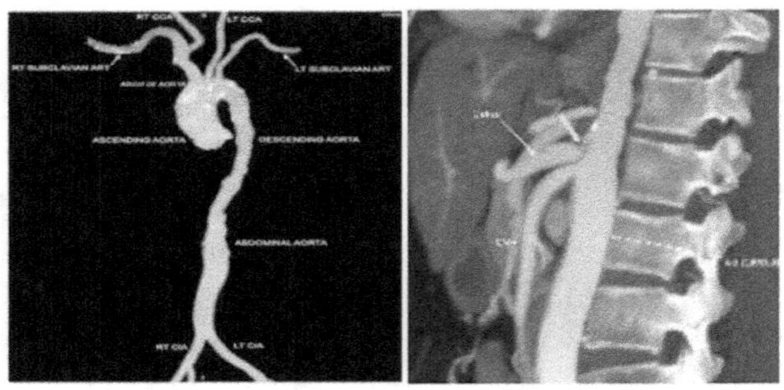

A. Post ductal coarctation of the aorta

B. Takayasu arteritis

C. Marfan syndrome

D. Ehler-Danlos syndrome

153. Fontaine grading is useful in

A. Angina severity

B. Claudication severity

C. Severity of cardiomyopathy

D. Childhood heart failure severity

154. Which is considered a contraindication for balloon mitral valvotomy

A. Pregnancy

B. Spontaneous echo contrast in LA

C. Bicommisural calcification

D. Mild MR

155. All of the following may cause cyanosis except

A. Unroofed CS

B. AP window in a 25-year-old

C. Gerbode defect

D. Common atrium

156. False about carcinoid heart disease
    A. Mitral valve is commonly involved
    B. Metastatic neuroendocrine tumours commonly underlie this condition
    C. Left-sided valves are involved in the presence of the foramen ovale
    D. Thickened and restricted valve mobility
157. Bypass tract is commonly associated with all except
    A. HCM
    B. Ebstein
    C. CCTGA
    D. Inlet VSD
158. Brockenbrough sign seen in
    A. HOCM
    B. Valvular AS
    C. Supravalvular AS
    D. Subaortic membrane
159. Drugs causing hypertension, all except
    A. Cyclosporine
    B. Erythropoietin
    C. NSAID
    D. Levodopa
160. IABP contraindicated in
    A. Aortic regurgitation
    B. Acute severe MR
    C. Post-MI ventricular septal rupture
    D. Acute MI with cardiogenic shock
161. Torsades may be treated with all except
    A. Pacing
    B. Beta blocker
    C. Intravenous magnesium sulphate
    D. Amiodarone

162. Equalisation of the diastolic filling pressure of all cardiac chambers is seen in

A. CCP

B. RV cardiomyopathy

C. RV MI

D. Amyloidosis

163. All of the following increase pulmonary vascular resistance except

A. Acidosis

B. Anaemia

C. Hypoxia

D. Atelectasis

164. All of the following echocardiographic parameters are used for the assessment of diastolic function except

A. Transmitral Doppler pattern

B. IVRT

C. Tissue doppler

D. GLS

165. Which of the following does not suggest a physiological range

A. Mean PA pressure- 15mm Hg

B. Cardiac index 1.7 l/min/m2

C. Right atrial pressure- 4 mmHg

D. PVR- 4 woods

166. Which is not an high-intensity statin

A. Atorvastatin 40mg

B. Atorvastatin 80mg

C. Rosuvastatin 20mg

D. Pitavastatin 2mg

167. Square wave response in Valsalva is seen in

A. Congestive heart failure

B. VSD

C. Coarctation of the aorta

D. CCP

168. During PCI, the effect of heparin is usually assessed by

    A. APTT

    B. ACT

    C. PT

    D. Bleeding time

169. RVH with early precordial transition seen in

    A. TOF

    B. Severe valvular PS

    C. DORV

    D. Tricuspid atresia

170. Heart transplantation is not indicated in

    A. HLHS

    B. Severe Ebstein

    C. DCMP

    D. VSD-Eissenmenger

171. A multislice cardiac CT scan is useful in all of the following scenarios except

    A. Left main stenosis

    B. Patency of bypass graft

    C. Instent restenosis

    D. Anomalous coronary origin

172. Reverse pulsus paradoxus is seen in

    A. Absent pericardium

    B. HOCM

    C. Hypovolemia

    D. Septic shock

173. Flash pulmonary oedema with hypertensive emergency suggests

    A. Renal artery stenosis

    B. Coarctation of the aorta

    C. Takayasu

    D. Pheochromocytoma

174. Pruning of the peripheral pulmonary arteries in CXR seen in
   A. Pulmonary artery hypertension
   B. Pulmonary venous hypertension
   C. Pulmonary edema
   D. Peripheral PS
175. All identify the morphological right ventricle except
   A. Moderator band
   B. Septal attachment of the tricuspid valve
   C. Coarse trabeculation
   D. Elliptical shape
176. A patent ductus is useful in all of the following conditions except
   A. TGA with intact ventricular septum
   B. Critical PS
   C. Persistent truncus arteriosus
   D. HLHS
177. Balloon atrial septostomy is useful in all except
   A. Primary pulmonary hypertension
   B. TOF
   C. Mitral atresia
   D. D-TGA
178. The wrong match is
   A. TGA- atrial switch
   B. ALCAPA- Takeuchi repair
   C. Tricuspid atresia- Fontan
   D. TOF- total correction
179. False statement regarding TOF
   A. The loudness of murmur is directly proportional to the degree of cyanosis
   B. P2 usually soft/absent
   C. VSD nonrestrictive
   D. Absent parasternal heave

180. Snowman's appearance in chest X-ray is seen in

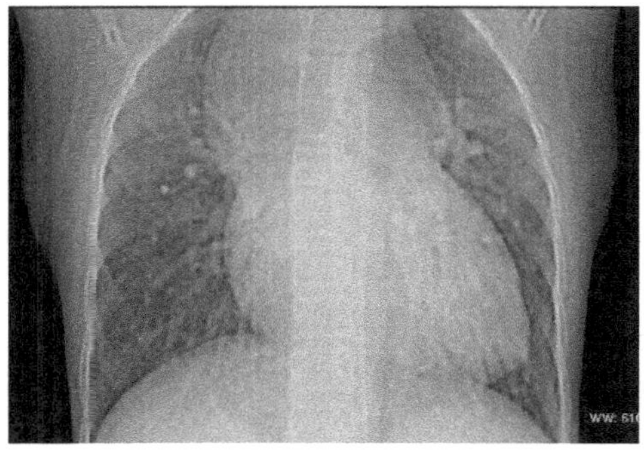

A. Supracardiac TAPVC

B. TGA

C. TOF with absent pulmonary valve

D. Tricuspid atresia

181. All are absolute contraindications of thrombolysis except

A. Pregnancy

B. Intracranial neoplasm

C. Whipple surgery 5days back

D. History of ICH

182. True statement regarding sinus venosus ASD is

A. Ideal for device closure

B. No RA/RV volume overload

C. Cyanosis may be seen in the absence of PAH

D. IVC type is more common

183. Patients with the following clinical condition (shown in the picture) usually present with

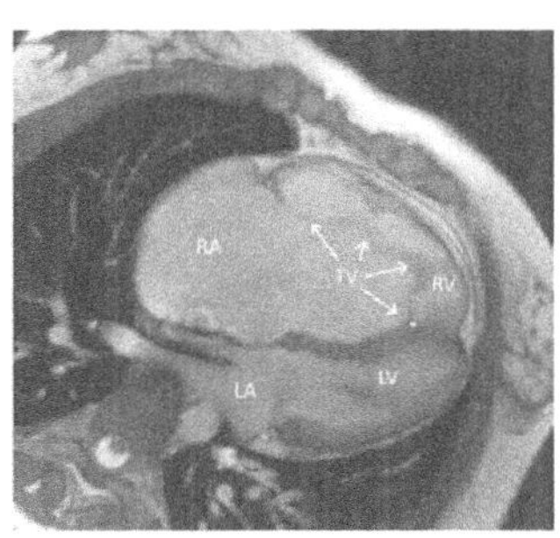

A. Heart failure

B. Cyanosis

C. Arrhythmia

D. All of the above

184. Supravalvular AS is usually associated with

    A. Elfin facies

    B. BAV

    C. Subaortic membrane

    D. Hyperkalemia

185. Cardiac allograft vasculopathy, all are true except

    A. Incidence 50% after 10 years

    B. A CT coronary angiogram is the investigation of choice

    C. Concentric atherosclerosis

    D. Invasive coronary angiography may be unremarkable

186. Senile cardiac amyloidosis results from the deposition of

    A. Transthyretin

    B. Calcitonin

    C. Fibrinogen

    D. Light chain

187. True about Eisenmenger Syndrome(ES), all except

    A. Cardiomegaly seen in VSD-ES

    B. Parasternal heave absent in VSD -ES

    C. Shunt murmur absent

    D. Flow murmur absent

188. Revascularisation in a patient with stable CAD mainly helps in

    A. Symptom relief

    B. Mortality reduction

    C. Prevention of MI

    D. Prevention of heart failure

189. False statement regarding Exercise ECG/TMT testing

    A. Duke score predicts prognosis

    B. Score ranges from +15 to -25

    C. Score -25 denotes the highest risk

    D. Exercise time is not used for score calculation

190. Which is not considered a contraindication for prasugrel

A. Age > 75

B. Weight < 60 kg

C. History of TIA

D. History of peptic ulcer disease

191. Ideal ACT range during PCI procedure

A. 200-300 S

B. 300-350 S

C. <200 S

D. No strict range required

192. A major disadvantage of the bioabsorbable vascular scaffold is

A. Scaffold thrombosis

B. Thick struts

C. ISR

D. Recurrent MI

193. Which of the following conditions is not associated with an increased BNP level

A. Obesity

B. Age >75yrd

C. Acute heart failure

D. Pulmonary embolism

194. Which of the following natriuretic peptide levels is not used for diagnostic purposes

A. MR pro ANP

B. BNP

C. NT pro BNP

D. CNP

195. False statement regarding natriuretic peptide

A. Beneficial effect in the pathophysiology of heart failure

B. Metabolised by neutral endopeptidases

C. Obesity decreases the blood level

D. NT pro BNP level is elevated with ARNI use

196. False statement regarding coronary intravascular imaging

A. IVUS has a better depth of penetration

B. IVUS better characterises plaque morphology than OCT

C. Mostly utilised for stent optimisation

D. Left main stenosis severity can be assessed

197. Which is not a cause of restrictive cardiomyopathy

A. Hemochromatosis

B. Sarcoidosis

C. Amyloidosis

D. Ethanol cardiomyopathy

198. A 60-year-old male with progressive dyspnea and low backache for the last 6 months. Ecocardiography revealed concentric ventricular hypertrophy and a dilated left atrium. ECG at presentation is shown below. Most probable diagnosis

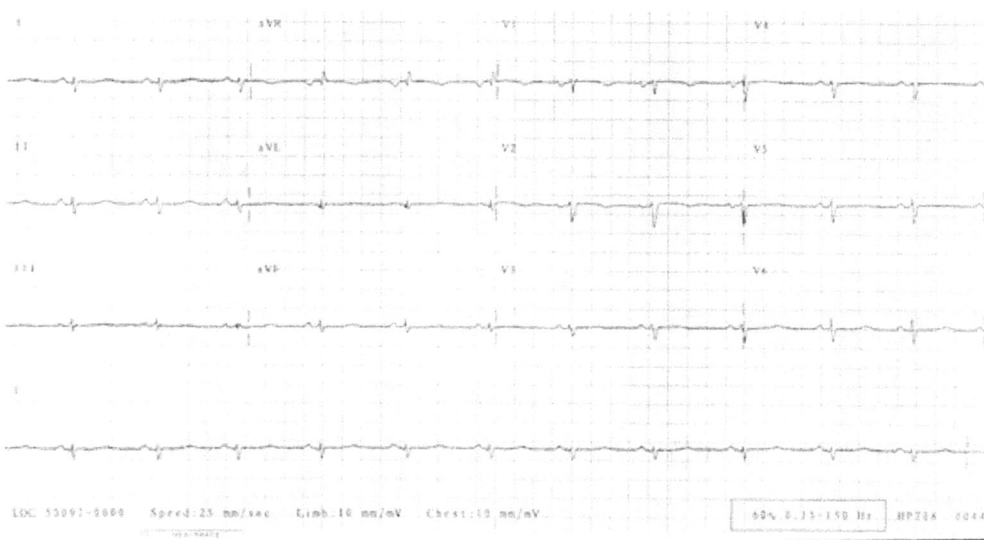

A. Cardiac amyloidosis

B. Idiopathic RCMP

C. Hemochromatosis

D. Pericardial tamponade

199. Which of the following drug is not used for the management of ATTR amyloidosis

A. Patisiran

B. Tafamidis

C. Inotersan

D. Daratumumab

200. The ATTRACT trial tested which drug

A. Patisiran

B. Tafamidis

C. Inotersan

D. Diflusinal

201. A 70-year-old male with chest pain of 1 hour duration with the following ECG. What should be the next step of management?

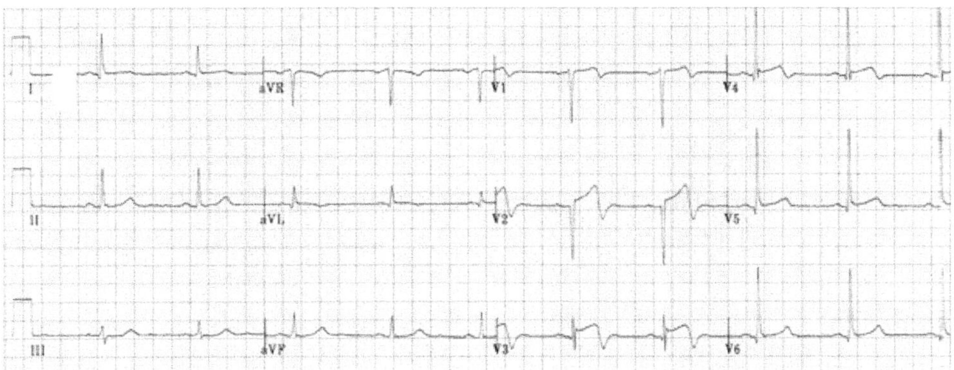

A. Emergency revascularisation

B. Thrombolysis

C. UFH

D. Medical stabilization

202. A 57-year-old smoker presented to the emergency room with the following ECG. Which of the following describes the ECG feature

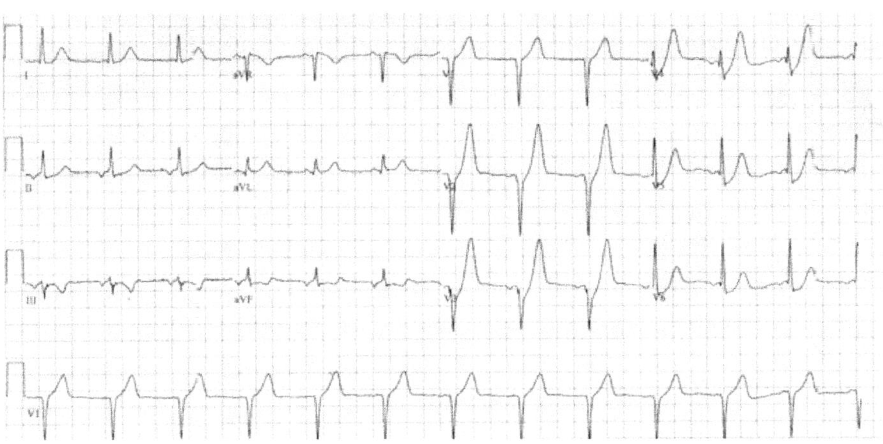

A. De Winter sign

B. Wellen sign

C. Brugada sign

D. AWMI

203. Which of the following ECG features suggest proximal LAD occlusion

A. qRBBB

B. ST elevation in lead avR

C. ST elevation in V1

D. All of these

204. Which of these is an IV antiplatelet agent

A. Ticagrelor

B. Cangrelor

C. Clopidogrel

D. Prasugrel

205. Which of the following investigation modalities is most useful for a patient undergoing TAVI

A. Multislice CT

B. Echocardiography

C. Cardiac MRI

D. Coronary angiography

206. Which of the following trial did not evaluate the role of TAVI

A. PARTNER

B. PARTNER II

C. MITRA FR

D. EVOLUT LOW RISK

207. Which of the following is not true about ECG changes during childhood

A. The normal heart rate of a neonate is 120-130/min

B. Dominant R in V1 is normal in an infant

C. T wave upright till 7 years of age

D. Presence of Q wave in the inferior leads

208. Which of the following conditions are not associated with congenital CHB

A. CCTGA

B. AV canal defect

C. Congenital rubella

D. Autoantibodies in the mother

209. Which of the following is not a cause of a short PR interval

   A. WPW pattern

   B. Fabry disease

   C. Low ectopic atrial rhythm

   D. AV nodal disease

210. Which of the following conditions are commonly associated with a bypass tract

   A. Ebstein

   B. HCM

   C. CCTGA

   D. All of the above

211. The most common cause of SVT in children

   A. WPW

   B. AVNRT

   C. EAT

   D. Junctional tachycardia

212. Which of the following statement is not true regarding RVH in ECG?

   A. QR pattern in V1 suggests pressure overload RVH

   B. The RSR pattern suggests volume overload

   C. An upright T wave during early childhood suggests RVH

   D. Right axis deviation is always present in RVH

213. Which of the following is not seen in the ECG of Tetralogy of Fallot

   A. RAD

   B. Sudden transition of R to S in V2

   C. RVH

   D. LAFB

214. False statement regarding Eisenmenger syndrome

   A. Estrogen-based contraception safe

   B. Pregnancy absolute contraindication

   C. Pulmonary vasodilators may be useful

   D. Non-cardiac major surgery should be avoided

215. Which is not a management option for Eisenmanger syndrome

A. Heart-lung transplantation

B. Pulmonary vasodilator

C. Routine phlebotomy

D. Iron supplementation

216. Eisenmenger syndrome is less common in

A. ASD

B. VSD

C. PDA

D. AP window

217. False regarding the hemodynamic effect of IABP

A. MAP decreased

B. Diastolic BP increased

C. Systolic BP decreased

D. Cardiac output increased

218. False statement regarding the Impella device

A. Percutaneously inserted into the LV cavity

B. Pumps blood from the left ventricle to the aorta

C. Improvement in cardiac output is less than that of IABP

D. Specially designed device for the right ventricle

219. Which of the following support systems provides both circulatory as well as respiratory support

A. Impella

B. VV ECMO

C. VA ECMO

D. Heartmate 3

220. Which of the following devices is used as long-term destination therapy for heart failure

A. Impella

B. Tandem heart

C. Heartmate 3

D. VA ECMO

221. Which of the following ECG features does not differentiate VT from SVT

    A. AV dissociation

    B. Fusion beat

    C. QRS duration >140ms

    D. Northwest axis

222. Pulmonary vasodilators are useful in

    A. PAH secondary to left heart disease

    B. Idiopathic PAH

    C. Eisenmenger syndrome

    D. Both B and C

223. Which of the following grafts is commonly used in CABG

    A. Left internal mammary

    B. Right internal mammary

    C. Right radial artery

    D. Dorsalis pedis artery

224. FFR assesses

    A. Physiological significance of coronary stenosis

    B. Anatomic significance of coronary stenosis

    C. Pathological properties of atherosclerosis

    D. All of the above

225. Which of the following trial evaluated the role of FFR in revascularisation

    A. PARTNER

    B. FAME

    C. ORBITA

    D. ISCHEMIA

226. Which is not a feature of an athlete's heart

    A. Low normal ejection fraction

    B. Dilated cardiac chambers

    C. Reduced GLS value

    D. Normal diastolic parameters

227. Which of the following drug is considered to be most suitable for statin-intolerant patients

   A. Bempedoic acid

   B. Ezetimibe

   C. Evolocumab

   D. Omega-3 fatty acid

228. Which of the following situations does statin therapy is indicated for all except

   A. Diagnosed ASCVD

   B. LDL >110

   C. Diabetic above 40yrs

   D. ASCVD score >20

229. Which is not included in the diagnosis of metabolic syndrome

   A. High TG level

   B. Low HDL level

   C. High LDL level

   D. Abdominal obesity

230. Which is not a part of the ASCVD risk assessment

   A. LDL cholesterol

   B. Total cholesterol

   C. HDL

   D. Race

231. False regarding ASCVD risk score assessment

   A. Used for secondary prevention statin therapy

   B. Should be assessed for all adults above 40 years

   C. Less than 5% suggest low risk

   D. Statin therapy is indicated if the score >20%

232. The Friedwald formula is used for the estimation of

   A. TG

   B. LDL cholesterol

   C. HDL

   D. Non-HDL cholesterol

233. Which of the following lipid parameters are usually not measured directly during routine lipid profile testing

   A. Total cholesterol

   B. LDL

   C. HDL

   D. Non-HDL

234. Which of the following drug is useful in the primary prevention of cardiovascular events

   A. Statin

   B. Aspirin

   C. Omega-3 fatty acid

   D. Bempedoic acid

235. Which of the following trial evaluated the role of aspirin in primary prevention of cardiovascular disease

   A. ASCEND

   B. ASPREE

   C. ARRIVE

   D. All of the above

236. Lake Louise criteria used for

   A. Histopathological criteria of myocarditis

   B. MRI diagnosis of myocarditis

   C. Echo diagnosis of myocarditis

   D. All of the above

237. Which of the following MRI features are NOT seen in cardiac amyloidosis

   A. Diffuse subendocardial LGE

   B. The amount of LGE corresponds with disease severity and prognosis

   C. Patchy LGE in myocardium

   D. Restrictive filling pattern

238. Myocardial oxygen demand depends upon

   A. Heart rate

   B. Contractility

   C. Wall tension

   D. All of these

239. Which of the following complications increased with the use of bioabsorbable coronary stents

A. Scaffold thrombosis

B. Stroke

C. Restenosis

D. All of these

240. Drug-coated balloons are useful in

A. Stent thrombosis

B. Instent restenosis

C. Calcific coronary stenosis

D. Tortuous coronary stenosis

241. The "cherry on top" apical sparing pattern in strain imaging is seen in

A. Cardiac amyloidosis

B. Fabry disease

C. Fulminant myocarditis

D. All of these

242. False statement regarding ARNI

A. Needs 4 weeks of ACEI trial before starting ARNI

B. The patient needs to stop ACEI for 36 hrs. before starting ARNI

C. Hyperkalemia is an adverse event

D. Increase in BNP level

243. Which drug has NO long-term mortality benefit in patients with HFrEF

A. Metoprolol succinate

B. Dapagliflozin

C. Digoxin

D. Spironolactone

244. Which of the following P2Y12 inhibitor agent is short-acting

A. Ticagrelor

B. Cangrelor

C. Prasugrel

D. Clopidogrel

245. Correct management of heparin reversal

A. Vit K 10mg IV bolus

B. Protamine sulfate 1mg for 100 units UFH

C. Protamine sulfate 10mg for 100 units UFH

D. 100 ml fresh frozen plasma

246. Which is not an advantage of Low molecular weight heparin (LMWH) over unfractionated heparin(UFH)

A. More potent anticoagulant

B. Monitoring not necessary

C. HITT is seen more frequently

D. Less plasma protein binding

247. Which of the antiplatelet agents can be used intravenously

A. Aspirin

B. Cangrelor

C. Ticagrelor

D. Prasugrel

248. Which of the following trial evaluated the role of Canakinumab in CAD

A. CANTOS

B. COLCOT

C. ISCHEMIA

D. All of these

249. The most common coronary anomaly seen in TOF

A. LAD from the right sinus/RCA

B. Single coronary artery

C. RCA from the left sinus

D. Absent RCA

250. The most common cause of secondary hypertension

A. Coarctation of the aorta

B. Primary hyperaldosteronism

C. Hyperthyroidism

D. Renovascular hypertension

251. A spike and dome pattern in LV pressure tracing is seen in

    A. Severe AS
    B. HOCM
    C. Severe MS
    D. Supravalvular AS

252. Antihypertensives of choice in patients with unilateral renal artery stenosis

    A. RAAS blocker
    B. MRA
    C. CCB
    D. Thiazide diuretics

253. Which is NOT an immunological phenomenon of infective endocarditis

    A. Osler node
    B. Roth spot
    C. Erythema marginatum
    D. Rheumatoid factor

254. Select the wrong match

    A. ALCAPA- Takeuchi repair
    B. Norwood- HLHS
    C. Pott shunt – TOF
    D. Fontan- TOF

255. A septal defect resulting in communication between the left ventricle and the right atrium is known as

    A. Raghib defect
    B. Gerbode defect
    C. Scimitar syndrome
    D. Holmes heart

256. The left atrium is differentiated from the right atrium by echocardiography

    A. Connection to LV
    B. PV drainage
    C. Left side of the heart
    D. Appendage

257. The second heart field gives rise to all except
    A. Left ventricle
    B. Right ventricle
    C. RV outflow
    D. Pulmonary trunk
258. Genetic testing in Long QT syndrome helps in
    A. Diagnostics
    B. Prognosis
    C. Therapeutic options
    D. All of these
259. False statement regarding Brugada syndrome
    A. ICD indicated for an asymptomatic Brugada pattern
    B. Quinidine for recurrent event
    C. Ajmaline can unmask the Brugada pattern
    D. SCD usually happen at rest
260. True statement regarding CPVT
    A. Bidirectional VT common
    B. ICD is considered in all symptomatic patients
    C. Abnormal Na handling by cardiac myocyte
    D. Cardiac sympathectomy for recurrent events
261. Which of the following drugs reverses the effect of NOAC and heparin
    A. Ciraparantag
    B. Idarucizumab
    C. Andexanet alfa
    D. All of these
262. Which of the following causes monomorphic VT
    A. CPVT
    B. Brugada
    C. Fascicular VT
    D. Early repolarisation syndrome

263. Which of the following auscultatory findings is consistent with severe MR

A. S3

B. Narrow split S2

C. Loud S1

D. All of these

264. A 15-year-old boy with recurrent palpitation, dyspnoea and cyanosis, with the following CXR. The likely diagnosis is

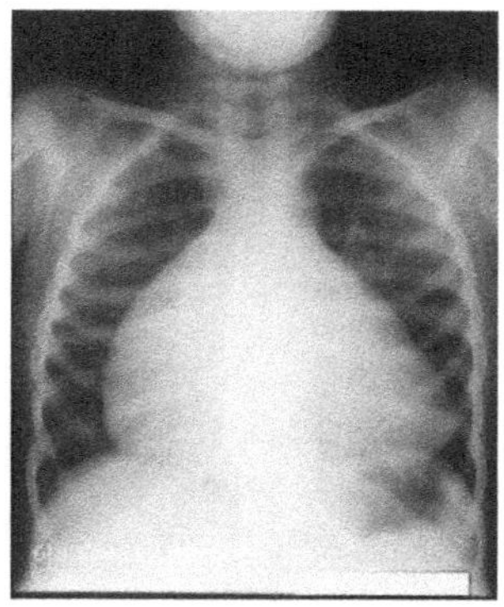

A. TGA

B. TAPVC

C. Ebstein

D. Tamponade

265. Best modality for risk stratification for sudden cardiac death of a young adult with the following ECG.

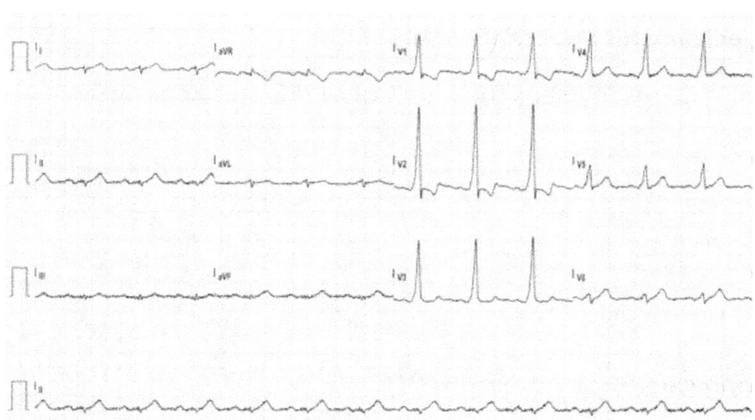

A. EP study

B. Exercise ECG

C. Holter

D. CAG

266. Congenital heart disease with equal saturation in all cardiac chambers and great vessels is

A. TGA

B. Ebstein

C. Tricuspid atresia

D. TAPVC

267. Which is considered an indication for tricuspid valve repair in a patient with severe mitral valve disease with tricuspid regurgitation

A. TV annulus > 40 mm

B. Severe PAH

C. Moderate TR

D. All of these

268. All of the following are correct regarding pulsus paradoxus except

A. Mostly seen in cardiac tamponade

B. Also seen in constrictive pericarditis

C. Exaggerated with severe AR

D. Absent in low-pressure tamponade

269. Equal A and V waves in JVP are seen in

A. Tamponade

B. CCP

C. Hypovolemia

D. ASD

270. 70-year-old male with BP 160/104 mm Hg. The initial antihypertensive of choice would be

A. Amlodipine+ perindopril

B. Amlodipine

C. Enalapril+ chlorthalidone

D. Telmisartan

271. SBP control causes maximum risk reduction in

A. CHF

B. Stroke

C. CAD

D. Nephropathy

272. The REVEAL 2 score used for risk stratification of PAH includes all except

   A. BNP

   B. Exercise desaturation

   C. Pericardial effusion

   D. WHO functional class

273. All are correct regarding coronary vasodilators except

   A. NO is endothelium-independent

   B. A G-protein-coupled receptor uses cAMP

   C. Adenosine acts via a G protein receptor

   D. Rhynodine is responsible for intracellular calcium release

274. All of the following drugs can be used in permanent AF except

   A. Ivabradine

   B. Flecainide

   C. Ibutilide

   D. Vernakalant

275. A 52-year-old male presented to the emergency department with a recent onset of shortness of breath and the following ECG. What is the next line of action?

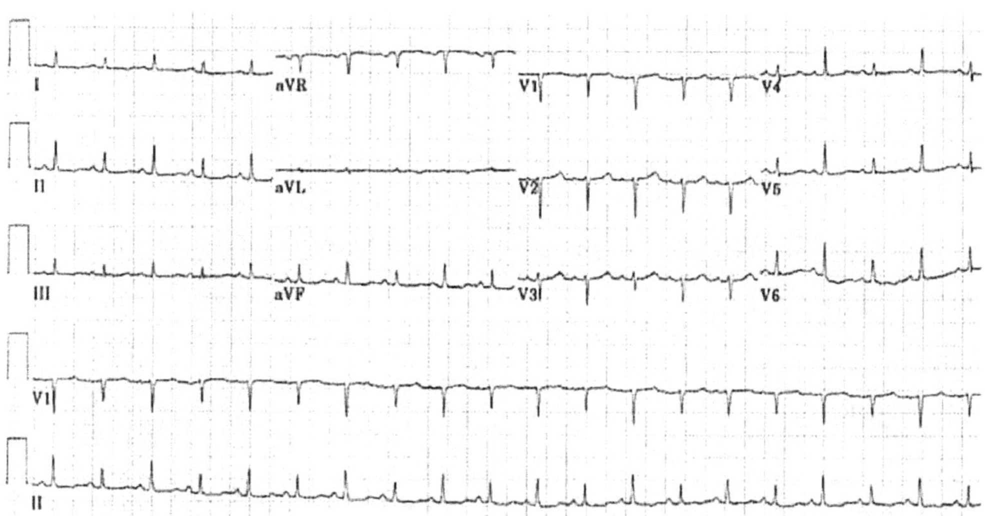

   A. Transthoracic echocardiography

   B. Cardiac MRI

   C. CXR

   D. Troponin

276. Rotablation contraindicated in

   A. dissection
   B. Tortuous lesion
   C. ACS
   D. All of the above

277. All are true regarding S3 except

   A. Suggestive of LV dysfunction in severe AR
   B. Can be heard intermittently in angina
   C. 100 ms after S2
   D. Presence rules out severe MS

278. Austin Flint murmur confused with

   A. MS
   B. MR
   C. AS
   D. None of these

279. Supravalvular AS is seen in all except

   A. Familial hypercholesterolemia
   B. Williams syndrome
   C. Post-transcatheter repair
   D. Post-surgical repair

280. Stroke volume decreased by all except

   A. IABP
   B. Impella
   C. Tandem heart
   D. ECMO

281. Correctly matched treatment options include all except

   A. RVOT VT- Verapamil
   B. Paroxysmal AF – ibutilide
   C. LQT3-Mexilitine
   D. Brugada- flecainide

282. An antihypertensive drug with a favorable effect on diabetes

A. Prazosin

B. Chlorthalidone

C. Metoprolol

D. Labetolol

283. The most common complication seen with diagnostic coronary angiography

A. Contrast allergy

B. Dissection

C. Thrombosis

D. Vascular complication

284. Best load-independent measure of cardiac contractility

A. ESPVR

B. Dp/dt

C. Ejection fraction

D. GLS

285. What are the properties of the Mahiam pathway

A. Can conduct retrogradely

B. Orthodromic conduction

C. Decremental conduction

D. All of these

286. The most common cause of SCD is

A. CAD

B. HOCM

C. Coronary anomalies

D. DCMP

287. The commonest cause of SCD in young athletes < 35 years of age

A. HCM

B. CAD

C. Coronary anomalies

D. Idiopathic

288. All are true regarding HFpEF except

   A. Hypertension is a common aetiology

   B. Can present with pulmonary oedema

   C. BNP levels elevated

   D. Can be differentiated from HFrEF by response to diuretics

289. Features of foetal heart failure, all except

   A. Hydrops

   B. Scalp edema

   C. Umblical venous pulsation

   D. Continuous flow in the umblical artery

290. The drug used in foetal tachycardia is all except

   A. Amiodarone

   B. Digoxin

   C. Sotalol

   D. Flecainide

291. The first selective coronary angiogram was done by

   A. Andreas gruentzig

   B. Frossmann

   C. Mason sones

   D. Momiz

292. ACE 2 receptor, which is the entry receptor for the COVID-19 virus in the lungs, causes

   A. Convert AT1 to AT2

   B. Convert angiotensinogen to AT1

   C. Convert AT2 to AT1

   D. Convert AT2 to AT 4

293. A young boy had dengue fever and had syncope when the phone bell rang, likely mutation is

   A. KCNH2

   B. KCNQ1

   C. KCNJ2

   D. SCN5A

294. Hypertrophy of the ventricular chamber in newborns in all except

A. Down

B. Noonan

C. Nesidioblastoma

D. Infant with a diabetic mother

295. A 35-year-old female with progressive dyspnoea for the last 5 years has recently had left-hand weakness. A chest X-ray of the patient is shown below. Most likely diagnosis is

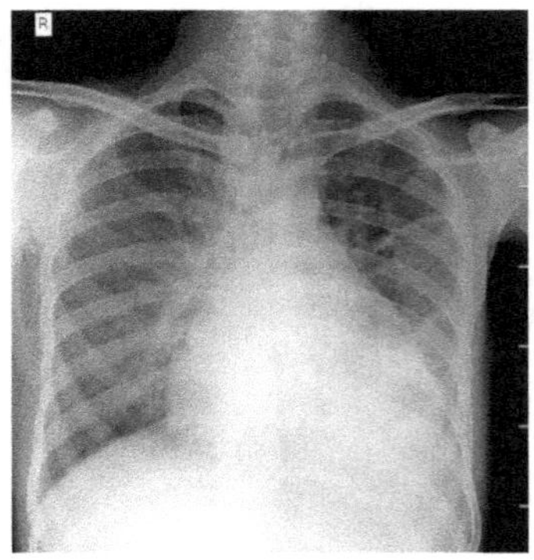

A. IPAH

B. Mitral stenosis

C. PFO

D. CTEPH

296. Which of the following statins is not metabolised by CYP

A. Lovastatin

B. Atorvastatin

C. Simvastatin

D. Rosuvastatin

297. A young female with Ebstein anomaly, with the following ECG, is likely to present with

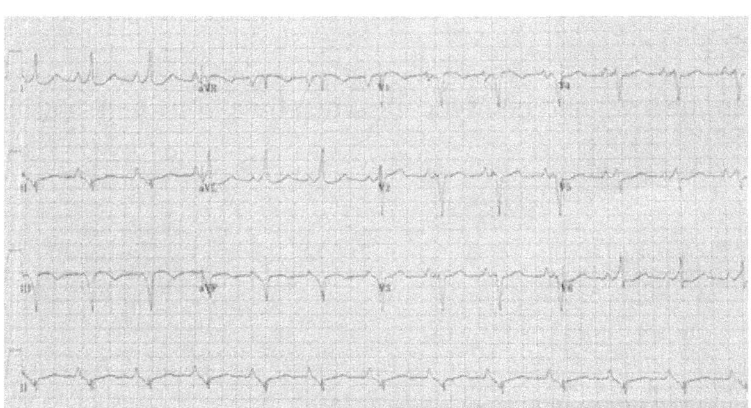

A. Intermittent palpitation

B. Cyanosis

C. Dyspnoea

D. None of these

298. Best marker of myocardial contractility

A. ESPVR

B. DP/DT

C. FCV

D. GLS

299. The wrong match is

A. DCMP- TITIN

B. LV noncompaction- Tafazzin

C. ARVD- Desmosome

D. Duchenne muscular dystrophy- Laminin

300. A 30-year-old male with h/o syncope and the following ECG. The next line cf management is

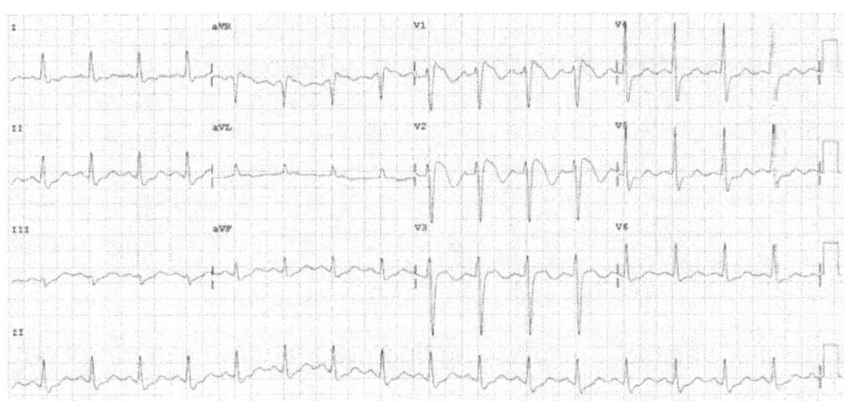

A. AICD

B. Beta blocker

C. CAG

D. Qunidine

301. Which is NOT a known side effect of statin

A. Myopathy

B. Diabetes mellitus

C. Cognitive dysfunction

D. Ischemic stroke

302. Which of the following features is not seen in a one-month-old child with coarctation of the aorta

A. Heart failure

B. Rib notching

C. Hypertension

D. Radiofemoral delay

303. The patient with the following CXR most likely had

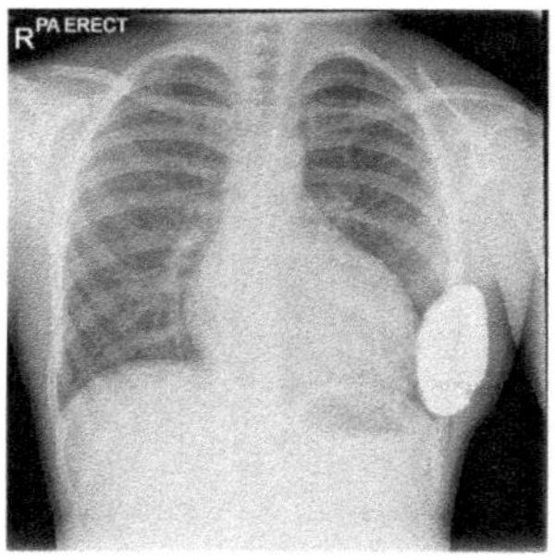

A. Pneumothorax

B. VT or aborted SCD

C. Cardiogenic shock

D. Heart failure

304. Thrombocytopenia is seen with all of the following drugs except

A. Amiodarone

B. Furosemide

C. Abciximab

D. Nicorandil

305. In a healthy young male, which of the following findings is abnormal during exercise ECG testing

A. VPC

B. BP 180/100

C. Rapid upsloping ST depression

D. LBBB

306. High chance of DVT in a patient with all except

A. Atrial fibrillation

B. Recent knee transplantation

C. Recent MI

D. Long air travel

307. What is the ideal time for balloon mitral valvotomy in mitral stenosis with pregnaancy

A. At conception

B. 32-34 weeks

C. Just before delivery

D. Second trimester

308. Pregnancy is absolutely contraindicated in

A. Severe PAH

B. Mitral regurgitation

C. HOCM

D. Severe PS

309. Type 2 MI is due to

A. Plaque rupture

B. Demand-supply mismatch

C. Stent thrombosis

D. SCD

310. False statement regarding the AV node

A. Subendocardial structure

B. Located at the apex of the triangle of Koch

C. L-type calcium channel blockade reduces conduction speed

D. The AV nodal artery predominantly arises from the circumflex artery

311. A young male with an ECG suggestive of 2:1 AV block and improved conduction after atropine suggests the site of block at

A. AV node

B. SA node

C. Bundle of his

D. Left bundle branch

312. Global subendocardial enhancement in MRI is seen in all except

A. Amyloidosis

B. Systemic sclerosis

C. Post-cardiac transplantation

D. CAD

313. True regarding IE, all except

A. PET CT is useful for implanted device infection

B. Mortality is the same now as in past

C. CT evidence of paravalvular leak is a major criterion for diagnosis

D. Oral antibiotics may be useful in selected cases

314. Drug of choice for resistant hypertension

A. Doxazocin

B. Amiloride

C. Spironolactone

D. Bisoprolol

315. Patient after Fontan surgery with ascites, serum protein 1.8 gm/dl, appropriate treatment for this condition

A. Octreotide

B. Medium-chain triglyceride

C. Creation of atrial fenestration

D. All of these

316. Air embolism after right heart catheterisation of a 5-year-old, causing stroke, can be seen in all except

A. Common atrium

B. Ebstein

C. TAPVC

D. Sinus venosus ASD

317. Normal in a well-trained athlete, all except

A. Sinus bradycardia

B. ST elevation in lateral leads

C. Increase in R wave amplitude

D. Mobitz type 1 AV block

318. A 50-year-old male with sick sinus syndrome and normal AV node function. The pacemaker mode of choice is

A. AAI

B. VVI

C. DDD

D. Any of these

319. The earliest indicator of low cardiac output

A. Increased A-V oxygen difference

B. Increased lactate

C. Increased urea

D. Increased SVR

320. Ivabradine is used in all except

A. JET

B. Inappropriate sinus tachycardia

C. AF with a fast ventricular rate

D. HFrEF

321. Wrong match

A. AIVR- enhanced automaticity

B. LQT- EAD

C. Digoxin toxicity- DAD

D. RVOT VT- re-entry

322. Cardiac catheterisation data of the patient reveal mean PA pressure 50 mmHg, PCWP 10mmHg and cardiac output 5 lt/min. calculate PVR

A. 8 woods

B. 18 woods

C. 10 woods

D. 5 woods

323. Echocardiography of a neonate born to of diabetic mother revealed biventricular hypertrophy without other congenital heart disease. What would be the next line of management?

A. Mavacampten

B. AICD

C. Surgical myectomy

D. Follow up with a periodic echo

324. LV to aorta Pull back pressure tracing of an 11-year-old revealed supravalvular aortic stenosis, most likely has

A. Elfin facies

B. HOCM

C. BAV with severe AS

D. PS

325. Unilateral rib notching confined to the left side suggests

  A. Coarctation distal to the left subclavian

  B. Anomalous origin of the right subclavian distal to the coA

  C. CoA at the orifice of the left SCA

  D. Abdominal coarctation

326. Which diuretic is safe in pregnancy

  A. Chlorthalidone

  B. Ethacrynic acid

  C. Spironolactone

  D. Furosemide

327. 70 yr old male 2yr following PCI with permanent atrial fibrillation. What is the best antithrombotic option

  A. Rivaroxaban + aspirin

  B. Aspirin alone

  C. Rivaroxaban + clopidogrel

  D. Rivaroxaban alone

328. ASD usually shunt left to right in all except

  A. Truncus arteriosus

  B. PAPVC

  C. TAPVC

  D. None of these

329. Pulsatile liver is seen in all except

  A. Tricuspid atresia

  B. ASD with MR

  C. PPAH

  D. Ebstein

330. Which of the following drug is not useful in CPVT

  A. Amiodarone

  B. Flecainide

  C. Verapamil

  D. Metoprolol

331. A 46-year-old male with chest pain for 4 hours visited a non-PCI capable centre, where thrombolysis was done with Tenecteplase. Patient's symptoms relieved and ST segment resolved. What is the next line of management?

A. Refer to a PCI-capable centre for coronary angiography

B. Medical management with DAPT and statin

C. Angiography after 6 weeks

D. Exercise ECG testing

332. A 37-year-old male with one episode of syncope while having a high-grade fever. ECG taken after the episode is shown below. What is the most likely diagnosis?

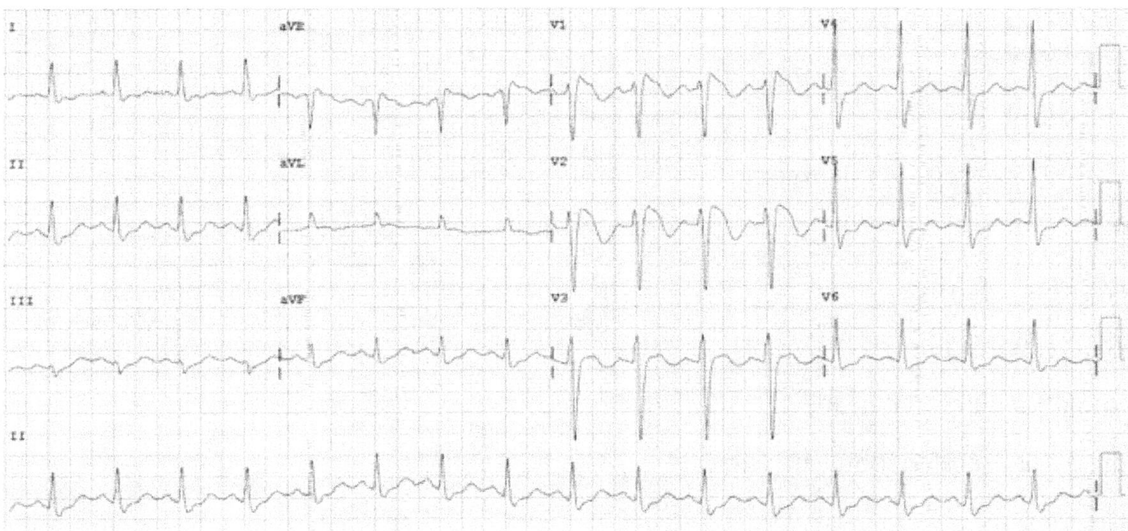

A. ARVC

B. Febrile seizure

C. Brugada syndrome

D. tachycardiomyopathy

333. True about Tangier disease

A. Decreased HDL

B. Increased LDL

C. Increased TG

D. All of these

334. The following image represents which shunt

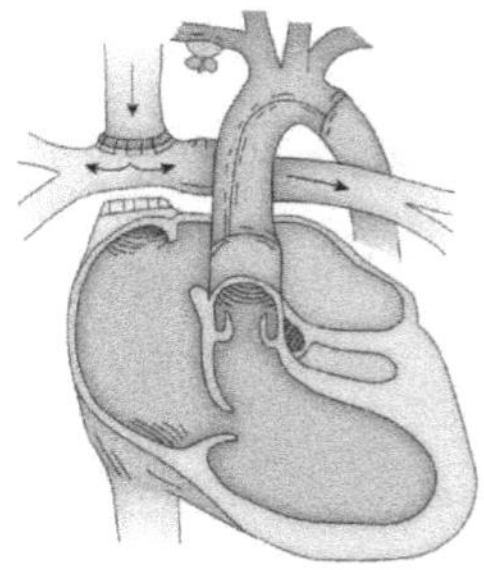

A. Glenn

B. BT shunt

C. Central shunt

D. Total shunt

335. Features of severe TS are all except

A. MDM

B. Peripheral cyanosis

C. No parasternal heave

D. Prominent y descent in JVP

336. The drug not useful in foetal arrhythmia

A. Amiodarone

B. Digoxin

C. Sotalol

D. Flecainide

337. The highest saturation of O2 is seen in

A. Vitelline vein

B. Umblical vein

C. Aorta

D. Umblical artery

338. All are risk factors for abdominal aortic aneurysm except

A. Tobacco smoking

B. Diabetes

C. CAD

D. Aneurysm elsewhere

339. The fourth branchial arch artery gives rise to

A. Arch of the aorta

B. Common carotid

C. Pulmonary artery

D. Ductus

340. False statement about heparin-induced thrombocytopenia

A. Risk of arterial and venous thrombosis

B. Need to stop LMWH also

C. Occurs within 24 hrs if previously used heparin

D. More common in the medical ICU than the surgical ICU

341. Precordial catch syndrome is (Texidor syndrome)

A. Sudden chest pain

B. Sudden cardiac death

C. Sudden breathlessness

D. Sudden palpitation

342. False about HDL

A. HDL cholesterol efflux capacity from macrophages better predictor of CV risk

B. HDL more than 60 mg/dl increases CV risk

C. Drugs targeting HDL have not shown CV benefit

D. Niacin decreases HDL levels

343. Which of the following does not cause tachycardiomyopathy

A. CHB with HR 60/min

B. Preexcitation

C. AF with controlled ventricular rate

D. Frequent PVC

344. Heart failure at birth is seen in all except

A. Large VSD

B. TGA

C. Obstructed TAPVC

D. Severe Coarctation of the aorta

345. Wrong match

A. Phenytoin-CYP2C9

B. Omeprazole- CYP 2C19

C. Quinidine- PGp

D. Propaphenone- CYP2D6

346. Sinus venosus ASD is commonly associated with the anomalous drainage of

A. RUPV

B. LUPV

C. RLPV

D. LLPV

347. B bump in M-mode echocardiography suggests

A. MS

B. MR

C. High diastolic pressure

D. All of these

348. Catheterisation data, as shown below, suggest

	Pressure (mm Hg)	Oxygen Saturation (%)
Superior vena cava		49
Inferior vena cava		55
Right atrium	4	
High		55
Medium		55
Low		55
Right ventricle	90/0–8	55
Main pulmonary artery	20/10	55
Left atrium	5	55
Left ventricle	96/0–8	56
Aorta	96/0–8	57

Vol. 10, No. 3, September 1983

A. VSD

B. ASD

C. PDA

D. TOF

349. A patient with ST-elevation MI develops the following rhythm after thrombolysis. Most likely explanation is

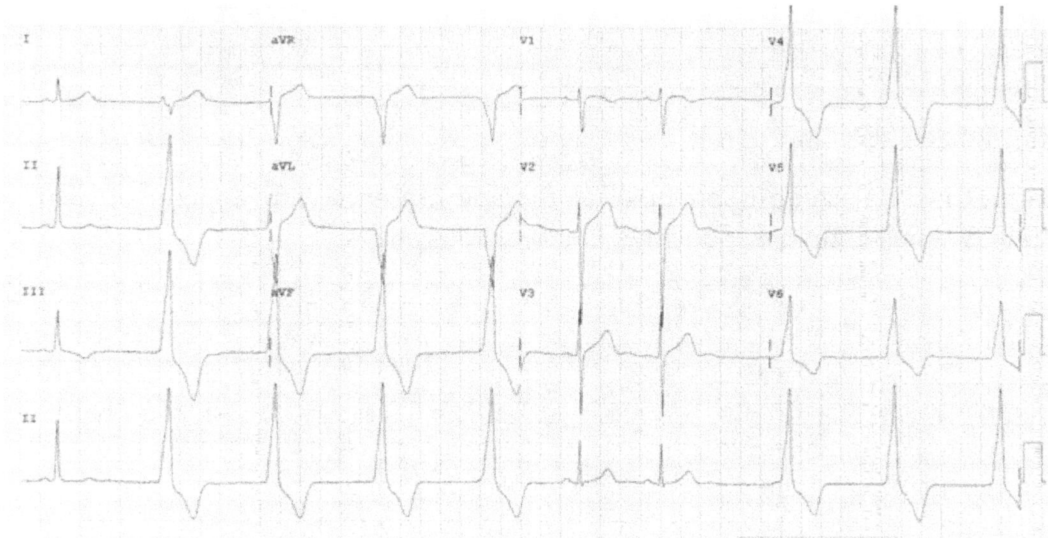

A. CHB

B. Junctional rhythm

C. AIVR

D. VT

350. NOAC should not be preferred in atrial fibrillation with

A. Bioprosthetic valve

B. TB on 4-drug ATT

C. HOCM

D. Severe MR

351. Echocardiographic features of HOCM are all except

A. Asymmetric septal hypertrophy

B. Increased EPSS >10mm

C. Systolic anterior motion of the mitral valve

D. Midsystolic closure of the aortic valve

352. False about the SGLT2 inhibitor

A. Increased risk of genital infection

B. Cardio protection

C. Low risk of ketoacidosis

D. Low risk of hypoglycemia

353. Intravenous iron therapy is useful in

A. HPpEF

B. HFrEF

C. Ferritin <200

D. Ferritin 100-200 with TSAT <20 %

354. A patient with mitral stenosis on medical therapy presents with abdominal pain, vomiting and dizziness. ECG at presentation is shown below. Most likely have

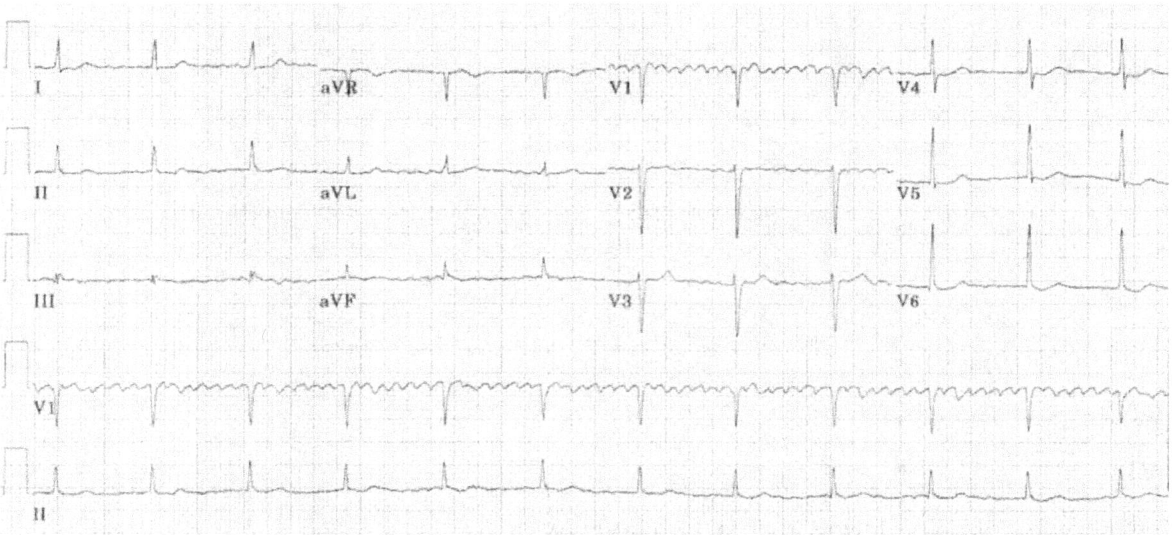

A. Digoxin toxicity

B. Sick sinus syndrome

C. Needs permanent pacing

D. Atrial fibrillation

355. Which of the following parameters is not calculated using Doppler echocardiography

A. PVRI

B. Mean pulmonary artery pressure

C. Systolic pulmonary artery pressure

D. VSD gradient

356. Nut-cracker syndrome represents

A. Left renal vein compression by the superior mesenteric artery

B. The right iliac artery compresses the left iliac vein

C. The superior mesenteric artery compresses the right renal vein

D. The left iliac artery compresses the right iliac vein

357. Tirzepatide is

A. SGLT2 inhibitor

B. Dual GLP and GIP receptor agonist

C. Causes weight gain

D. Useful only in diabetes

358. Pulse wave velocity is an indicator of

A. Endothelial function

B. Arterial stiffness

C. Cardiac inotropy

D. Peripheral arterial resistance

359. Which is a measure of vascular endothelial function

A. Flow-mediated dilation

B. Pulse wave velocity

C. Augmentation index

D. Pulse pressure

360. Which of the following trials evaluated the role of SGLT2 inhibitors in heart failure patients

A. DAPA-HF

B. DELIVER

C. EMPOROR-PRESERVED

D. All of these

361. Which is an indication for intravenous iron therapy in patients with heart failure

A. Ferritin <100 ng/ml

B. Recurrent HF hospitalisation

C. Hb <11 g/dl

D. All of the above

362. Which is not an echocardiographic method to assess the ejection fraction of the left ventricle

A. Simpson

B. Visual eyeballing

C. M-mode

D. TAPSE

363. Which of the following actions of SGLT2 inhibitors helps in heart failure patients

   A. Diuresis

   B. Antiinflammatory

   C. Efficient energy metabolism of the myocardium

   D. All of these

364. ARNI has a survival benefit in which of the following patients

   A. HFrEF

   B. Hypertension

   C. HFpEF

   D. Post-MI patients

365. Which of the following stress test has the highest specificity to detect myocardial ischemia

   A. Stress MPI

   B. Stress ECG

   C. Stress echocardiography

   D. CTCA

366. Which of the following findings is considered normal during exercise ECG testing (TMT)?

   A. Upsloping ST depression

   B. Sustained VT

   C. Hypotension

   D. LBBB

367. Acetazolamide in decompensated heart failure was evaluated in which of the following trial

   A. ADVOR

   B. ASSIST

   C. COLCOT

   D. APOLLO

368. Which is not a calcium modification method during coronary angioplasty?

   A. rotablation

   B. Orbital atherectomy

   C. lithotripsy

   D. OCT

369. Which of the following antianginal targets cardiac metabolism?

   A. Ivabradine

   B. Trimetazidine

   C. Nicorandil

   D. Statins

370. Which of the following shunt lesions is least likely to develop Eisenmenger syndrome

   A. ASD

   B. VSD

   C. PDA

   D. AP window

371. Rosuvastatin 40mg is likely to reduce serum LDL level by?

   A. 20%

   B. 50%

   C. 95%

   D. 90%

372. Which is not considered a contraindication for balloon mitral valvotomy

   A. Pregnancy

   B. LA thrombus

   C. Bicommisural calcification

   D. Moderate MR

373. False statement regarding JVP

   A. Absent a wave in atrial fibrillation

   B. CV wave in severe MR

   C. Kussmaul sign seen in RV infarction

   D. Rapid Y descent in constrictive pericarditis

374. Reverse pulsus paradoxus is seen in

   A. HOCM

   B. Hyperventillation

   C. Constrictive pericarditis

   D. Hemopericardium

375. False statement regarding hangout interval

A. Longer for pulmonary circulation

B. Hangout interval is the cause of the physiological splitting of the first heart sound (S1)

C. Depend upon vascular resistance

D. Delayed closure of the pulmonary semilunar valve

376. A fixed split second heart sound is heard in

A. ASD

B. VSD

C. PDA

D. RSOV

377. Which is not a cause of a continuous murmur

A. PDA

B. Lutem Bacher syndrome

C. VDS with AR

D. RSOV

378. RV cardiomyopathy associated with cutaneous manifestations is seen

A. Naxos syndrome

B. Taffazin syndrome

C. Titin syndrome

D. Timothy syndrome

379. False statement regarding cardiac involvement in Carcinoid Syndrome

A. The mitral valve is involved if associated with PFO

B. Metastatic neuroendocrine tumours commonly underlie this condition

C. Aortic valve involvement is the most common

D. Thickened and restricted valve mobility

380. Which is not an example of a major drug interaction?

A. Digoxin and verapamil

B. Pravastatin and ketoconazole

C. Sildenafil and NTG

D. Amiodarone and digoxin

381. Which of the following trials involved a sham procedure for the evaluation of coronary revascularisation

A. ORBITA

B. COURAGE

C. ISCHEMIA

D. STITCH

382. Which of the following does not require exercise testing for provoking arrhythmia?

A. CPVT

B. Brugada

C. LQT

D. SQT

383. Which of the following is most frequently seen in children with long RP tachycardia

A. AVNRT

B. PJRT

C. JET

D. AVRT

384. A patient of DCMP with CHF was admitted with worsening dyspnea. Investigation reveals Na 128, K 3.4, and urea 69. All are correct except

A. Chronic hyponatremia has a poor prognosis

B. 3% saline can be infused slowly

C. Diuretics can be given

D. Can be volume repleted or depleted

385. Treatment options for diltiazem toxicity, all except

A. Inj calcium gluconate

B. Inj glucagon

C. Inj insulin

D. Inj aminophylline

386. Drug of choice for beta-blocker intoxication

A. Inj glucagon

B. Inj sodabicarbonate

C. Specific monoclonal ab

D. Idarucizumab

387. Relative risk of which of the following is highest with hypertension

A. Heart failure

B. Stroke

C. MI

D. Death

388. SGLT2 inhibitors – all are true except

A. Reduce mortality in HFrEF

B. Reduce mortality in HFpEF

C. Reduce stroke incidence

D. Should be avoided when very low GFR

389. A 70-year-old type 2 DM, all are considered useful preventive measures except

A. Aspirin

B. Atorvastatin

C. Ramipril

D. SGLT2 inhibitor

390. Best time of POG to do foetal echo

A. 16-20 weeks

B. 20-24 weeks

C. After 30 weeks

D. First trimester

391. Use of Lithium in the mother is associated with which of the following congenital anomaly in the baby

A. Ebstein

B. TGA

C. ASD

D. AVSD

392. The most common benign cardiac tumour in children

A. Papillary fibroelastoma

B. Atrial myxoma

C. Rhabdomyoma

D. Lipoma

393. In heterotaxy, peripheral blood smears are most likely to show

A. Howel Jolly bodies

B. Sickle cell

C. Lymphoblast

D. Spherocyte

394. New onset LBBB during peak exercise suggest

A. Phase 3 block

B. Old MI

C. Coronary spasm

D. Circus movement tachycardia

395. Zilebesiran-False statement is

A. Newer antidiabetic

B. RNA interference of angiotensinogen

C. Six-monthly subcutaneous injections

D. Long-term BP control

396. Which anti-hypertensive agent has been shown to worsen heart failure

A. Doxazocin

B. Lisinopril

C. Chlorthalidone

D. Amlodipine

397. The desmoplakin mutation responsible for

A. Arrhythmogenic cardiomyopathy

B. Dilated cardiomyopathy

C. Cardiac sarcoidosis

D. Ventricular non-compaction

398. Lorundrostat is

A. Aldosterone synthase inhibitor

B. Aldosterone receptor antagonist

C. Newer ACE inhibitor

D. Newer ARB

399. Lorundrostat is evaluated for the management of

A. Resistant hypertension

B. ATTR amyloidosis

C. Adrenal adenoma

D. Heart failure

400. Wilkins' echo score is useful in

A. Mitral valvotomy suitability

B. Aortic valvotomy suitability

C. Mitral valve replacement

D. TAVI

Answer Key Level I

1. A (Ref summary-23)
2. A (Ref summary- 43)
3. D. All of these etiologies affect the ascending aorta, causing ostial narrowing of LMCA/RCA
4. C (Ref summary-20)
5. C (Ref summary-20)
6. C (Ref summary-20)
7. D (Ref summary-21)
8. D (Ref summary-20)
9. C. Digoxin shortens QT interval (Ref summary-8)
10. A (Ref summary-21)
11. A (Ref summary-21)
12. D (Ref summary-21)
13. A (Ref summary-8)
14. D (Ref summary-8)
15. A (Ref summary-8)
16. A (Ref summary-8)
17. B (Ref summary-13)
18. C (Ref summary-13)
19. A (Ref summary-13)
20. A (Ref summary-13)
21. A (Ref summary-13)
22. D, all of these are common causes of diastolic dysfunction
23. D (Ref summary-9)
24. D, both systolic/diastolic dysfunction increase the value of MPI.
25. C (Ref summary 6)
26. D (Ref summary 34)
27. D (Ref summary-20)
28. C (Ref summary-25)
29. B, hypoglycemia uncommon with SGLT2 inhibitors (ref summary 8)
30. A (Ref summary-8,9)
31. B (Ref summary-32)

32. A (Ref summary-23)
33. D, Plaque rupture is the commonest cause of ACS, followed by plaque erosion and rarely calcium nodule
34. A
35. A, Global Cardiovascular Risk Consortium (NEJM 2023)
36. A
37. C (Ref summary- 5)
38. A (Ref summary-22)
39. B, TAPVC involves a cardiac structural abnormality of anomalous pulmonary venous drainage to the right atrium
40. B (Ref summary-30)
41. D, closure of the shunt is contraindicated in Eisenmenger syndrome
42. A, valvular regurgitant lesions are relatively well tolerated in pregnancy compared to stenotic pathology (Ref summary-39)
43. A (Ref summary-40)
44. D (Ref summary-25)
45. D (Ref summary-25)
46. B (PARADIGM-HF trial Ref summary- 8)
47. A (Ref summary-8)
48. C. RCC-LCC fusion common (Ref summary-16)
49. A (Ref summary-1)
50. B. Alters myocardial energy source substrate from fatty acid to glucose (Ref summary-1)
51. A. Gerbode defect from LV to RA is a purely left-to-right shunt
52. A (Ref summary-29)
53. B (Ref summary-12)
54. D, RV faces systemic circulation and fails early (Ref summary-25)
55. A
56. B (Ref summary-18)
57. A (Ref summary-24)
58. A (Ref summary-37)
59. B (Ref summary-23)
60. A, progressive worsening of PR and RV dysfunction is a long-term sequela of TOF repair (Ref summary-25)

61. A (Ref summary-)
62. D (Ref summary-16)
63. D (Ref summary-25)
64. A (Ref summary-18)
65. A
66. A. Acute TR following trauma is usually acute and a/w short early systolic murmur
67. D, Ranolazine reduces HbA1c. All other drugs in the options are known to increase blood sugar.
68. C Exercise decreases peripheral resistance.
69. A (Ref summary-1)
70. B
71. A, CAD remains the major cause of sudden cardiac death worldwide
72. B (Ref summary-5)
73. A
74. C, Pneumothorax is a possible complication during permanent pacemaker implantation. This is secondary to injury of the lung apex during venous puncture. High flow O2 and tube drainage are indicated for this complication (Ref summary- 42)
75. D ECG s/o bidirectional VT (Ref summary-20)
76. D. Pulmonary sympathetic denervation has been tried for idiopathic PAH (Ref summary-31)
77. D. One of the subclavian can be involved in Takayasu or aortic dissection, causing upper limb pulse disparity. Higher BP/pulse in the right arm in supravalvular aortic stenosis due to preferential streaming (Coanda effect)
78. B (Ref summary-44)
79. A, ejection click is secondary to the opening of aortic/pulmonary valve and heard immediately after S1 (Ref summary-40)
80. A, common causes of renal artery stenosis are atherosclerotic, fibromuscular dysplasia, Takayasu arteritis and neurofibromatosis
81. B, Monoarthritis is included in major criteria (Ref summary-13)
82. A (Ref summary-21)
83. B, the most common cyanotic heart disease at birth is TGA
84. A. To avoid the issue of renal dysfunction and acidosis
85. A
86. A, pulse pressure is usually wide secondary to a stiff aorta
87. A, (Ref summary 19)

88. D (Ref summary-2)
89. A (Ref summary-5)
90. B (Ref summary-36)
91. A. EMF is characterised by apical obliteration of ventricles with thrombus (Ref summary-12)
92. A, ST elevation in lead III is more than lead II, with reciprocal ST depression in I, avL, suggestive of RCA occlusion. II>III indicate LCX stenosis
93. B (Ref summary-19)
94. D
95. D
96. A (Ref summary-25)
97. A
98. A
99. C (Ref summary-37)
100. A (Ref summary-34)
101. C (Ref summary-1)
102. D compression ventilation ratio 30:2 recommended (ACLS guideline)
103. D
104. B
105. A, X-ray suggestive of supracardiac TAPVC with a figure 8 sign and an arrow representing vertical vein connecting the pulmonary vein to the innominate vein
106. D (Ref summary-40)
107. A. LQT3 precipitated by sleep (Ref summary-21)
108. A (Ref summary-14)
109. B (Ref summary-23)
110. A
111. C. automatic tachycardia usually do not respond to cardioversion
112. C (Ref summary-22
113. D. Hilar waterfall sign seen in persistent truncus arteriosus
114. D Myxoma is usually associated with constitutional symptoms
115. A (Ref summary-26)
116. A (Ref summary-20)
117. D (Ref summary-32)

118. C (Ref summary-11)
119. A (Ref summary-32)
120. A (Ref summary-32)
121. A (Ref summary-19)
122. B, fascicular VT is an idiopathic VT that responds well to RF ablation. (Ref summary-20)
123. C (Ref summary-8)
124. C (Ref summary-36)
125. C (Ref summary-32)
126. A, deep T inversion v4-6 is characteristic of apical HCM (Ref summary-10)
127. A, Biphasic T waves v2-3 with minimal ST elevation suggest Wellens pattern indicating underlying critical LAD stenosis
128. A, should be managed like STEMI
129. A, Left-sided pneumothorax following a pacemaker needs ICTD
130. C, suggestive of atrial flutter, which responds well to catheter ablation
131. A (Ref summary-44)
132. D (Ref summary-32)
133. C (Ref summary-32)
134. C, statins are first line (Ref summary-32)
135. D (Ref summary-37)
136. A, dehydration worsens hyperviscosity symptoms and stroke risk (Ref summary-25)
137. D (Ref summary-34)
138. D, dilated aortic root, causing aortic regurgitation, is common in Marfan syndrome.
139. D, presence of ASD decompresses LA pressure in mitral stenosis
140. B (Ref summary-40)
141. B, Pulmonary vascular resistance (PVR) is increased in Eisenmenger
142. B, LA size increased in HFpEF due to an increase in filling pressure
143. A, hemoptysis and pleuritic chest pain are common with distal segmental small PTE secondary to pulmonary infarction. Hypotension and hypoxia are common in massive PTE.
144. B (Ref summary-22)
145. A, congenital CHB usually involves the AV node (Ref summary-30)
146. A. Mitral annular calcification is an age-related degeneration of the mitral annulus, which hampers the constricting function of the mitral valve and MR

147. C (Ref summary-38)

148. D (Ref summary-15)

149. A

150. C. ECG classic of Torsades, which usually results from prolonged QTc. Long QT syndrome is secondary to loss of loss-of-function mutation of KCNQ1

151. A (Ref summary-22)

152. B, diffuse narrowing, irregularity and calcification are characteristic of Takayasu

153. B

154. C (Ref summary-14)

155. C. Gerbode defect is a purely left-to-right shunt

156. A. Right-sided valves are commonly involved.

157. D

158. A (Ref summary-7)

159. D (Ref summary 29)

160. A, IABP increase diastolic aortic pressure, worsening AR

161. D (Ref summary-20)

162. A (Ref summary-12)

163. B

164. D (Ref summary-26)

165. D. Normal PVR should be less than 2 woods

166. D (Ref summary-32)

167. A (Ref summary-43)

168. B (Ref summary-5)

169. A (Ref summary-25)

170. D. Lung transplantation or combined Heart-lung transplantation can be considered in Eisenmenger

171. C. CT scan is not a good modality for assessment of stent restenosis due to metallic artefacts (Ref summary-27)

172. B (Ref summary-40)

173. A

174. A (Ref summary-31)

175. D

176. C

177. B (Ref summary-25)
178. A. Arterial switch for TGA, not atrial (Ref summary-25)
179. A. Loudness of murmur denotes pulmonary blood flow, so inversely proportional to cyanosis (Ref summary-25)
180. A (Ref summary-25)
181. A (Ref summary-4)
182. C (Ref summary-23)
183. D. MRI image of Ebstein anomaly showing apical displacement of the tricuspid valve. (Ref summary-25)
184. A. Associated with Williams syndrome (Ref summary-35)
185. B. Coronary angiogram with intravascular imaging is the investigation of choice (Ref summary-38)
186. A (Ref summary-11)
187. A. Cardiomegaly usually reverses with the development of Eisenmenger and a decrease in left-to-right shunt (Ref summary-24)
188. A (Ref summary-1)
189. D (Ref summary-2)
190. D (Ref summary-3)
191. A (Ref summary-5)
192. A (Ref summary-5)
193. A (Ref summary-8)
194. D (Ref summary-8)
195. D. BNP levels are elevated with ARNI use. NT-pro BNP is used for monitoring patients with HF taking ARNI (Ref summary-8)
196. B (Ref summary-5)
197. D. Ethanol abuse usually leads to dilated cardiomyopathy (Ref summary-12)
198. A. low low-voltage QRS complex in the presence of ventricular hypertrophy suggests myocardial infiltration. Clinical scenario here hints possibility of AL amyloidosis with bone pain
199. D (Ref summary-11)
200. B (Ref summary-11)
201. A. ECG suggestive of Wellen syndrome, indicating underlying critical LAD stenosis
202. A. De Winter sign- upsloping ST depression in precordial leads. Usually denoted critical stenosis of proximal LAD
203. D
204. B (Ref summary-3)

205. A (Ref summary-16)
206. C (Ref summary-16)
207. C (Ref summary-44)
208. C (Ref summary-30)
209. D. AV nodal disease usually leads to a prolonged PR interval
210. D (Ref summary 19)
211. A (Ref summary-19)
212. D (Ref summary-44)
213. D (Ref summary-25)
214. A (Ref summary-24)
215. C (Ref summary-24)
216. A (Ref summary-24)
217. A (Ref summary-41)
218. C (Ref summary-41)
219. C (Ref summary-41)
220. C (Ref summary-41)
221. C (Ref summary-20)
222. D (Ref summary-31)
223. A (Ref summary-44)
224. A (Ref summary-5)
225. B (Ref summary-5)
226. C (Ref summary-10)
227. A (Ref summary-32)
228. B (Ref summary-32)
229. C
230. A (Ref summary-44)
231. A. ASCVD score used for cardiovascular risk stratification and primary prevention statin therapy (Ref summary-44)
232. B (Ref summary-32)
233. B. LDL cholesterol is usually estimated from other parameters and is usually not measured directly (Ref summary-32)
234. A (Ref summary-32)

235. D (Ref summary 44)
236. B (Ref summary-27)
237. C (Ref summary-27)
238. D
239. A (Ref summary-5)
240. B (Ref summary-5)
241. A (Ref summary-11)
242. A (Ref summary-8)
243. C (Ref summary-8)
244. B (Ref summary-3)
245. B (Ref summary-44)
246. C (Ref summary-44)
247. B (Ref summary-3)
248. A (Ref summary-33)
249. A (Ref summary-25)
250. B (Ref summary-29)
251. B (Ref summary-7)
252. A. RAAS blockers are contraindicated in bilateral renal artery stenosis (Ref summary-29)
253. C (Ref summary-37)
254. D (Ref summary-25)
255. B (Ref summary-23)
256. D (Ref summary-44)
257. A (Ref summary-34)
258. D (Ref summary-21)
259. A (Ref summary-21)
260. D (Ref summary-21)
261. A. Ciraparantag is a universal antidote for heparin and DOAC
262. C (Ref summary-20)
263. A (Ref summary-40)
264. C. Cyanosis with cardiomegaly is common in Ebstein anomaly (Ref summary-25)
265. A. EP study assesses the refractory period of accessory pathway (Ref summary-19)

266. D. Admixture of both systemic and pulmonary venous return happen in the right atrium, and then the same blood circulates to both circulations. Oxygen saturation is equal in all chambers. (Ref summary-25)

267. A

268. C. Pulsus paradoxus is absent in the presence of severe AR and ASD (Ref summary-40)

269. D

270. A (ACCOMPILSH trial)

271. A (SPRINT Trial)

272. B (Ref summary-31)

273. A

274. A

275. A. Electrical alternans in ECG suggestive of cardiac tamponade. So, echocardiography should be done as the next best step.

276. D (Ref summary-5)

277. A. S3 indicate turbulence during the rapid filling phase. Severe AR even without LV dysfunction produces S3.

278. A.

279. C (Ref summary-44)

280. A (Ref summary-41)

281. D. Quinidine is the treatment of choice for Brugada

282. A. Beta blockers and thiazide diuretics cause hyperglycemia as an adverse event.

283. A (Ref summary-5)

284. A (Ref summary-43)

285. C (Ref summary-19)

286. A

287. A

288. D. Decongestion with diuretics improve symptoms in both HFrEF and HFpEF

289. D. Normally, there is continuous forward flow in both systole and diastole in the umbilica artery. In foetal heart failure, there is reversed or absent diastolic flow.

290. A

291. C (Ref summary-6)

292. C

293. A. Auditory stimuli precipitate syncope in LQT2 with KCNH2 mutation (Ref summary-21)

294. A

295. A. A straight left heart border with dilated LA is classic of mitral stenosis. Progressive dilation of LA leads to the development of AF and cardioembolic stroke.

296. D. CYP enzymes do not metabolise Pravastatin and rosuvastatin. (Ref summary-32)

297. A. AVRT secondary to preexcitation

298. A (Ref summary-43)

299. D. Dystrophin mutation in DMD

300. A (Ref summary-21)

301. D (Ref summary-32)

302. B. Rib notching develops late with the formation of collaterals

303. B (Ref summary-20)

304. D

305. D. Upsloping ST depression is normal during stress test. Horizontal or down-sloping ST depression indicates ischemia.

306. A

307. D (Ref summary-14)

308. A (Ref summary-39)

309. B (Ref summary- 44)

310. D. AV nodal blood supply predominantly from RCA. (Ref summary-34)

311. A (Ref summary-30)

312. D. Regional subendocardial LGE in CAD (Ref summary-27)

313. B (Ref summary-37)

314. C (Ref summary-29)

315. D (Ref summary-25)

316. D. Systemic air embolism happens mostly in patients with right-to-left shunts. SV ASD is predominantly left to right

317. B

318. A (Ref summary-40)

319. A. Arerio (aorta) -venous (mixed venous) oxygen difference indirectly suggests cardiac output during a cardiac catheterisation study. Normally it is aound 25%. A higher difference suggests a low cardiac output or increased demand at the tissue level.

320. C (Ref summary-8)

321. D (Ref summary-44)

322. A (Ref summary-7)

323. D. usually reverses with age

324. A. William syndrome

325. B. Collaterals only from the left subclavian formed.

326. A

327. D

328. C. ASD acts as an obligatory shunt from right to left in TAPVC (ref summary 25)

329. A. No TR in tricuspid atresia to cause pulsatile liver.

330. A (Ref summary-21)

331. A. Routine angiography (pharmacoinvasive strategy) is recommended for all patients after thrombolysis. (Ref summary-4)

332. C (Ref summary-21)

333. A (Ref summary-32)

334. A. SVC to PA anastomosis is a Glenn shunt (Ref summary-25)

335. D. High RA pressure and right-to-left shunt via PFO may cause cyanosis in TS.

336. A

337. B (Ref summary-34)

338. B

339. A (Ref summary-34)

340. D (Ref summary-44)

341. A

342. D (Ref summary-32)

343. A (Ref summary-44)

344. A. left-to-right shunt in VSD is low due to high PA pressure at birth. CHF develops after days to weeks once PA pressure drops. All other causes are CHF at birth (ref summary 25)

345. C

346. A (Ref summary-23)

347. C (Ref summary-26)

348. D. Reduced aortic saturation indicates a cyanotic condition. Equal pressure in RV and LV suggests a large VSD. Pressure gradient between RV and PA suggests pulmonary stenosis. Overall, the most likely diagnosis is TOF. (Ref summary-25)

349. C. Accelerated idioventricular rhythm/slow VT is a regular wide complex tachycardia at a slower rate. Common after reperfusion in MI.

350. B. Rifampicin is an enzyme inducer and has drug interaction with NOAC. (Ref summary-22)

351. B. Cardiac contractility usually increases in HCM with reduced EPSS. (Ref summary-10)

352. C. Ketoacidosis is a side effect of the SGLT2 inhibitor (Ref summary-8)

353. B. Role of IV iron is not clear in HFpEF as of now (Ref summary-8)

354. A. Regularised AF or AF with complete AV block is characteristic of digoxin toxicity. Patients with mitral stenosis are frequently prescribed digoxin for rate control of atrial fibrillation (Ref summary-8)

355. A. PVRI is calculated from cardiac catheterisation data (Ref summary-7)

356. A. Left renal vein compressed by the superior mesenteric artery, presenting as hematuria, flank pain and left-sided varicocele.

357. B. Dual GLP1 and GIP receptor agonist useful for diabetes and obesity.

358. B. Carotid femoral pulse wave velocity is an indicator of arterial stiffness (Ref summary-44)

359. A. (Ref summary-44)

360. D (Ref summary-8)

361. A (Ref summary-8)

362. D. TAPSE is used for RV function assessment (Ref summary-26)

363. D (Ref summary-8)

364. A. (Ref summary-8)

365. C (Ref summary-2)

366. A (Ref summary-2)

367. A. ADVOR trial showed better decongestion with acetazolamide in decompensated HF (Ref summary-8)

368. D. OCT is a type of intravascular imaging (Ref summary-5)

369. B (Ref summary-1)

370. A (Ref summary-24)

371. B (Ref summary-32)

372. A (Ref summary-14)

373. B. CV wave seen in severe TR (Ref summary-40)

374. A (Ref summary-40)

375. B. Longer hangout interval of pulmonary valve leads to physiological splitting of S2 (Ref summary-40)

376. A (Ref summary-40)

377. C (Ref summary-40)

378. A (Ref summary-35)

379. C. The tricuspid valve is commonly involved in carcinoid syndrome as inflammatory cytokines reach the right heart via the venous route.

380. B (Ref summary-44)

381. A (Ref summary-1)

382. B (Ref summary-21)

383. (Ref summary-)

384. B

385. A

386. A (Ref summary-)

387. (Ref summary-)

388. C (Ref summary-44)

389. A (Ref summary-44)

390. B

391. A (Ref summary-25)

392. C (Ref summary-36)

393. A. Seen due to lack of spleen in rt isomerism/asplenia (Ref summary-25)

394. A (Ref summary-30)

395. A (Ref summary-29)

396. A (Ref summary-29)

397. A (Ref summary-21)

398. A (Ref summary-29)

399. A (Ref summary-29)

400. A (Ref summary-14)

SUMMARIES

1. Chronic Coronary Syndrome (CCS)

- The 2019 ESC guideline suggested the term Chronic Coronary Syndrome (CCS) to refer to all patients with stable CAD in a non-acute presentation.

> - Stress ECG (TMT) is **NOT** a first-line test to rule out obstructive CAD when an imaging stress test is available
> - Mostly done to assess functional capacity and risk stratification

Approach to suspected CCS/stable chest pain

- Patients with chest pain should first be assessed for the clinical likelihood of obstructive CAD based on symptom characteristics and CV risk factors (smoking, DM, HTN, Dyslipidemia and family history)
- Further evaluation is based on the clinical likelihood of obstructive CAD, as in the following flow diagram-
  - Very Low <5%- no further testing
  - Intermediate- CTCA/stress testing (stress ECHO, Nuclear scan, MRI)
  - Very high >85%- Invasive angiogram
- Indications of invasive coronary angiogram in CCS
  - Very high clinical likelihood
  - Low threshold angina
  - Severe ischemia in non-invasive tests
  - CTCA with LM stenosis> 50%, proximal LAD >70% with DVD, TVD

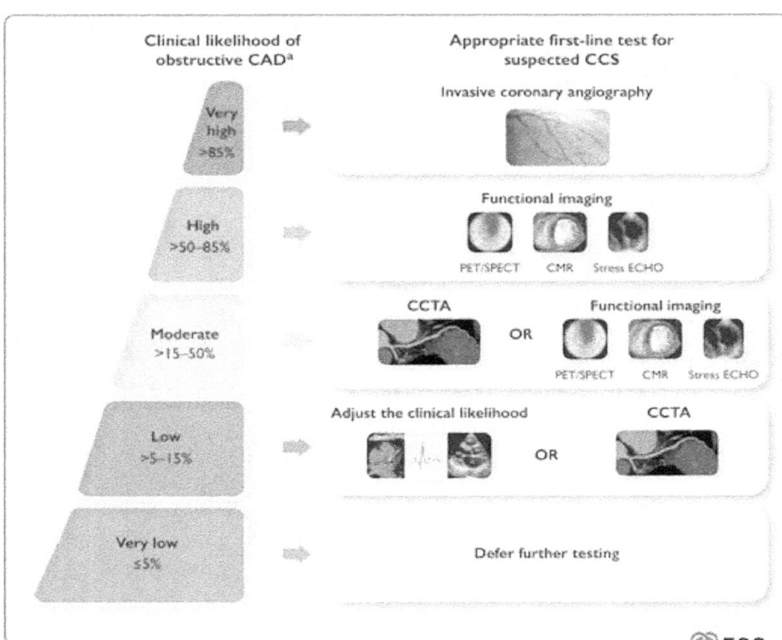

Nitrate

Short-acting

- Nitroglycerin

  Sublingual for rapid angina relief

Long acting

- Isosorbide dinitrate

  Isosorbide mononitrate

- Tolerance is common, and a drug-free period of 8-12 hrs should be ensured

Contraindications

- HOCM or severe aortic stenosis
- Along with a PDE inhibitor (sildenafil), it causes severe hypotension

Ranolazine **decrease HbA1c** and is useful in diabetic patients

Management of CCS

- **Risk factor control**
- **Antiplatelet**
  - Single antiplatelet therapy (either Aspirin or Clopidogrel) is recommended for secondary prevention
  - Dual antiplatelet therapy after PCI
- **Lipid lowering**
  - Lipid-lowering therapy to achieve an LDL goal (< 55mg/dl) is recommended. (statin, ezetimibe, PCSK9inhibitors)
- **Antianginal**
  - **First line anti-anginal-** beta blocker, CCB,
  - **Second line-** Long-acting nitrate, Trimetazidine, Ranolazine, Nicorandil, Ivabradine
  - No trial showed superiority of one drug over another
  - Antianginal does not improve long-term cardiovascular outcomes

Antianginal	Mechanism of action	Side effects
Nitrate	Venodilation and decrease preload	Headache, tachycardia, Methhemoglobinemia
Beta blocker	Decrease HR and contractility, reduce demand	Erectile dysfunction
CCB	Decrease HR and afterload	
Nicorandil	K+ channel opener and Nitrate effect (vasodilation)	Headache
Ranolazine	Inhibit Late Na+ channel → decrease intracellular calcium and improve relaxation	QT prolongation
Trimetazidine	Inhibit 3 Ketoacyl CoA Thiolase (3-KAT) in fatty acid oxidation → change myocardial substrate from fatty acid to glucose	Parkinsonism-like symptom GI upset

Metabolic anti-anginal- Trimetazidine and Ranolazine

- Affects myocardial metabolism- inhibits fatty acid oxidation and changes myocardial substrate from fatty acid to glucose
- Glucose metabolism is more energy efficient (requires less oxygen) and reduces myocardial oxygen demand
- These drugs do not affect HR and BP

Coronary Revascularisation in CCS (PCI/CABG)

- Multiple trials evaluated the role of medical therapy only Vs medical therapy with revascularisation (PCI/CABG)
- However, the majority of landmark trials showed NO mortality benefit of revascularisation over medical therapy

Landmark trials

ORBITA (2018)- PCI does not improve exercise time/angina over medical therapy in patients with stable angina. (compared with a placebo/sham procedure)

ORBITA 2 (2023)- coronary revascularisation with PCI in patients with stable angina resulted in a decrease in angina score compared to placebo

- Mortality benefit of PCI in CCS is questioned in various trials
- The primary goal of PCI in CCS is to improve symptoms

COURAGE (2007)- Initial management with PCI does not decrease death, MI or MACE when added to medical therapy

ISCHEMIA (2020)- Initial invasive strategy over medical therapy does not reduce mortality or CV events in patients with moderate to severe ischemia. It excluded patients with LMCA stenosis. (3.2 yr follow-up)

ISCHEMIA Extend (2023)- lower risk of CV mortality in the PCI arm. No difference in all-cause mortality. (5.7 yr follow-up)

Indications of revascularisation in CCS

- Left main stenosis (even if asymptomatic)
- Triple vessel disease
- Single/double vessel disease involving proximal LAD
- Persistent angina refractory to medical therapy in functionally significant coronary stenosis (FFR positive)

CABG is preferred over PCI

- LMCA/complex coronary anatomy
- Diabetes with triple vessel disease
- LVEF <35%

2. Stress Testing in CAD

Patients with symptoms suggestive of stable CAD / chronic coronary syndrome during OPD visit should first be assessed for pretest probability of CAD, and further evaluation is advised accordingly

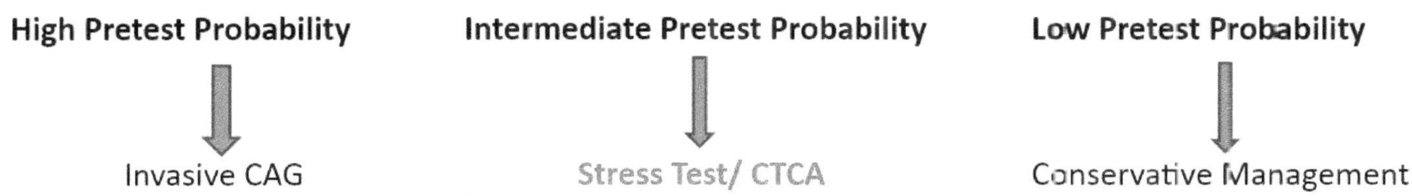

The pretest probability of CAD is assessed based on

- Age
- Sex
- Symptoms (anginal vs non-anginal chest pain)
- Risk factors for CAD (Hypertension, diabetes, dyslipidemia, smoking and family history)

What is a stress test?

- Non-Invasive test, where the heart is exposed to stress (exercise/pharmacological) to identify underlying significant coronary stenosis

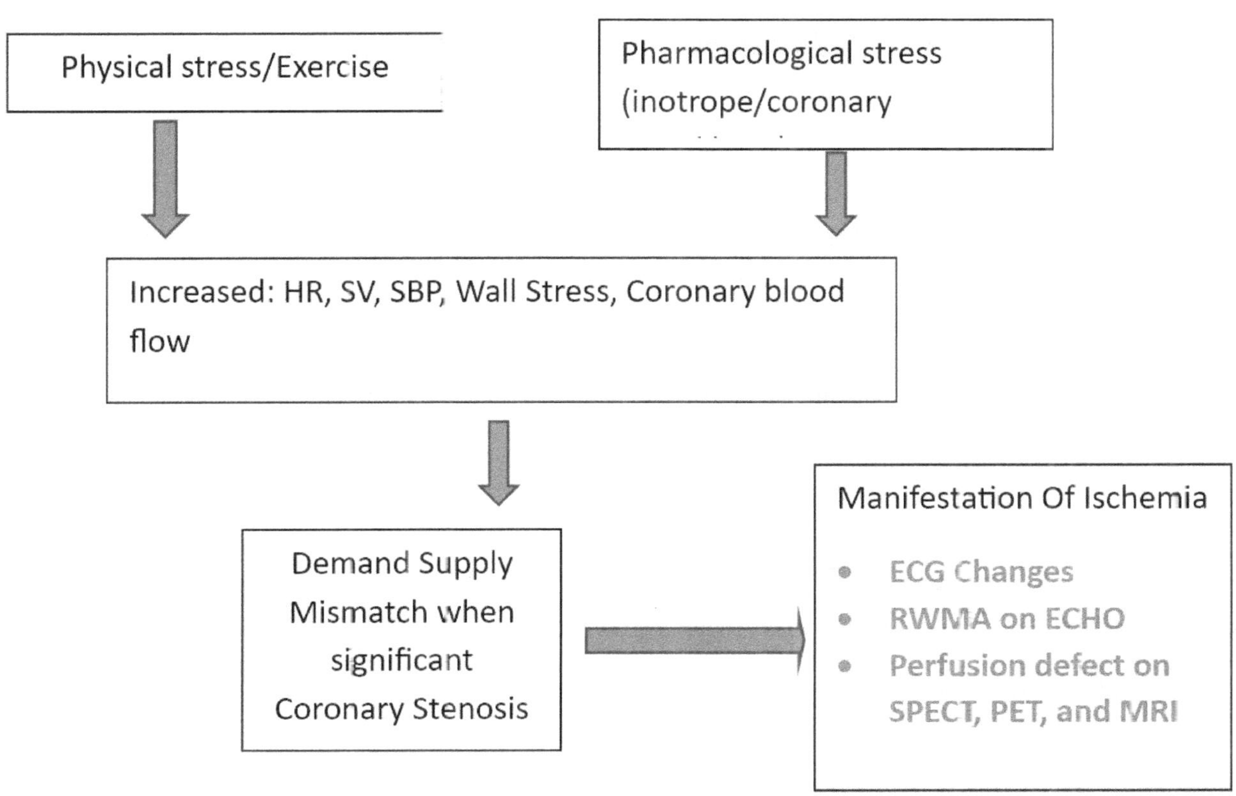

Types of stress

Physical Stress (exercise)	Pharmacological Stress
More physiological	Non-Physiological
Functional capacity can be assessed	Cannot be assessed
• Commonly preferred • pharmacological stress when one cannot perform exercise	Limitation: Side effect of drugs • Adenosine: AV Block, Bronchospasm • Dobutamine: Ventricular Arrythmia • Interaction with drugs e.g., Beta Blockers

MET (Metabolic Equivalents)

- An Objective Measure of expressing functional capacity (exercise capacity)

  1 MET = 3.5 ml O2/kg/min (Suggests the amount of energy used at rest)
- MET involved in any exercise = $\frac{\text{Metabolic rate during Activity}}{\text{Resting Metabolic rate (3.5 ml O2/Kg/min)}}$
- E.g., while running, one uses 8-9 METs

  Climbing 2 flights of stairs involves 4 METS
- Functional capacity during stress test expressed in terms of METS
- Functional capacity assessed during a stress test is the most important prognostic indicator.

How to choose between stress tests?

Stress test modalities

- Stress ECG (TMT)
- Stress ECHO
- SPECT MPI
- Stress PET
- Stress MRI

- Stress ECG (TMT) has poor diagnostic accuracy (sensitivity 60%, Specificity 60%) compared to Stress Echo (Sensitivity, Specificity) and SPECT MPI (Sensitivity, Specificity) when compared with angiography.
- Stress MPI and Stress Echo are preferred over stress ECG
- A stress ECG is usually not done in patients with baseline ECG changes
- For functional capacity assessment, TMT is better

Newer Modalities

- Stress MRI
- Stress PET

Normal Predicted maximal exercise capacity (METs)

MEN: 18 – (0.15 X Age)

WOMEN:14.7 – (0.13 X Age

EXERCISE/ STRESS ECG TEST (TMT)

- Real-time ECG recording, while the patient performs exercise (treadmill walking is a common mode of exercise)
- The Bruce/modified Bruce protocol exercise is commonly performed, which involves a graded increase in speed and inclination of the treadmill

High-risk features during Exercise ECG test (TMT)

- Hypotension
- Poor HR recovery (persistent high HR after exercise)
- Ventricular arrhythmia
- LBB at low heart rate

Normal findings during exercise

- VPCs
- Upsloping ST depression
- Increased BP
- SVT/NSVT

- ECG changes, BP, HR and symptoms monitored during exercise
- **Assess-**
  - Functional capacity (Most important for prognosis)
  - ECG changes suggestive of stress-induced ischemia

Absolute contraindications	Relative contraindications
• Unstable angina/MI within 2 days • Severe symptomatic AS • Ventricular arrhythmia • Hemodynamic instability • Decompensated heart failure • Pulmonary embolism	• Moderate to severe AS • Left main stenosis • Acquired complete AV block • Tachyarrhythmia with uncontrolled ventricular rate

Peak heart rate

- Suggest the adequacy of the exercise test

  Maximal Predicted HR (MPHR) = 220 – Age

  Should achieve 85% of MPHR, to call an adequate study (If < 85% of MPHR achieved, test results are non-diagnostic)
- Persistent high HR (Slow recovery) is associated with poor Prognosis.

ST- T Changes

- Down-sloping / horizontal ST depression in three consecutive beats is considered positive. Upsloping ST depression can be physiological during tachycardia.
- ST depression doesn't localise ischemia / identify the culprit artery (ST elevation does)
- ST elevation ≥ 1 mm in aVR is a predictor of LM / Multivessel CAD

BP Response

- Normally, SBP should increase (usually > 140), and diastolic BP remains the same / slightly decreases with exercise.

- Functional capacity **estimated** (METS) during the exercise ECG test
- Functional capacity is **accurately measured** in cardiopulmonary testing **(CPT)**

- Exercise-induced hypotension (20 mmHg fall from resting) suggests underlying severe CAD (normally multivessel CAD with LV dysfunction)

DUKE Treadmill Prognostic Score

To access the prognosis, combining three parameters

- **Score** = **Exercise time** – (5 X **ST deviation**) – (4 X **Angina Index**)
  - ST deviation: Max ST elevation/depression, except in aVR.

- Angina Index:
  - 0 = None
  - 1 = Non-limiting Angina
  - 2 = Exercise limiting angina
- Score ranges from -25 to +15, where:
  - ≥ + 5 = low risk
  - - 10 to + 4 = moderate risk
  - ≤ - 11 = high risk

STRESS ECHO/DOBUTAMINE STRESS ECHO (DSE)

- Pharmacological stress using dobutamine (5 μg/kg/min to 20-40 μg/kg/min) is commonly done.
- Real-time assessment of ventricular contractility and RWMA is evaluated with increasing dobutamine doses.
- Stress echo has the **highest specificity** for assessing ischemia among other ischemia tests.

DSE is also used for the assessment of low-flow low-gradient aortic stenosis to differentiate true AS from pseudo-severe AS

Rest	Stress	interpretation
Normal	Hyperdynamic	Normal
Normal	Hypokinetic	ischemia
Akinetic	Akinetic	infarct
hypokinetic	Improves and then deteriorate (Biphasic response)	hibernating

STRESS MPI (SPECT)

- Assessment of myocardial ischemia by injecting radioactive contrast at peak exercise/ pharmacological stress and comparing perfusion images at rest and stress
- Details in the Nuclear cardiology **summary 28**

3. Management of NSTEMI

A. General Measures

Anti-ischemic management (O2, nitrate and beta blockers)

Dosing of P2Y12

- Ticagrelor 180mg stat f/b 90mg BD
- Prasugrel 60mg stat f/b 10 mg OD
- Clopidogrel 300-600 mg stat f/b 75 mg OD

B. Antiplatelet therapy

a. Aspirin 162-325 mg to all patients.

Non-enteric-coated tablets are preferred for rapid absorption

Enteric-coated 75-100 mg OD for maintenance.

b. P_2Y_{12} Inhibitors- Ticagrelor/prasugrel preferred over clopidogrel

Thienopyridine	Non Thienopyridine
• Clopidogrel Prasugrel • Irreversible P_2Y_{12} Inhibition • Pro Drug, Needs hepatic CYP for activation	• Ticagrelor • Reversible P_2Y_{12} Inhibition • Direct acting

- Usually given once the coronary anatomy is evaluated by CAG and planned for PTCA.
- P_2Y_{12} Inhibitors are not given if planning for CABG. (high risk for bleeding)
- It can be given simultaneously with aspirin if an early invasive strategy (PCI/CABG) is not planned.

Cangrelor

Short-acting intravenous P2Y12 inhibitor

Mostly used when surgery is planned

C. Anticoagulation

a. Parenteral anticoagulation should be given to all patients till revascularisation is done.

b. 3 commonly used agents:

i. UFH: - 60 Units /kg IV bolus f/b 12 Units/kg/hr Infusion

i. LMWH(Enoxaparin): - 1 mg/kg S/C every 12 hourly

ii. Bivalirudin: - 0.1 mg/kg IV bolus f/b 0.25 mg/kg/hr Infusion

Contraindications of Prasugrel

- History of TIA
- Age > 75
- Weight <60kg

Revascularisation in NSTEMI (ESC guideline 2023)

- Routine invasive approach (CAG and Revascularisation) recommended in all patients with confirmed NSTEMI/ high index of suspicion of unstable angina to reduce mortality

- **Early invasive (<24 hr)** is usually preferred for **high-risk NSTEMI**
  - A confirmed diagnosis of NSTEMI with positive hsTroponin
  - Dynamic ST-segment or T wave changes.
  - Transient ST-segment elevation.
  - A GRACE risk score >140.

> Risk stratification of NSTEMI is done using
> - **GRACE score**
> - **TIMI score**

- **Immediate invasive** strategy for **very high-risk NSTEMI**
  - Haemodynamic instability or CS.
  - Recurrent or ongoing chest pain refractory to medical treatment.
  - Acute HF secondary to ongoing myocardial ischaemia.
  - Life-threatening arrhythmias or cardiac arrest after presentation.
  - Mechanical complications.
  - Recurrent dynamic ECG changes suggestive of ischaemia (particularly with intermittent ST-segment elevation)
- PCI with drug eluting stent is preferred mode of revascularization and is usually successful in 90%-95% of patients.
- CABG considered in:
  - DM with triple vessel disease
  - Poor LVEF (<35%)
  - Contraindications to DAPT
  - Coronary anatomy not suitable for PCI
  - Other indications of surgery, e.g. valvular disease.

Long-term therapy (for all patients after ACS, including NSTEMI/STEMI)

> **REBOOT CNIC trial**
> - Beta blocker therapy after MI without reduction in EF (EF >40%) does not reduce reinfarction, death or hospitalisation

A. Antiplatelets

a. In most patients with ACS with or without revascularisation, DAPT (Aspirin + P2Y12 Inhibitors) is needed for 6-12 months.

b. Duration of antiplatelet therapy can further be individualised according to ischemic and bleeding risk.

c. In high bleeding risk, 1-3 months DAPT followed by a single antiplatelet (preferably Ticagrelor) is appropriate. (**TWILIGHT Trial)**

B. Beta Blockers and ACE Inhibitors

a. Beta blockers

   i. If LVEF <40% regardless of symptoms (Class I)

   ii. To all patients, irrespective of EF (Class IIa)

- LDL target after ACS < 55 mg/dl
- If recurrent ACS within 2 years,
- target <40 mg/dl

Causes of troponin elevation

- ACS/MI,
- Heart failure
- Severe hypertension
- Myocarditis
- Pulmonaryembolism
- Cardiacprocedures
- Arrhythmias
- Renal failure, sepsis, critical illness

b. ACE Inhibitors

 i. If LVEF <40%, symptomatic HF, DM, CKD (Class I)

 ii. To all patients, irrespective of EF (Class IIa)

c. MRA- If LVEF <40% and symptomatic HF/ DM

C. Statins and lipid-lowering Drugs

a. High intensity statin started to all and assessed after 4-6 weeks with a target LDL < 55mg/dl

b. Addition of Ezetimibe and PCSK9 inhibitors, if the target LDL is not achieved after 4-6 weeks.

c. LDL target < 40mg/dl if recurrent ACS (recurrence within 2 yrs)

High-sensitivity troponin (hs troponin)

- Newer method of detecting very low levels of troponin in the blood **(ng/L range)**
- Detects very early after myocardial injury/MI (within 1-3 hours)
- Very high negative predictive value and useful in an emergency setting to rule in/rule out MI
- **Rise and/or fall** of hs-cTn values with at least **one value above the 99th percentile upper reference limit (URL)** is considered diagnostic for MI

4. Management of STEMI

The goal of management in STEMI is to initiate revascularisation therapy early to protect the myocardium from irreversible damage.

Pre-Hospital Thrombolysis

1. Meta-analysis shared 17% mortality reduction with prehospital mediated thrombolysis
2. Pre-hospital thrombolysis is considered reasonable when there is a significant delay in transportation (greater than 60-90 minutes) to a PCI-capable centre and adequate paramedical support is available.

Initial medical management

> - Ticagrelor (PLATO trial), or Prasugrel (TRITON TIMI 38), are preferred over Clopidogrel in patients with ACS undergoing PCI
> - Clopidogrel is used in patients undergoing thrombolysis

- Pain relief: Morphine 4-8mg, anti–anginal (nitrates, beta–blockers)
- Oxygen: Only when there is hypoxia(spo2<90%)
- Nitrates: Used for pain relief

  avoided when IWMI with RV infarction, hypotension, or

  bradycardia
- **Beta blockers**
  - Routine use of IV beta blocker is not recommended, may be detrimental in some patients(COMMIT TRIAL).
  - Can be given to patients with hypertension and ongoing ischaemia (IV metoprolol 5MG bolus)
  - Avoid if heart failure, SBP < 90mmHg, HR < 60 BPM, or AV block.
  - Oral beta blockers should be started early within 24 hours and continued unless contraindicated.
- **Antiplatelet**
  - Loading of aspirin 162-325mg (chewable non-enteric coated tablet for rapid absorption), maintenance dose of 75-162 mg afterwards
  - P2Y12 inhibitor-
    - TICAGRELOR (180mg stat followed by 90 mg BD)
    - PRASUGREL (60 mg stat followed by 10mg OD)
    - CLOPIDOGREL preferred in patients undergoing thrombolysis (COMMIT TRIAL)

Cangrelor is a potent IV antiplatelet agent with very rapid action, and can be given to patients undergoing PCI.

Anticoagulation

Patients undergoing thrombolysis

- UFH
- Enoxaparin (30 mg IV bolus followed by 1mg/kg s/c 12 hourly)

Patient undergoing PCI

- UFH is preferred during PCI, and no prior anticoagulant is needed.
- Monitored by the point of care ACT (activated clotting time)

  Target ACT 250-300

  200-250 (if GPIIb/IIIa needed)

GPIIb/IIIa inhibitors are contraindicated in those receiving thrombolysis

Revascularisation in STEMI

- Overall, PCI is superior to fibrinolysis in terms of clinical outcome.
- Few trials showed that very early thrombolysis (<3 hours) is as effective as primary PCI. (**STREAM trial**)

A. Thrombolysis in STEMI

- Should be considered in patients when shifting to a PCI-capable centre takes more than 120 minutes.
- Fibrin-specific agents (alteplase, reteplase, tenectiplase) preferred over streptokinase.

Ideal

Door-to-needle time < 30min

Door-to-balloon time < 90min

Drug	Dose	Specificity	Patency Rate	TIMI III flow rate
Streptokinase	1.5 MU over 30-60 min	Non-Specific	60% - 68 %	~30%
Alteplase (tPA)	15 mg bolus 0.75 mg/kg (50 ml) over 20 min 0.5 mg/ kg (35 mg) over 1 hr	Fibrin specific	73 % - 84 %	~54%
Reteplase	10 unit + 10 unit Double bolus 30 min apart	Fibrin specific	84%	~54%
Tenecteplase	Bolus: wt based 0.5 mg / kg	Fibrin specific	85%	~54%

Referred to PCI capable centre even if delay >120 mins, if

- Contraindication to thrombolysis
- Late presentation (>12 hours)
- Shock/ acute severe heart failure

Contraindications to thrombolysis

- Previous history of intracranial bleed
- Structural lesion/ intracranial neoplasm
- Ischaemic stroke (within <3 months)
- Suspected aortic dissection,
- Acute bleeding
- Closed facial trauma
- Intracranial/ spinal surgery within 6 months.

- Ticagrelor, Prasugrel, GpIIb/IIIa inhibitors are contraindicated in patients undergoing thrombolysis
- Very high bleeding risk

The overall rate of intracranial bleed after thrombolysis is 1 %

Resistance to STK with recent exposure to Streptococcus

Should not use STK if STK has been used within the last 6 months.

- **Pharmacoinvasive PTCA** is routinely done after thrombolysis
- **Rescue PTCA** immediately after thrombolysis if failed PTCA / hemodynamic instability
- **Facilitated PTCA** to all patients immediately after thrombolysis not recommended

After thrombolysis → Pharmacoinvasive PCI

- All patients should be transferred to a PCI-capable centre for CAG and revascularisation (**pharmacoinvasive strategy**) within 3 to 24 hours.
- Emergency transfer for **Rescue PTCA** PCI-capable centre as early as possible when:
    - Failed thrombolysis
    - Severe heart failure/ cardiogenic shock
    - Persistent angina/ischaemia.

B. Primary angioplasty/PTCA

- Standard of care in patients with STEMI
- High rate of achieving TIMI-III flow (>=90%) and very low bleeding risk compared to thrombolysis
- Wiring of the culprit artery, followed by balloon angioplasty and stenting.
- Routine use of aspiration thrombectomy is not recommended (class III)

Facilitated PTCA

- Routine thrombolysis followed by PTCA immediately
- Increases mortality and is not recommended now (class III)
- PCI should not be done within 2-3 hours of thrombolysis in stable patients, as there is increased bleeding risk.

In patients with multivessel CAD

- When we find one culprit artery and significant stenosis in other vessels
- In stable patients, complete revascularisation (both culprit and other vessels) can be done in same hospitalization.
- In hemodynamically unstable/ shock, culprit vessel revascularisation only recommended (CULPRIT SHOCK trial)

5. Coronary Intervention

> **Contrast agents**
>
> - High osmolar (1400-1800 mOsm/kg)
>   - Urograffin
> - Low osmolar (500-850)
>   - Iohexol (Omnipaque)
> - Iso-osmolar (290)
>   - Iodixanol (Visipaque)
> - Non-ionic is less nephrotoxic than ionic
> - Osmolarity of Iodixanol is almost similar to plasma and is the least nephrotoxic
> - Urograffin is not used now

A. Coronary angiography (CAG)

- Selective injection of coronary arteries with iodinated contrast agent with real-time X-ray imaging (fluoroscopy) to assess coronary anatomy
- Femoral or radial access is commonly used (radial most preferred)
- A thin, flexible tube (**diagnostic catheter**) is inserted via this access and selectively engaged with the right and left coronary arteries
- Contrast agent injected and imaged using multiple views
- Angiography views
  - As the arteries are oriented three-dimensionally around the heart, they are imaged in multiple oblique views
  - Views are named as per the **position of the image-intensifier**
  - Four standard views of CAG are-
    - LAO cranial
    - RAO crania
    - LAO caudal
    - RAO caudal
  - Caudal views best visualise the proximal part of the arteries, and cranial views are for the distal part of the arteries

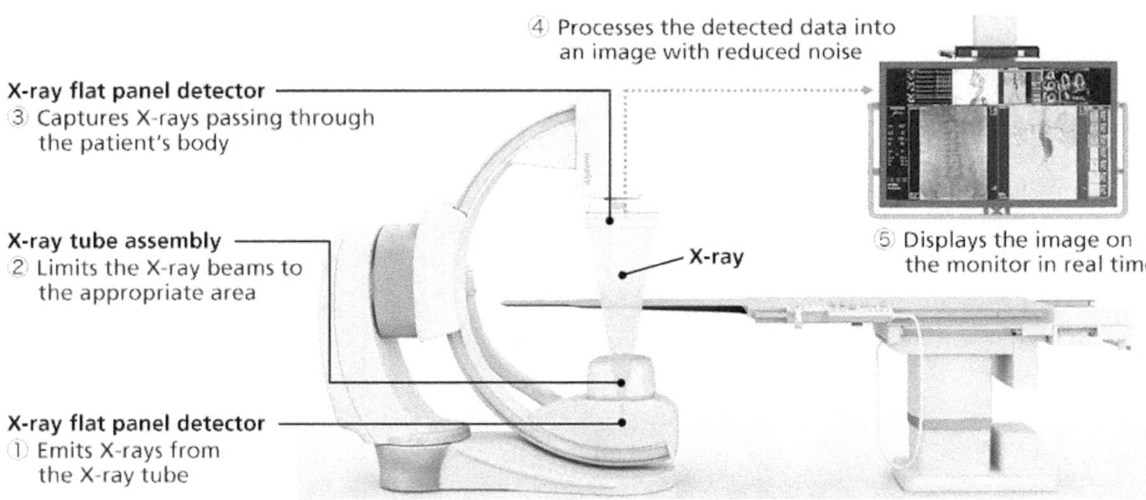

Fig 5.1 Standard Cardiac Catheterization Lab (Cath-lab)

- **Normal coronary angiogram**

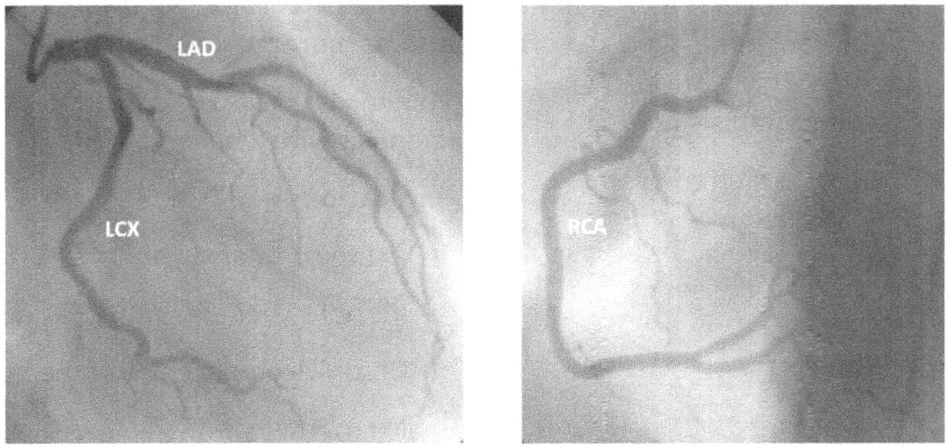

- **Significant coronary stenosis (Obstructive CAD)**
  - Angiographically diametric **stenosis of > 70 %** considered significant for major epicardial arteries
  - For **left main >50%** stenosis is considered significant

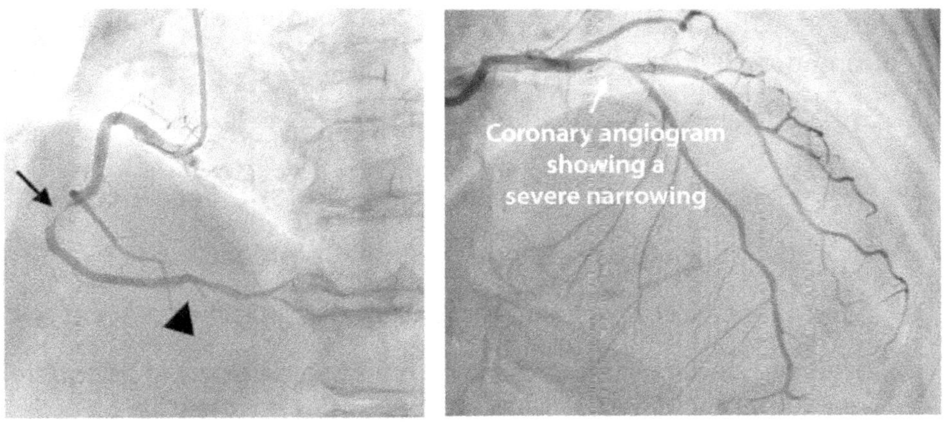

SYNTAX score

- Objective assessment of the anatomic complexity of coronary stenosis in multivessel disease
- Used for decision making between revascularization methods (CABG Vs PTCA) in multivessel CAD
- Total score- 60

High Score (> 32) CABG is preferred

Low or intermediate score (<22, 22-32) suitable for PTCA

- Types of coronary lesion/stenosis based on the anatomic complexity of stenosis

  Type A- Discrete (<10mm), concentric, non-ostial, no calcification, thrombus, angulation or major side branch involvement

  Type B- Tubular (10-20 mm), eccentric, moderate angulation, moderate to heavy calcification, ostial lesion

  Type C- diffuse (>20 mm), CTO, bifurcation stenosis, excessive tortuosity, degenerated venous graft stenosis

  The chances of successful PTCA are higher with type A and lowest with type C

- Revascularisation is indicated for significant left main stenosis (<50%) even if asymptomatic
- CABG is preferred over PTCA for left main stenosis

- ACT (activated clotting time) is measured during PTCA to assess adequate anticoagulation during PTCA
- Desired ACT range during procedure: 250-350

B. Coronary angioplasty

Percutaneous coronary intervention (PCI) or Percutaneous transluminal coronary angioplasty (PTCA)

- Minimally invasive procedure to open a significant coronary stenosis with a balloon/stent
- **Indications of PTCA**
  - Acute coronary syndrome (STEMI, NSTEMI, Unstable angina)

    Mortality benefit with PTCA over medical management only
  - Chronic coronary syndrome/stable CAD

    No mortality benefit. Improved quality of life and symptomatic relief. Medical therapy is equally good. PTCA considered in high risk or angina refractory to medical therapy.
- **Procedure**
  - Access- femoral/radial
  - Anticoagulation- Unfractionated heparin (UFH) is used for anticoagulation during the procedure (dose: 100 units/kg IV)
  - Hardwares
    - Guide catheter- to engage the desired coronary artery
    - Coronary guide wire- passed across the desired coronary stenosis
    - Balloon catheter- stenotic segment is predilated
    - Stents- deployed across the dilated segment to prevent re-occlusion
- Stenosis with severe calcification may not be opened adequately with ballooning only and may require additional **calcium modification methods**
- Complex stenosis, such as CTO (chronic total occlusion) and stenosis at the coronary bifurcation, requires additional hardware and procedural expertise

CTO (Chronic Total Occlusion)

- Complete occlusion of coronary artery for more than 3 months
- Revascularisation with PTCA requires additional hardware (guide and wires)

Bifurcation stenosis

- When stenosis involves the branching point of two major epicardial arteries
- Involved the risk of occluding one branch while opening the other
- Medina classification for better naming of bifurcation stenosis
- Techniques for bifurcation PTCA

- Provisional stenting
- Dedicated two-stent strategy- Mini Crush, DK crush, Cullote, T and TAP technique

Calcium modification methods

Stenosis with severe calcification requires additional calcium modification methods before stenting for adequate vessel opening

- **Cutting balloon/scoring balloon**
  - Small blades over the balloon device to give microincisions in fibrocalcific stenosis. Wolverine, Flextome cutting balloon
- **Rotablation**
  - A rotating burr mounted with diamond particles is used for modifying and debulking vascular calcium
- **Orbital atherectomy**
  - Rotating crown similar to Rotablation
- **Intravascular lithotripsy**
  - A balloon device using sonic pressure waves to break calcium in the vessel wall, helping in better balloon dilation and stenting
- **LASER**
  - Excimer LASER coronary angioplasty

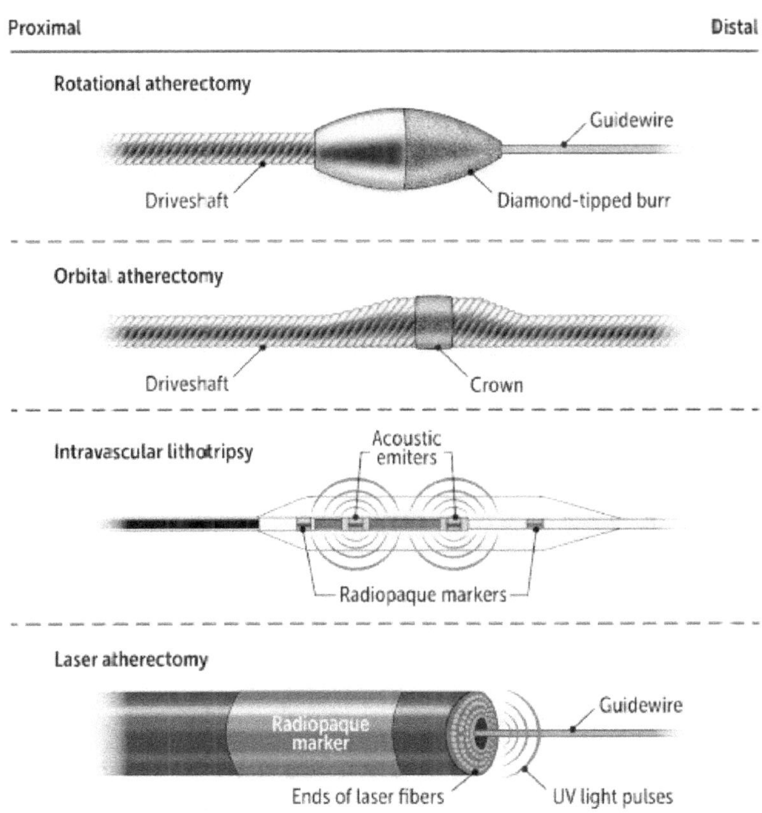

Coronary stents

- **Stent thrombosis-**

  Acute occlusion of the stent with thrombus formation

- **Restenosis-**

  chronic occlusion secondary to intimal hyperplasia

- Issues with balloon angioplasty
  - Acute vessel closure (secondary to dissection, thrombus)
  - Recoil after balloon dilation and residual stenosis
  - Long-term restenosis
- All these issues with balloon angioplasty led to the introduction of metallic stents after balloon dilation of stenosis

Bare metal stent (BMS)

- metallic frames made of stainless steel/alloy (cobalt-chromium/platinum-chromium)

  Approved BMS- R stent, Express 2, Omega, Matrix

  Disadvantage- High state of long-term stenosis secondary to intimal hyperplasia.

- Late stent thrombosis increases after 1st-generation DES compared to BMS.

Drug-eluting stent (DES)

- An antiproliferative drug coated over a metallic frame to reduce reactionary intimal hyperplasia, resulting in a lower restenosis rate compared to BMS
- DES is the standard of care now in PTCA. BMS are no longer used.
- 3 components of DES
  - **Metallic stent**
  - **Drug** (Sirolimus, everolimus, zotarolimus, paclitaxel)
  - **Polymer** - helps in the sustained release of the Drug
- Antiproliferative drugs inhibit intimal hyperplasia over the stent, reducing the restenosis rate
- However, very late stent thrombosis increases after 1st-generation DES compared to BMS. It was attributed to the polymer used for drug delivery.
- Subsequently, with improvement in polymer and stent technology/strut thickness stent thrombosis rate decreased significantly.
- 1st generation DES- CYPHER, TAXUS

  2nd generation DES- XIENCE, PROMUS, ENDEAVOR

- There is ongoing evolution in stent technology to reduce stent failure

Newer developments

- **Drug-coated balloons**- mostly used for stent restenosis
- **Bioabsorbable vascular scaffold (BVS)**- A biopolymer-based stent that would degrade completely and is designed to avoid a foreign metal inside the artery.

ABSORB_BVS-made of PLLA, resorbs completely at 3 years. Increased incidence of scaffold thrombosis.

- FFR less than 0.8 is significant
- Revascularisation guidelines-class I-in patients with angina without any evidence of ischemia, and intermediate angiographic stenosis, FFR/ IFR should be done before PCI.

FFR & IFR

- Issues with angiographic assessment of coronary stenosis
  - Diametric assessment has interobserver variability (60% vs 70%)
  - Angiographically significant appearing stenosis may not always cause myocardial ischemia

1. FFR

- The concept of FFR was introduced to assess the **functional significance** of coronary stenosis, i.e. whether stenosis is causing myocardial ischemia
- Helps in decision-making for revascularisation (PTCA) for angiographically borderline stenosis (40-80%)

Procedure

- An invasive procedure
- Performed by a pressure wire placed across the coronary stenosis, and the ratio of distal pressure **Pd** and proximal pressure **Pa** (pressure in the aorta) is calculated.
- Adenosine (infusion/ bolus) is used for coronary hyperemia (pressure directly proportional to flow when resistance in the coronary bed is minimal by using vasodilation)
- FFR = Pd/Pa at maximal hyperemia
- FFR (Pd/Pa ratio) value **less than 0.8** is considered significant

Evidence-

- **FAME trial** in patients with multivessel CAD planned for PCI, FFR-guided PCI is better than angiographic guided PCI.
- **FAME II trial** in patients with stable CAD, initial FFR-guided revascularisation is better than OMT alone for urgent revascularisation.
- **FAME III trial** in patients with triple vessel disease FFR FFR-guided PCI is non-inferior to CABG for death, MI, and repeat revascularisation at one year.

2. IFR (Instantaneous wave-free ratio)

- Pd /Pa ratio measured similar to FFR but without the use of adenosine for coronary hyperemia.
- Pressure is measured at wave wave-free period of the cardiac cycle when
- **Cut off 0.89** correlates with 0.8 in FFR

Coronary intravascular imaging (IVUS and OCT)

- An invasive coronary angiogram is a luminogram and doesn't characterise atherosclerotic plaque well
- This led to the development of intravascular imaging to better characterise the vessel wall and atherosclerotic plaque
- IVUS (Intravascular ultrasound) and OCT (optical coherence tomography) are two different modalities with different principles and imaging, summarised in the following table

	IVUS	OCT
Principle	Sound wave/ Ultrasound	Light wave/ near infrared
Resolution	Poor (70-200μ)	Good 10-20 μ
Depth of penetration	More 5-10 mm Depth of calcium not assessed	Less 1-3.5 mm Better assessment of depth of calcium
Need of contrast	No	Yes (Blood free space required)
Plaque characterization	Fibrofatty calcific Not a good modality for fatty plaque detection Plaque burden	Better delineate fibrofatty, calcific plaque Better delineate plaque erosion Vs rupture Vulnerable plaque macrophage

Current use of intravascular imaging during coronary intervention

- To assess the severity of left main stenosis [lumen area <6 mm2 considered significant], [Angiographic diameter stenosis>50% considered significant]
- Stent optimisation (sizing, apposition, expansion, complications). Intravascular imaging-guided PTCA/stents have better long-term results compared to angiographically guided stent implantation

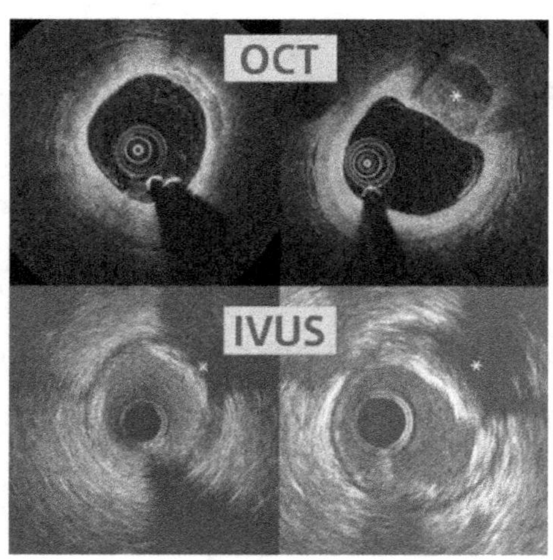

Upper panel showing an OCT image of calcific coronary stenosis with better resolution and assessment of the depth of calcification. Lower panel showing IVUS image of the same.

6. Landmark History

1929 – First human cardiac catheterisation

- **Werner Forssmann** catheterised his own right atrium, proving the feasibility.
- He used a ureteric catheter and inserted it into his arm vein, then advanced it to the right atrium, and then took an X-ray to confirm its position.

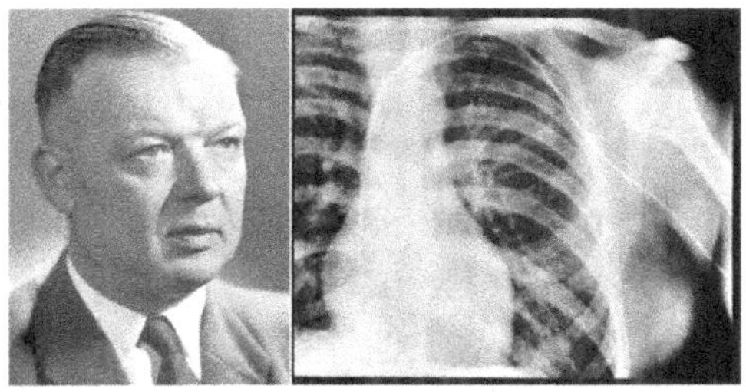

1964 – First coronary angiography

- **Mason Sones** accidentally injected contrast into the right coronary artery while performing an aortic root angiogram in a patient with RHD
- Although it was accidental, it laid the feasibility of selective coronary angiography

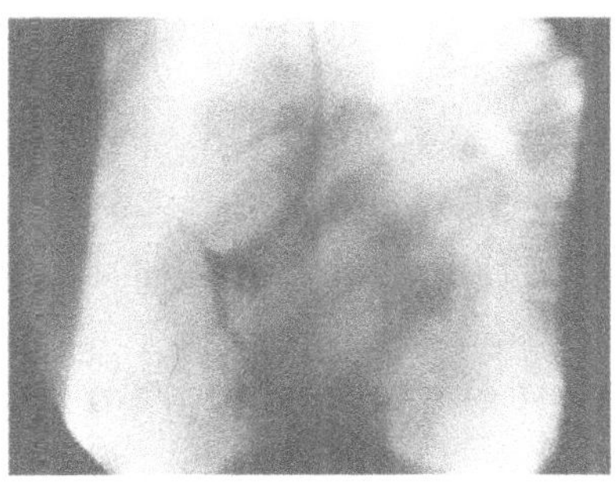

1977 – First percutaneous coronary angioplasty (PTCA)

- **Andreas Gruentzig** performed the first successful **balloon angioplasty** in Zurich, revolutionising CAD treatment.

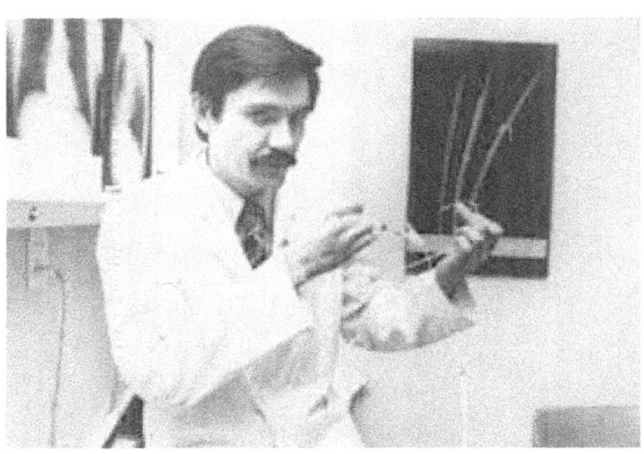

1986 – First coronary stent

- **Sigwart and Puel** placed the first coronary stent (Wallstent) to prevent restenosis post-angioplasty.

2002 – Introduction of Drug-Eluting Stents (DES)

- The first, sirolimus-eluting stent (CYPHER), reduced restenosis dramatically.

2002- The first TAVR (Transcatheter Aortic Valve Replacement),

- **Alain Cribier** performed TAVR via transseptal antegrade approach in a patient with severe AS and end-stage heart failure

Other notable history

1958: **Åke Senning and Rune Elmqvist** implanted the **first pacemaker** to treat Stokes-Adams attacks.

1970: **Michel Mirowski** invents the automatic implantable cardioverter-defibrillator **(AICD),** designed to abort life-threatening ventricular arrhythmias.

1953: John Gibbon performed the first open-heart surgery using a heart-lung machine, revolutionising surgical procedures

1967: **Christiaan Barnard** performed the first successful human heart transplant.

1944: **Helen Taussig and Alfred Blalock** developed the first corrective surgery for Tetralogy of Fallot.

1960: **Albert Starr and Lowell Edwar**ds introduced the first mechanical heart valve, revolutionising the treatment of valvular heart disease.

1961: The **Framingham Study** publishes its first report, identifying key risk factors for heart disease, including high blood pressure, smoking, and high cholesterol levels.

1903: **Willem Einthoven** develops the first **electrocardiogram (ECG),** transforming the study of cardiac electrical activity into a clinically useful tool.

7. Cardiac Cathetrization

- Cardiac catheterisation literally means putting a catheter (plastic pipe) percutaneously into any cardiac chamber for the diagnosis of structural heart disease
- With the advancement of imaging (2D, Doppler echocardiography, CT and MRI), diagnosis is made non-invasively in the majority of cardiac diseases
- However, cardiac catheterisation remains the **gold standard** in the diagnosis of structural heart disease and is used mostly when there is diagnostic confusion with imaging

Cardiac catheterization

Assessment of structure + Assessment of function

- Selective angiogram

- Pressure, waveform, gradient
  Calculation of shunt, Qp, Qs

↓

Final diagnosis

- Example: catheterisation in aortic stenosis

  Left ventricular angiogram showing doming and restricted opening of the aortic valve. Pressure measurement shows high LV systolic pressure and a significant gradient between LV and the aorta during systole. Combining all this information leads to the diagnosis of aortic stenosis.

Normal pressures and waveforms of cardiac chambers

- Before diagnosing abnormalities, we should know the normal pressure and waveform of various cardiac chambers

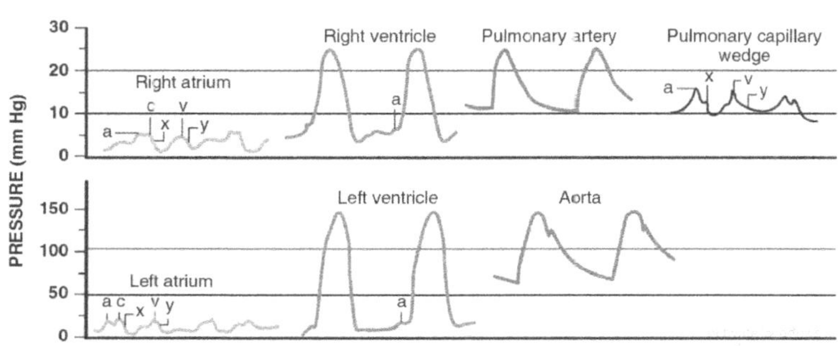

Cardiac Chamber	Pressure in mmHg
RA	0-4
RV	18-25/3-8
PA	15-30/3-12
LA	4-12
LV	100-140/4-12 (ED)
AO	100-140/60-80
PCWP	4-12

PCWP (Pulmonary capillary wedge pressure)

- Indirect measure of LA pressure (commonly taken as entering LA via trans-septal puncture is cumbersome.
- Measured via venous access/right heart catheterisation
- An end-hole catheter is wedged in a small PA branch, so that no forward flow is allowed, and measures distal pressure from LA.
- Balloon-tipped (Swan Ganz Catheter) is also used for this purpose
- However, PCWP can over/underestimate LA Pressure
- Normal value: 4-12 mmHg
    - **Mean LA pressure ~ LVEDP ~ PCWP**

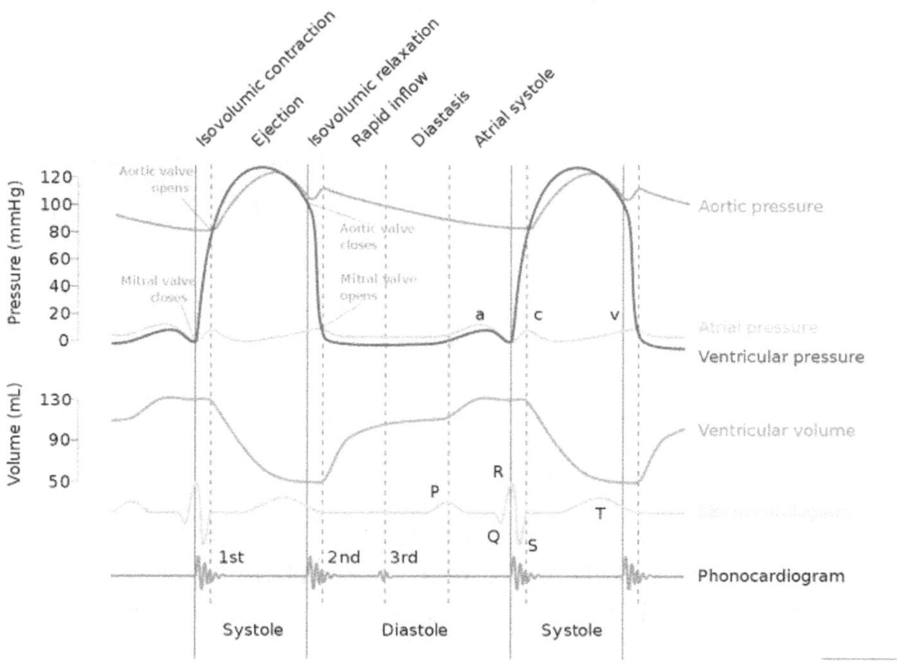

Keep in mind **Wiggers' diagram** of the cardiac cycle to have a comprehensive idea of the pressure change in different chambers during the cardiac cycle

Indications of cardiac catheterisation

- Pressure measurement in various chambers
- CO (Cardiac Output) measurement
- PCWP measurement
- Evaluation of valvular heart disease
- HOCM
- Shunt Lesion
- CCP VS RCMP

Coronary Angiogram- is a part of left heart catheterisation with selective angiogram of coronary tree to diagnose coronary stenosis

Right heart catheterization	Left heart catheterization
Catheter put via Venous access (commonly Femoral vein) to access right side chambers	Catheter put retrogradely from arterial access (femoral artery) to access left side chambers
Measure pressure/ SpO2 of SVC, IVC, RA, RV, PA, PCWP	Measures pressure/ SpO2 of Aorta, LV, may be LA
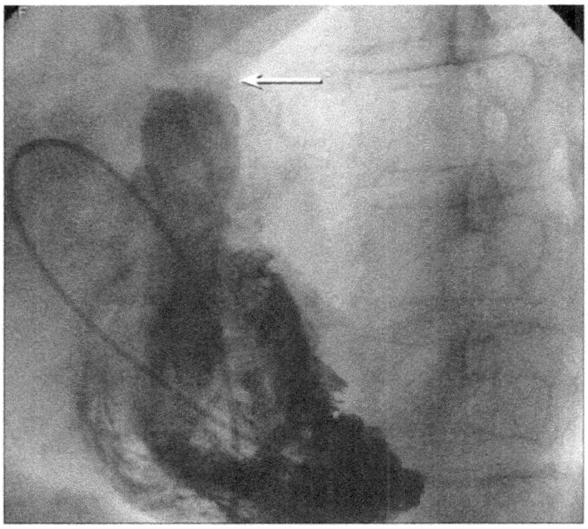 RV Angioram showing pulmonary stenosis	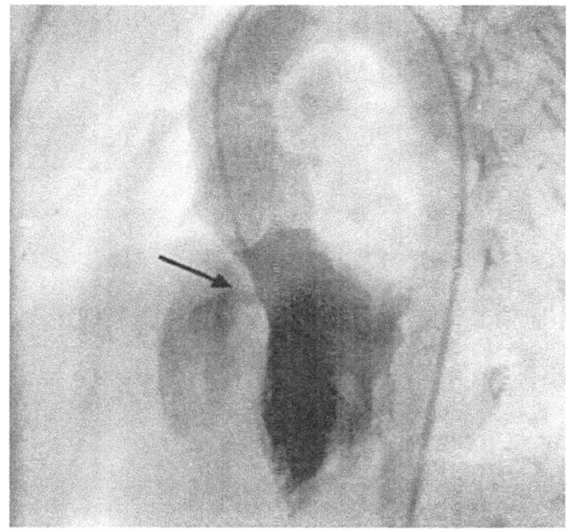 LV Angiogram showing VSD

Calculations

After measuring pressures and saturation of various cardiac chambers and great vessels, the following calculations can be done.

Cardiac Output (Based on Fick's Principle)

$$\textbf{CO} = \frac{\text{VO2 (O2 Consumption) ml/min}}{\text{(A-V) O2 Content}}$$

Where: VO2 –based on age, sex, HR

O2 Content: SpO2 X 1.36 X Hb (g/dl)

SpO2 is measured by doing blood gas analysis of a blood sample from the desired chambers (SVC, RA, PA, Aorta)

E.g. VO2=210 ml/mim, Hb 13 g/dl, SpO2 of Ao= 95%, Mixed Venous SpO2 = 65%

$$\text{CO} = \frac{210}{(0.95 - 0.65)\ 1.36 \times 13 \times 10} = 3.96 \text{ L/min}$$

Qp/Qs: 1-1.5 Mild Shunt

1.5-2 Moderate Shunt

>2 Large Shunt

>1.5-2 usually require shunt closure

Shunt Calculation

Qp = Cardiac output of RV = Pulmonary Blood Flow (PBF)

Qs = Cardiac output of LV = Systemic Blood Flow (SBF)

$$\textbf{Qp/Qs} = \frac{VO2/\ (PVO2 - PAO2)\ Hb \times 1.36 \times 10}{VO2/\ (SaO2 - MVO2)\ Hb \times 1.36 \times 10}$$

$$= \frac{SaO2 - MVO2}{PVO2 - PAO2}$$

Where: **SaO2:** SpO2 of Aorta

PVO2: SpO2 of PV (usually assumed to be 99%)

PAO2: SpO2 of Pulmonary Artery

MVO2: Mixed Venous SpO2 = $\frac{3\ SVC\ O2 + 1\ IVC\ O2}{4}$ **(FLAMM Formula)**

- Normally Qp/Qs ~ 1
- When L→R shunt (ASD, VSD, PDA): Qp/Qs >1
- When R→L Shunt (TOF): Qp/Qs <1

Vascular resistance

$$\textbf{PVR} = \frac{\text{LA Mean} - \text{Mean PA Pressure}}{Qp}$$

PVRI = PVR X BSA

$$\textbf{SVR} = \frac{\text{Aortic Mean} - \text{Mean RA Pressure}}{Qs}$$

SVRI = SVR X BSA

Expressed in Woods Unit

1 wood unit = 80 dyne-second cm -5

Normal Value

Vascular Resistance	Mean (Dyne-Sec-cm-5)	Range (Dyne-Sec-cm-5)
Systemic Vascular Resistance	1100	700-1600
Total Pulmonary Resistance	200	100-300
Pulmonary Vascular Resistance	70	2-130

Valve Orifice Area of Stenotic Valve (Gorlin Formula)

Aortic Valve Area (AVA)

$$\frac{CO/SEP \times HR}{44.3 \times \sqrt{\text{mean pressure gradient}}}$$

SEP: Systolic Ejection Period

Mitral Valve Area (MVA):

$$\frac{CO/DFP \times HR}{37.7 \times \sqrt{\text{mean pressure gradient}}}$$

DFP: Diastolic filling Period

Normal AVA: 2.6-3.5 cm2 **Severe AS** <1 cm2

Normal MVA 4-6 cm2 **Severe MS** <1 cm2

Common structural heart disease and cardiac catheterisation

1. Aortic Stenosis:

The gradient between LV and Aorta can be measured by pulling back the catheter from LV to Aorta or putting two catheters simultaneously in Aorta and LV

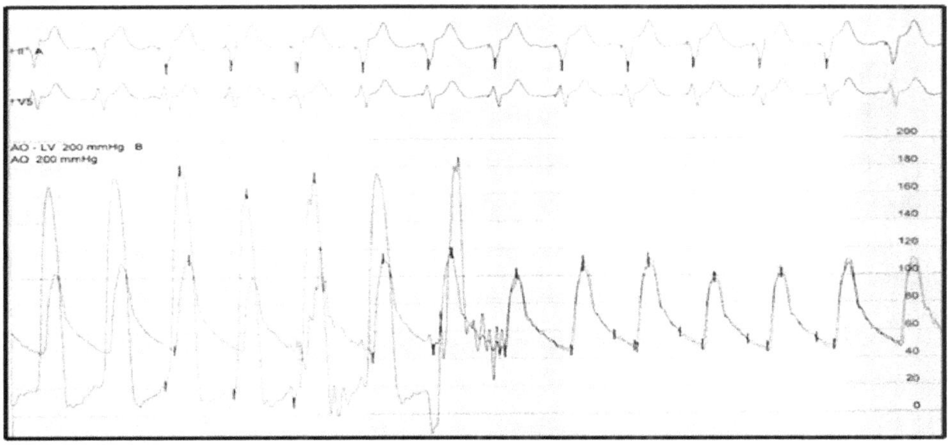

Pullback tracing in AS

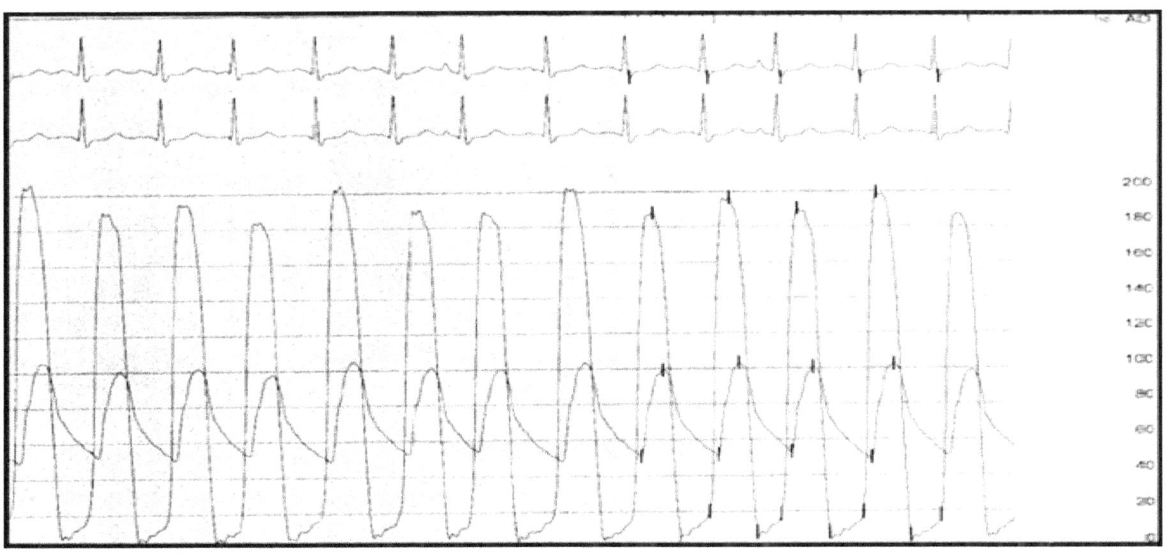

Simultaneous tracing in AS

2. HOCM:

- Obstruction at the subvalvular level and dynamic in nature (increases with Increase in Contraction and Load dependent)
- While pulling back the catheter from the LV apex to the Aorta, a gradient noted before the aortic valve (marked by a persistent ventricular pressure waveform with similar diastolic pressure and systolic gradient)

- Typical spike and dome pattern in aortic waveform, as there is initial rapid ejection followed by slowing secondary to dynamic obstruction

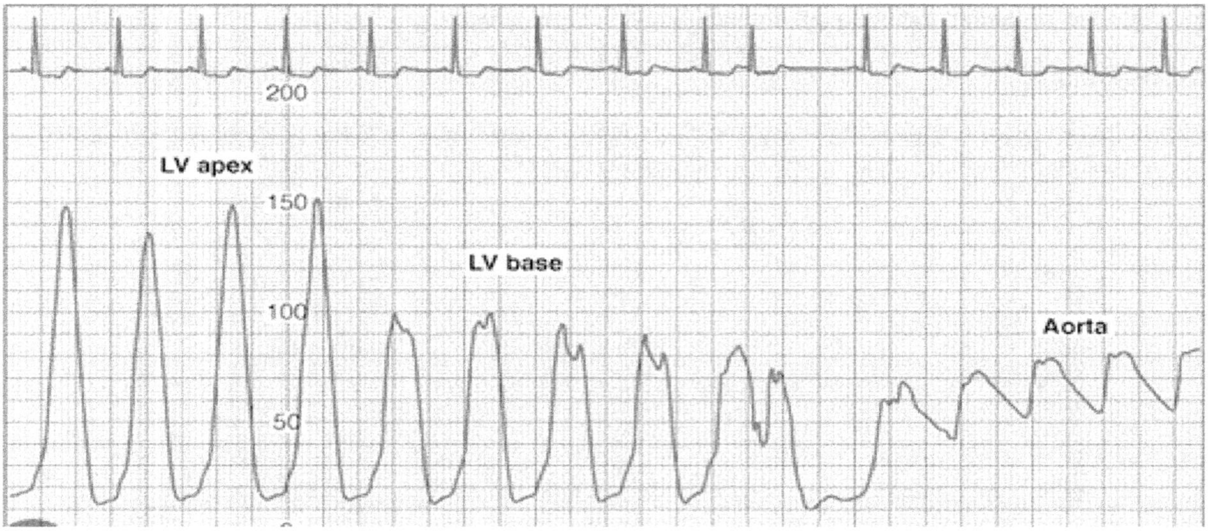

Pullback Tracing in HOCM

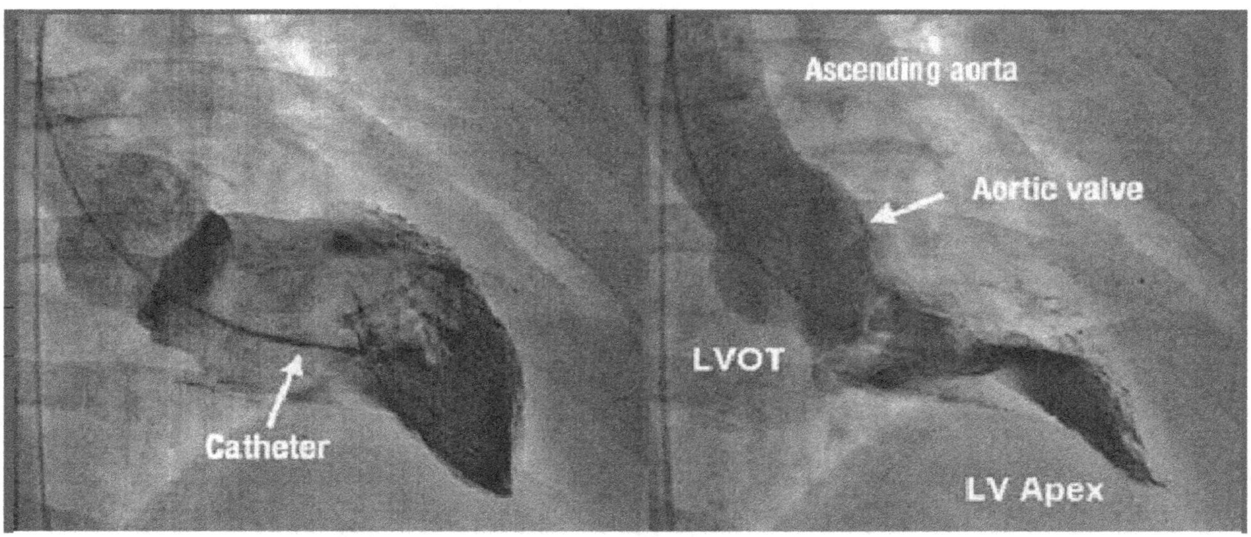

Angiogram of HOCM

Post PVC Waveforms

- Following PVC, there is an increase in the gradient in both AS and HOCM as LV contracts more vigorously, with a rise in LV pressure
- However, pulse pressure decreases following PVC in HOCM (**Brockenbrough Braunwald Morrow Sign**), pathognomonic of dynamic LVOT obstruction.
- Pulse pressure remains normal or increased in AS

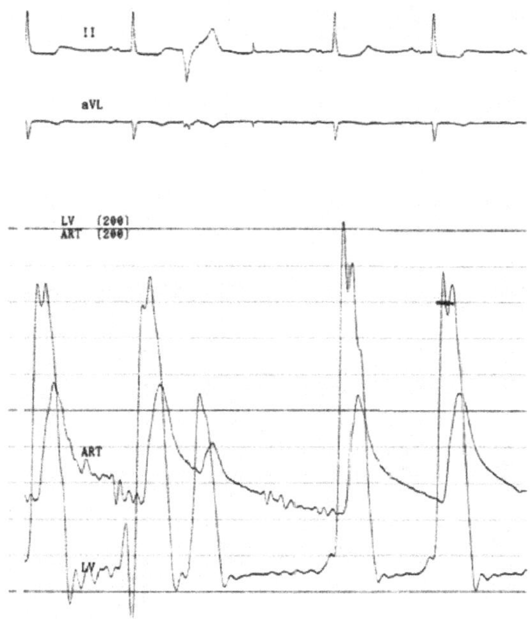

Post PVC tracing in AS

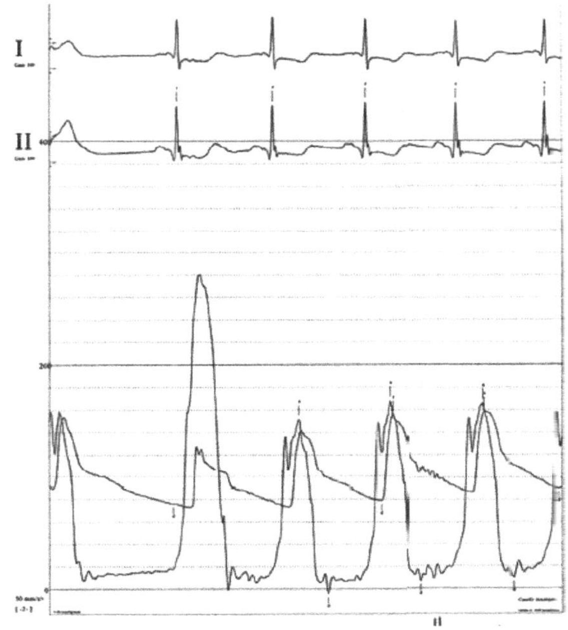

Post PVC tracing in HOCM

Explanation: Following PVC LV contracts more vigorously, leading to more dynamic LVOT obstruction, leading to less stroke volume and low systolic BP. However, in Valvular Aortic stenosis, there is fixed stenosis and stroke volume and systolic BP improve with vigorous contraction.

3. Mitral Stenosis

- LA pressure: elevated mean and Large a wave and slow X and Y descent
- Normal LV Pressure
- Significant Gradient between LA/ PCWP and LV pressure
- The mean gradient can be calculated by computer software or following formula

  Mean Gradient: LA Mean Pressure – LVEDP/2

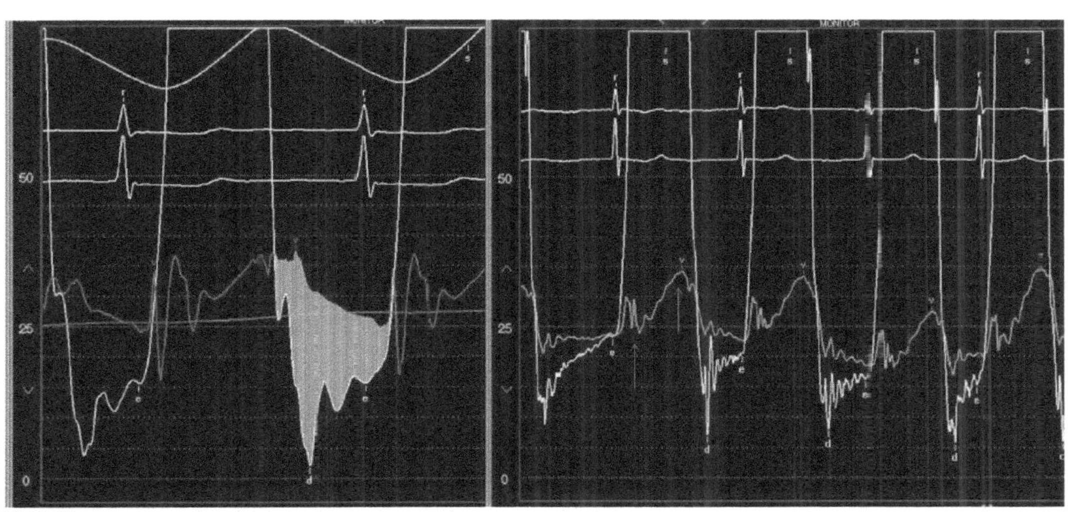

FIGURE 22.22 **Hemodynamic tracings in a patient with mitral stenosis.** *Left,* LV and PCW tracings show a large mitral valve gradient of approximately 20 mm Hg (pressure scale is 0 to 50 mm Hg). *Right,* LV and directly measured LA pressures (via transseptal approach) show higher fidelity pressure waveforms and marked reduction in the mitral pressure gradient (6 mm Hg). On the LA pressure, the *c* notch and *v* wave are distinct compared with the waveforms on the PCW.

4. Pulmonary Stenosis

- Gradient during pullback from PA to RV
- Can be valvular/subvalvular/supravalvular

5. CCP vs RCMP

- Cath study is considered the gold standard to differentiate between the two.
- Differentiation is very important, as there is a surgical cure with CCP and medical management in the RCMP

CCP	RCMP
Initial part of relaxation not impaired, sudden cessation of later part of diastole	Relaxation defect throughout diastole
Ventricular interdependence as both ventricles caged inside a common pericardium which is stiff and non-compliant	No ventricular dependence
Equalization of filling pressure LVEDP- RVEDP <5 mm Hg Square root pattern in ventricular waveform	LVEDP- RVEDP > 5 mm Hg Not seen
Systolic area index >1.1	Systolic area index < 1.1
PASP <55 mmHg	PASP >55 mmHg
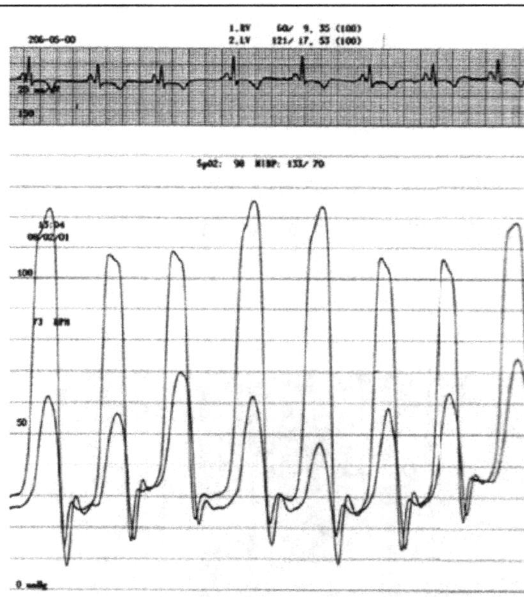	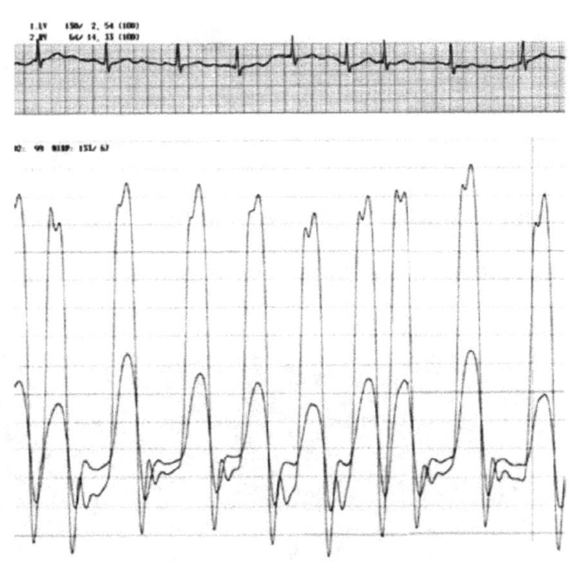

- Square root pattern in the early diastolic ventricular waveform in the CCP due to the sudden cessation of relaxation and rise in pressure

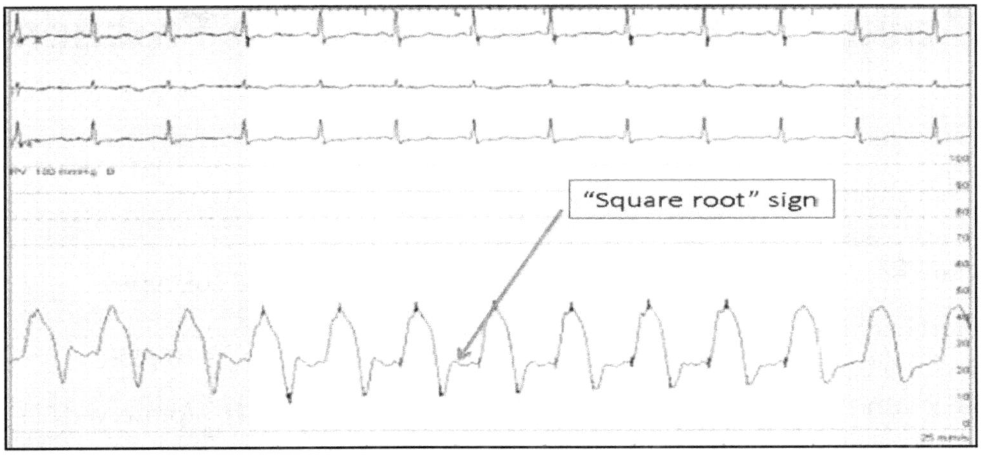
"Square root" sign

8. Heart Failure with Reduced Ejection Fraction (HFrEF)

HF with improved EF

- Improvement in LVEF from less than 40% to more than 40% with therapy
- Continue therapy even after improvement to prevent relapse

Classification of heart failure

Heart failure is currently classified into 3 subtypes

HFrEF (reduced EF)	**HFmrEF** (mildly reduced EF)	**HFpEF** (preserved EF)
LVEF < 40 %	**41 - 49 %**	**≥ 50 %**
Symptoms + signs	Symptoms + signs	Symptoms + signs
		• Cardiac structural or functional abnormality with diastolic dysfunction • Elevated BNP

Drug therapy for HFrEF

- The modulation of RAAS and sympathetic stimulation to reduce the detrimental effects of these compensatory mechanisms underlies the foundation of HF therapy

- Metoprolol tartarate is a short-acting beta-blocker not useful in chronic therapy

Four pillars of treatment of chronic heart failure(HFrEF) are- beta blockers, ARNI, SGLT2 inhibitors and Mineralocorticoid receptor antagonist

Beta blocker

- Four cardioselective beta blockers showed mortality benefit in patients with HFrEF
    - Metoprolol succinate (long-acting)
    - Carvedilol
    - Bisoprolol
    - Nebivolol
- Started at low dose in euvolemic and hemodynamically stable patients and uptitrated the dose to maximum

- The mortality benefit of ARBs is inconsistent in studies
- Recommended in patients intolerant to ACEI/ARNI

ACEI

- First class of drugs to show mortality benefit in HFrEF
- ACEI and beta blocker can be started simultaneously after diagnosis of HFrEF
- ARNI (Valsartan + Sacubitril) is considered first-line therapy and preferred over ACEI

ARNI (Angiotensin Receptor Neprilysin Inhibitor)

Mechanism

- **Sacubitril:** inhibits neprilysin, increasing levels of natriuretic peptides → vasodilation, natriuresis, diuresis, and anti-fibrotic effects.
- **Valsartan:** angiotensin II receptor blocker (ARB) → reduces vasoconstriction, aldosterone release, and myocardial remodelling.

  Dual action provides superior neurohormonal modulation compared to ACEi or ARB alone.
- Must **withhold ACEi for ≥36 hours** before starting ARNI to avoid angioedema

Evidence

- **PARADIGM HF-** Sacubitril/Valsartan superior to Enalapril in HFrEF in terms of mortality and worsening heart failure
- Renal dysfunction and hyperkalemia are less common, and hypotension is more common than enalapril
- **PIONEER-HF** and **TRANSITION Trials:** Safe and effective initiation in hospitalised patients with acute decompensated HF.

PARAGON HF

- No benefit of ARNI compared to ARB in HFpEF

MRA

- Spironolactone and eplerenone are MRAs recommended for all patients with HFrEF
- Eplerenone is more specific and has less gynaecomastia compared to spironolactone

SGLT2 inhibitors

- Recent trials showed the mortality benefit of SGLT2 inhibitors in HFrEF irrespective of diabetes status
  - **DAPA HF-** Dapagliflozin
  - **EMPORER REDUCED-** Empagliflozin
- Combined SGLT1 and SGLT2 inhibitor- Sotagliflozin showed a favourable outcome in patients with diabetes and worsening HF **(SOLOIST HF)**

Adverse events with SGLT2 inhibitors

- Urinary tract infection
- Bone fracture
- Ketoacidosis
- Limb amputation (canagliflozin)

Hydralazine/isosorbide dinitrate combination has a mortality benefit in the **Black population**

Hydralazine+ Isosorbide dinitrate

- May be considered in patients who do not tolerate or are contraindicated for ACEI/ARB/ARNI
- The African-American Heart Failure Trial (A-HeFT) showed a favourable outcome of this combination in the **black population**

Ivabradine

- Ivabradine slows the heart rate by inhibition of the *If* channel in the sinus node.
- Considered in symptomatic patients, EF<35 %, sinus rhythm with HR>70 on maximal tolerated beta blocker **(SHIFT trial)**
- New-onset AF is an adverse event

Drugs with mortality benefit in HFrEF

- ACEI
- ARNI
- Beta blocker
- SGLT2 inhibitor
- Hydralazine/isosorbide dinitrate

Vericiguat

- Oral guanylyl cyclase inhibitor
- **VICTORIA Trial**- showed favourable results in terms of CV death/HF hospitalisation with Vericiguat in patients with recent decompensation
- Vericiguat may be considered in patients who have **worsening HF** despite all other drugs (Class IIb)

Omecamtiv mecarbil

- Cardiac myosin activator
- **GALACTIC-HF** trial: The primary endpoint of a first HF event or CV death was reduced by 8%. There was no significant reduction in CV mortality.
- Current guidelines do not recommend routine use

Digoxin

- Na-K ATPase inhibitor. Improves myocardial contractility by increasing intracellular calcium
- **DIG trial**-Digoxin did not reduce overall mortality, but it reduced the rate of hospitalisation with worsening heart failure
- May be considered in symptomatic HF despite being on ACE inhibitors/ beta blockers to reduce HF hospitalisation
- Not safe in acute coronary syndrome
- ECG changes during digoxin therapy- prolonged PR, short QT interval, reverse tick ST segment, inverted T wave
- **Digoxin toxicity**
  - Risk factors-renal impairment, hypokalemia, hypercalcemia, hypomagnesemia
  - Drug interaction- amiodarone, verapamil, quinidine
  - Arrhythmias during toxicity
    - Atrial tachycardia with block **(most specific)**
    - AV block, VPC, VF, **regularised AF** (AF with CHB), bidirectional VT

- **Digoxin** improves the quality of life and has **NO** mortality benefit in patients with HFrEF

- **Digitoxin**- showed reduction in composite of mortality and HF hospitalisation in HFrEF **(DIGIT-HF trial)**

- Nausea, vomiting, abdominal pain
- **Xanthopsia** (yellow/ green vision)
- **Management**
  - **Digibind/DigiFab** (digoxin-specific Ab)
  - Correction of electrolyte disturbance
  - Phenytoin/lidocaine for ventricular arrhythmia

Iron therapy in HF

- In patients with HF, iron deficiency is defined as either a serum ferritin concentration <100 ng/mL or 100–299 ng/mL with transferrin saturation (TSAT) <20%
- IV iron (ferrous carboxymaltose) is considered in patients with HFrEF with iron deficiency to improve symptoms

- ICD therapy has a significant benefit in ICMP compared to non-ischemic DCMP

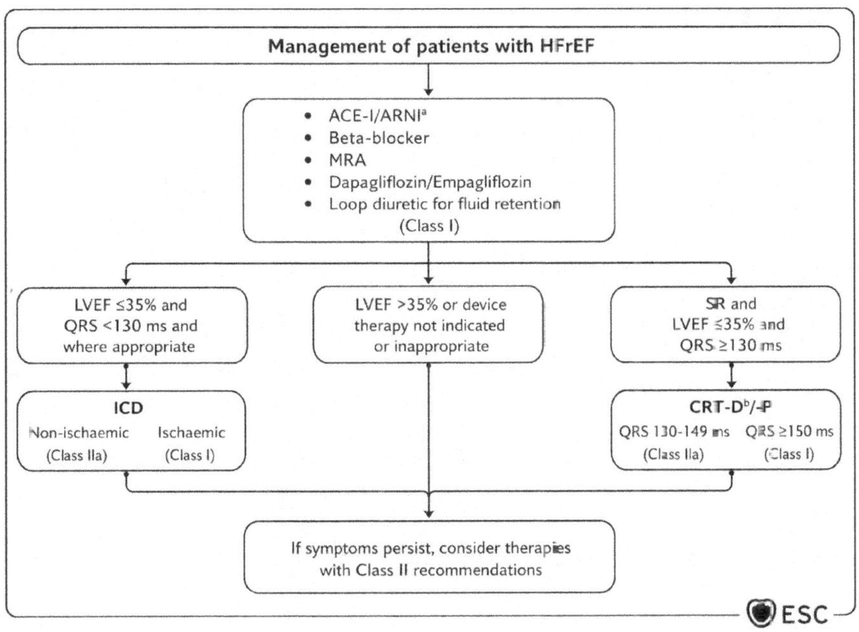

HF with mildly reduced EF (EF 41-49%)

- SGLT2 inhibitors are recommended for HFmrEF (Class I)
- ARNI, Beta blocker, MRA may be considered (Class IIb)

Implantable cardioverter defibrillator (ICD) in HFrEF

- In HFrEF NYHA II-III with ischemic aetiology (ICMP) with EF<35 % despite optimal medical therapy for 3 months (Class I)
- In HFrEF NYHA II-III with non-ischemic aetiology (DCMP) with EF<35 % despite optimal medical therapy for 3 months (Class IIa)
- ICD implantation not recommended within 40 days of MI (Class III)
- ICD therapy is contraindicated for NYHA IV and severe symptoms refractory to drug therapy

CARDIAC RESYNCHRONIZATION THERAPY (CRT)

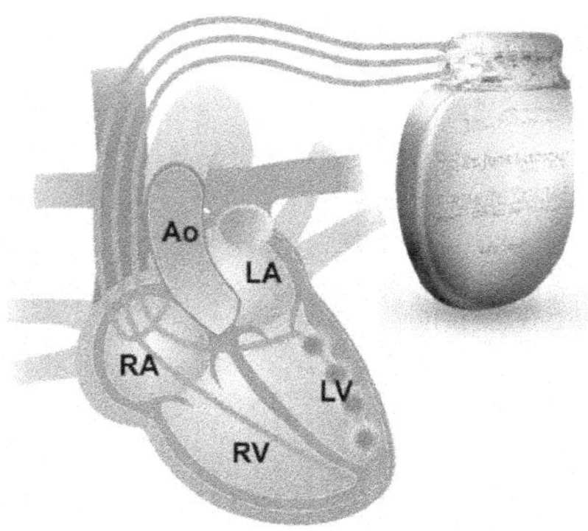

- In patients with chronic heart failure, with a wide QRS complex, there is significant mechanical desynchrony
- Differential contraction of the septum and the lateral wall (mechanical dyssynchrony) leads to low cardiac output and worsening heart failure
- CRT/ biventricular pacing aims to pace septum and the lateral wall simultaneously to restore synchronisation
- RV lead placed at RV septum and LV lead placed in the coronary sinus tributary at the site of the latest activation (last) of LV, and both paced simultaneously
- Pacing is only called as CRTP, and when a defibrillation lead is placed in the RV, it's called CRTD

Benefits of CRT

- Improve LV remodelling and increase LVEF by 5-10%
- Reduce LV size
- Increase cardiac output
- Reduce secondary MR
- Improve HF symptoms
- Reduce mortality

Indications of CRT (ESC guideline 2021)

- Recommended in symptomatic heart failure despite OMT with LVEF<35%, LBBB, **QRS duration > 150ms,** sinus rhythm (Class I)
- Should be considered in symptomatic heart failure despite OMT with LVEF<35%, LBBB, **QRS duration 130-149ms,** sinus rhythm (Class IIa)
- Should be considered in symptomatic heart failure despite OMT with LVEF<35%, **non-LBBB morphology, QRS duration > 150ms,** sinus rhythm (Class IIa)

CRTD is considered over CRTP, given the primary prevention of SCD in patients with LVEF<35%. CRTD is preferred more in patients post-MI

Factors determining optimal benefit from CRT

Although CRT is put in all patients with HFrEF with EF <35, % following parameters predict a better response

- LBBB
- QRS>150 ms
- Female sex
- DCMP>ICMP
- Small LA volume

In contrast to traditional pacing (where pacing is delivered when required), in the case of CRT, all beats are paced, even when in sinus rhythm (pacing should be> 97%)

Natriuretic peptides (BNP and NT pro BNP)

- Natriuretic peptides (ANP, BNP, CNP, DNP and Urodilatin) are released in response to increased cardiac filling pressure
- They have favourable cardiac effects in terms of natriuresis, diuresis, vasodilation and decrease in cardiac fibrosis
- Metabolised by neutral endopeptidases (Neprilysin), and drugs inhibiting neprilysin preserve the beneficial effects of natriuretic peptides

Pro-hormone ANP → ANP + NT-pro ANP

Prohormone BNP → BNP + NT pro BNP

(active) (inactive)

Clinical implications

- BNP and NT pro BNP are used for the diagnosis, monitoring of therapy and prognosis of heart failure
- Most useful to rule out heart failure in the setting of acute dyspnea in the emergency department
- Cut off for diagnosis for HF: BNP >100 pg/ml, NT pro BNP >300 pg/ml
- Elevated BNP in
  - Heart failure
  - PAH, pulmonary embolism
  - Cardiac arrhythmia
  - Non-cardiac- sepsis, renal dysfunction
  - Increased level with higher age
  - ARNI use- BNP level is falsely elevated as its metabolism is inhibited with ARNI use. NT pro BNP is useful for monitoring patients on ARNI.
- Obesity causes a decrease in BNP level

9. Heart Failure with Preserved Ejection Fraction (HFpEF)

The usual patient profile of HFpEF is older age, usually female, with hypertension, CKD and atrial fibrillation.

Cut-off for heart failure

- **BNP**

> 35 (sinus rhythm), > 105 (AF)

- **NT Pro BNP**

>125 (sinus rhythm),

> 365 (AF)

Diagnosis of HFpEF (ESC 2021)

- Symptoms and signs of heart failure
- LVEF > 50 %
- Cardiac structural or functional abnormality consistent with diastolic dysfunction or elevated filling pressure
- raised biomarker (BNP/ NT Pro BNP)

Echocardiographic evidence of LV diastolic dysfunction

- LV mass index >= 95 gm/ m2 (Female), => 115 gm / m2 (Male)
- LA volume index – 34 ml / m2
- E / E' > 9 at rest
- TR velocity > 2.8 m/sec , PASP>35

Management of HFpEF

The following drugs have failed to show a survival benefit as the primary end point.

- **ACEI**- Perindopril (PEP-CHF)
- **ARB**- CHARM Preserved (CANDESARTAN)

  I PRESERVED (Irbesartan)
- **MRA**- TOPCAT (Spironolactone)
- **Digoxin** -DIG PRESERVED
- **ARNI**- PARAGON HF
  - No reduction in the primary end point of HF hospitalisation or CV death
  - Trend toward heart failure hospitalisation reduction with ARNI

- **SGLT 2 inhibitor**- the only class of drug that showed a reduction in the primary endpoint of HF hospitalisation or CV death

SGLT 2 inhibitors

Recent trials showed a reduction in the composite of worsening heart failure and CV death with SGLT2 inhibitors.

- **EMPEROR preserved(** EMPAGLIFLOZIN)
- **DELIVER** (DAPAGLIFLOZIN)

Guideline recommendation (ESC update 2023)

- Diuretics for decongestion and symptom control (class I)
- Management of etiologies and comorbidities (e.g. Hypertension, CAD)
- SGLT2 inhibitors (Dapagliflozin/Empagliflozin) to reduce HF hospitalisation or CV death (class I) (based on results of EMPEROR preserved and DELIVER trials)

FINEARTS HF – Finerenone in HFpEF and HFmrEF

- **Finerenone,** a non-steroidal mineralocorticoid receptor antagonist, has shown a reduction in heart failure worsening and CV mortality in patients with HF with preserved or mildly reduced EF

SUMMIT Trial - Tirzepatide in HFpEF and obesity

- **Tirzepatide**- dual agonist of glucagon-like peptide 1 and glucose-dependent insulinotropic polypeptide receptor, reduces HF hospitalisation and CV mortality in HfpEF and obesity

HFimpEF (Heart failure with improved EF)

- These are the patients in whom the EF improved to normal ranges after therapy.
- GDMT should be continued to prevent the relapse of heart failure

10. Hypertrophic Cardiomyopathy (HCM)

Unexplained LV Hypertrophy in the absence of pressure overload (AS, HTN) or infiltrative condition (amyloidosis/hemochromatosis)

MYBPC3 is the **most common** sarcomeric mutation associated with HCM

Epidemiology & Genetics

- **Prevalence:** 1 in 500 adults (the most common monogenic heart disease)
- **Inheritance:**
  - Inherited Sarcomeric mutations are seen in almost **60%**

    Sarcomeric genes commonly mutated are **MYBPC3** (Myosin Binding Protein C3), **MYH7** (Myosin Heavy Chain 7), **Troponin T** (TNNT2), **TNN13, MYL2**
  - Sporadic (40%)
- **Key Differential Diagnoses:**
  - **Storage diseases:** Fabry, Pompe, amyloidosis
  - **Syndromic:** Noonan syndrome, mitochondrial disorders

ECG LVH Criteria

- SV1 +R V5/6 >35 mm

  (Sokolow Lyon)
- SV3 +RavL >28 (male) 20 (female) (Cornell voltage criteria)
- Romhilt Estes' point score system
- R wave peak time in v5/6 >50 msec
- ST depression and T inv lateral leads (strain pattern)
- LAD
- LAE

Diagnosis

1. Clinical Presentation

- Symptoms: Dyspnea (70%), angina (30%), syncope (15%)
- Harsh systolic murmur (increases with Valsalva/ standing)
- Double apical impulse

2. Diagnostic Testing

ECG: Evidence of LVH

Deep T inversion V4-V6 in patients with apical HCM **(Figure 10.1)**

Evidence of preexcitation (WPW pattern)

Echocardiography:

- LV Wall thickness >15 mm (>13 mm with family history), considered diagnostic.
- Asymmetry in septal hypertrophy
- Increased cardiac contractility (EF usually more than 70% and EPSS <10mm)

- Systolic anterior motion (SAM) of the anterior mitral leaflet (AML) in M-mode echocardiography **(Figure 10.2)**
- Classified into obstructive HCM and Non-Obstructive HCM depending upon LV outflow obstruction assessed by Doppler echocardiography.
- LVOT gradient ≥30 mmHg (obstructive HCM)

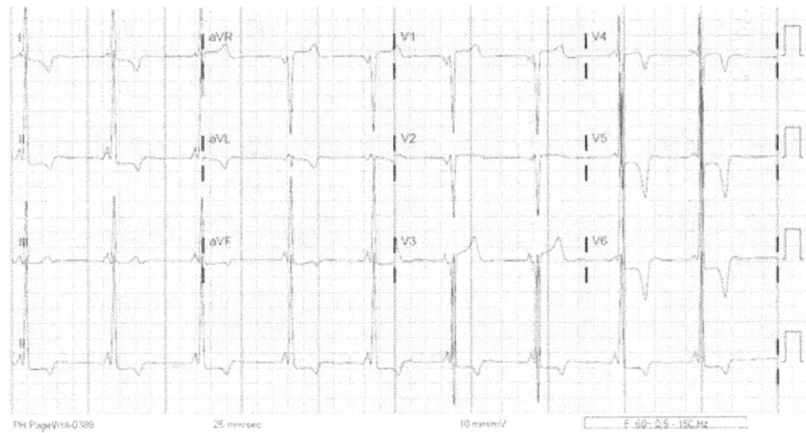

Figure 10.1. Deep T inversion in v4-6, I, avL suggestive of apical HCM

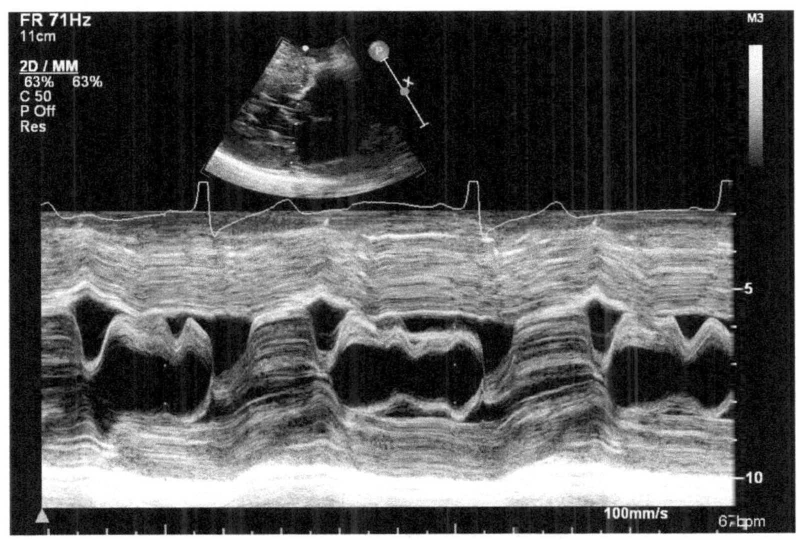

Figure 10.2. Systolic anterior motion of AML in obstructive HCM

Cardiac MRI:

- For an accurate assessment of LV hypertrophy and pattern (apical, midventricular hypertrophy)
- To assess the LGE (Late Gadolinium Enhancement) burden suggestive of myocardial fibrosis

  LGE burden >10-12% predicts SCD risk

> **Cardiac MRI in HCM**
>
> 1. LGE burden >10-12% predicts SCD risk and is an indication for ICD

Genetic testing

- Recommended for first-degree relatives (Class I, ESC 2023)

Myocardial Biopsy

- To rule out storage disease (e.g., Fabry) that mimics HCM.

3. Management

A. Symptomatic Management for Dyspnea / HF

- General measures- avoiding dehydration, alcohol, and stimulants, and intense exertion, which can increase cardiac contractility or reduce left ventricular cavity size.

New drugs for HCM symptom control

- Mavacamten
- Aficaamten

- Avoid high-dose diuretics, vasodilators and inotropes.
- Beta blockers: mainstay of management: - reduce LVOT obstruction and contractility
- Calcium Channel Blockers: Verapamil
- Disopyramide: Potent negative inotrope

Should always be combined with CCB/βB (increases AV conduction in AF)

Mavacamten

- **A cardiac myosin inhibitor** that directly targets sarcomere hypercontractility to alleviate left ventricular outflow tract (LVOT) obstruction
- **VALOR-HCM- phase 3 study showed improved symptoms and decreased eligibility for SRT (US FDA approval 2022)**
- **ODYSSEY-HCM-** No improvement in symptoms in non-obstructive HCM

Septal reduction therapy (SRT)

- NYHA III/IV symptomatic with LVOT gradient >50 mmHg, despite maximum tolerated medical treatment.
- Methods- surgical myectomy

  Alcohol septal ablation

Surgical Myectomy	Alcohol Septal Ablation
Proximal septum resected via transcatheter approach	Absolute alcohol instilled into one of major septal artery supplying LVOT area
High success rate	Lower success rate
More chance of developing **LBBB.** (develop CHB if patient has preexisting RBBB) Left Bundle has dual supply from LAD and RCA-PDA	High chances of developing **RBBB** (develop CHB if patient has preexisting LBBB) Right Bundle has single blood supply from LAD.
Preferred in severe hypertrophy, young individuals, other surgical indications	More preferred in view of percutaneous procedure.

B. Prevention of SCD

- ICD is indicated in all patients who have had an episode of VT or aborted SCD (secondary prevention).
- For Primary prevention, all patients should be risk-stratified. The following risk factors predict SCD and ICD is indicated if present:
    - Family history of SCD
    - Unexplained syncope
    - Multiple NSVT on Holter
    - Massive LVH (>30mm)
    - LGE burden >15% of LV mass (MRI)
    - Abnormal exercise BP response (failure to increase BP by 20 mmHg or a drop in BP during exercise).

High LVOT Gradient alone does not predict the risk of SCD and is not an indication for ICD

C. Family screening

- Screening of first-degree relatives with ECG, echo and genetic study

Athletes Heart

- LV hypertrophy in trained atheletes mimic HCM and need to be differentiated for furter management and risk stratification. HCM increases risk of sudden death in athletes.

Features	Athletes Heart	HCM
LV Cavity	Enlarged (>55 mm)	Normal to reduced size (<45 mm)
LV Systolic Function (LVEF)	Low normal (LVEF ~50%)	Usually high >60%
Diastolic function	Normal	Abnormal
GLS Echo	Normal	Abnormal
LGE on MRI	Absent	Present
Sarcomeric Mutation	Absent	Present
ECG	• Normal • Sinus Bradycardia • Ectopic atrial rhythm • Junctional escape rhythm • 1st degree and Mobitz type 1, 2o AV block (Wenckebach) • Incomplete RBBB • LVH by QRS Voltage criteria • Early Repolarization • Convex ST elevation with T inversion in V1-V4 in black/ African athlete.	• Abnormal • Pathological Q wave • LBBB • WPW Pattern • Marked Left axis deviation or Right axis deviation • Type 1 Brugada

- The Wenckebach pattern is considered physiological in athletes because of high vagal tone

11. Cardiac Amyloidosis

Infiltrative cardiomyopathy secondary to interstitial deposition of abnormal proteins (AL/ATTR)

AL amyloidosis (deposition of light chain)

- Distinct from multiple myeloma
- 10-15% of patients with multiple myeloma and 1% of patients with MGUS have AL amyloidosis
- Cardiac involvement occurs in around 70% of patients with AL amyloidosis

ATTR amyloidosis (deposition of Transthyretin)

- Two variants- senile (wild type ATTR) and hereditary (mutant ATTR)
- Prevalence of senile ATTR increases with age
- Also, associated with aortic sclerosis
- Polyneuropathy is common in the hereditary variant

Clinical features

> Polyneuropathy is commonly associated with ATTR amyloidosis

- Progressive diastolic dysfunction leading to symptoms of heart failure as the initial manifestation
- Elderly males are commonly affected
- Early presentation in hereditary ATTR amyloidosis
- Features of right heart failure [ascites, pedal oedema] in the late stage of the disease
- Features of other systemic involvement—
  - ATTR –neuropathy (pain, sensory loss)
  - AL-proteinuria(kidney), neuropathy, macroglossia, back pain, peri-orbital ecchymosis (raccoon eye) secondary to increased capillary fragility

ECG

- Low-voltage QRS complexes are seen in 50% of AL amyloidosis
- Low voltage QRS in the setting of LV hypertrophy should raise suspicion of cardiac amyloidosis
- Pseudo-infarct pattern (Q wave) in anterior and inferior leads
- Conduction disturbance (AV block) is more common in ATTR
- Atrial fibrillation/flutter is more common, and VT/VF is uncommon

- The 'cherry on top' pattern in the strain imaging bull's-eye map is characteristic of cardiac amyloidosis due to relative sparing of the cardiac apex

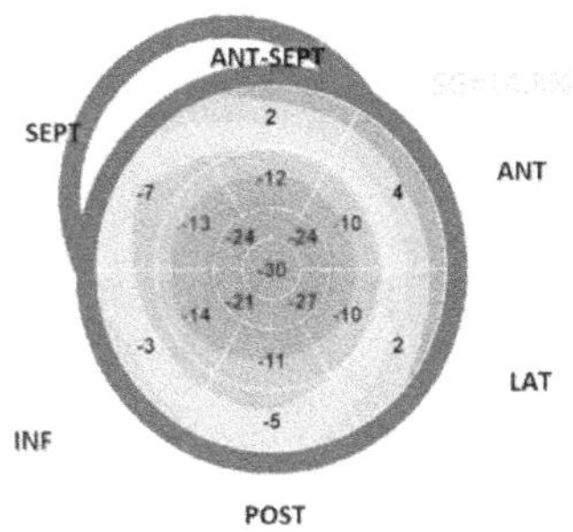

- PYP scan / Pyrophosphate scintigraphy using Tc99m PYP is diagnostic for ATTR cardiac amyloidosis

Echocardiography

- Increased wall thickness of ventricle, IVS, IAS
- Hyperrefractile interventricular septum
- Evidence of diastolic dysfunction
- Systolic dysfunction (low LVEF) in late stages
- Impaired GLS with apical sparing [cherry on top in bull eye map]

Diagnosis

- High index of clinical suspicion in an elderly patient with unexplained LV hypertrophy with diastolic heart failure
- Discordant ECG voltage [low voltage with LVH in echo]
- Endomyocardial biopsy = gold standard for diagnosis
  - Mostly not done nowadays with advanced imaging, with cardiac MRI and SPECT
- AL amyloid – cardiac MRI (diffuse subendocardial LGE) with evidence of AL

  [serum electrophoresis/bone marrow]
- ATTR amyloid- pyrophosphate nuclear scintigraphy [PYP scan/SPECT]

Management

- Supportive treatment of heart failure and arrhythmia
- Poor tolerance to beta blocker and ACE inhibitor [orthostatic hypotension and secondary autonomic neuropathy]
- Low-dose diuretic, maintain euvolemia
- Non-DHP CCB (verapamil, diltiazem) contraindicated (binds to myeloid proteins leading to significant negative ionotropic and chronotropic effects)
- DHP CCB preferred for HTN management
- Digoxin also binds to amyloid – should be used cautiously

Device therapy

- Permanent pacing in patients with significant conduction disturbance
- Role of ICD not clear [VT/VF less common, pulseless electrical activity common terminal event]

Targetted therapy

AL amyloidosis

- Chemotherapy similar to multiple myeloma (Bortezomib, cyclophosphamide, dexamethasone)

- Patchy myocardial inflammation in sarcoidosis
- AV block in the young is common
- Basal septal thinning in the echo is characteristic

- Daratumumab (anti-CD38 Ab) (Dara-CyBorD regimen) is the standard of care chemotherapy.
- Autologous stem cell transplantation
- Fibril depleters (Doxycycline, Birtamimab)

ATTR amyloidosis

- TTR gene silencer (siRNA)- Patisiran (APOLLO trial), Inotersan
- TTR stabiliser- Tafamidis (ATTRACT trial), Acoramidis, Diflusinal (NSAID)
- Liver transplantation

CARDIAC SARCOIDOSIS

Inflammatory cardiomyopathy, characterised by granulomatous inflammation and patchy myocardial involvement

- Mostly associated with systemic sarcoidosis, with evidence of other organ involvement
- Cardiac involvement in sarcoidosis is associated with high morbidity and mortality
- Common clinical presentation- AV block, ventricular arrhythmia and heart failure
- Echo- basal septal thinning, RWMA, reduced EF
- Cardiac MRI -Usually diagnostic with patchy LGE and evidence of oedema
- Endomyocardial biopsy- poor diagnostic yield due to patchy myocardial involvement
- Look for involvement of extracardiac organs (lungs, lymph nodes, eye, skin lesions)
- Management

  -Device therapy (PPI/AICD)

  - Immunosuppressant (Corticosteroid, Methotrexat

12. Restrictive Cardiomyopathy (RCMP)

Restrictive cardiomyopathy (RCM)

- Group of myocardial diseases characterised by near-normal Ejection Fraction and predominantly diastolic dysfunction

Etiology

- Infiltrative disorders- Amyloidosis, Sarcoidosis
- Storage disorders- Glycogen storage diseases, Fabry, Hemochromatosis
- Endomyocardial disorders- Loefler's endocarditis, Endomyocardial fibrosis (EMF), Radiation-induced.
- Idiopathic

Pathophysiology and clinical features

Diastolic Dysfunction

↓

Increased End Diastolic Pressure

↓ ↓

features of biventricular failure | Biatrial Enlargement

↓

AF

- Features of LV failure (Dyspnea) and RV Failure (Ascites and Pedal Oedema)
- Elevated JVP and Anasarca in Late Stages
- Atrial Fibrillation is common, secondary to biatrial enlargement
- Echo: Biatrial Enlargement, Normal EF, Normal to Increased LV wall thickness, Evidence of Diastolic Dysfunction

Diagnosis and management

- Endomyocardial Biopsy: Myocyte hypertrophy, Interstitial Fibrosis, Endomyocardial Fibrosis

Loefler's endocarditis

- RCMP caused by eosinophilic infiltration and progressive fibrosis of the endocardium
- Common etiologies: Hypereosinophillic syndrome, parasitic infection

Endomyocardial fibrosis (EMF)

- Characterised by progressive fibrosis of the ventricular endocardium, obliteration of the apex with thrombus
- Seen in tropical countries, southern India

Fabry disease

- X-linked glycogen storage disease
- Deficiency of alpha-galactosidase

Cardiac manifestations

- Concentric LVH with diastolic dysfunction
- Short PR interval
- Conduction disturbance in late stages

- Cardiac MRI: Characterisation of myocardium, LGE
- Management mostly symptomatic
  - Diuretics
  - Targeted therapy for the underlying aetiology (e.g. Amyloidosis, Hemochromatosis)
- Overall poor prognosis

  Survival Rate 64% at 5 yrs. and 37% at 10 yrs

Chronic Constrictive Pericarditis (CCP)

Thickened, fibrotic, and sometimes calcified, leading to impaired diastolic filling of the heart due to external constraint.

Tuberculosis is the **most common** cause of CCP in India

Etiology:

- In developing countries, Tuberculosis (the most common)
- In developed countries, Post-viral, idiopathic, post-cardiac surgery, radiation therapy, and connective tissue disorders.

Pathophysiology:

- Rigid pericardium prevents normal diastolic expansion → Elevated & equalised diastolic pressures in all chambers.
- Ventricular interdependence: As one ventricle fills, the other is compressed (due to non-compliant pericardium).
- "Dissociation between intrathoracic and intracardiac pressures"

Clinical Features:

- Symptoms of Right Heart Failure: Ascites, pedal oedema
- Elevated JVP with prominent **x and y descents**
- **Kussmaul's sign:** Rise in JVP on inspiration
- Pericardial knock (early diastolic sound, earlier than S3)

Investigations:

- ECG: Non-specific ST-T changes, low voltage; atrial fibrillation
- Chest X-ray: Pericardial calcification (especially in tubercular CCP).
- Echocardiography:
  - Thickened pericardium
  - Septal bounce (abrupt interventricular septal motion)
- Dilated IVC with poor inspiratory collapse
- CT/MRI: Best for pericardial thickness (>4 mm suggests constriction); detects calcifications.

- Cardiac catheterisation:
    - Equalisation of diastolic pressures
    - Dip-and-plateau (square root) sign in ventricular pressure tracing
- Definitive treatment: Pericardiectomy (surgical removal of pericardium)

CCP Vs RCMP

- Clinically mimic each other with signs of right heart failure and systemic congestion.
- Differentiating is challenging and important for management. CCP has a good outcome with surgical pericardiectomy and medical management for RCMP
- **Cath study** is considered the **gold standard** to differentiate between the two.

CCP	RCMP
Initial part of relaxation not impaired, sudden cessation of later part of diastole	Relaxation defect throughout diastole
Ventricular interdependence as both ventricles caged inside a common pericardium which is stiff and non-compliant	No ventricular dependence
Equalization of filling pressure LVEDP- RVEDP <5 mm Hg Square root pattern in ventricular waveform	 LVEDP- RVEDP > 5 mm Hg Not seen
Systolic area index >1.1	Systolic area index < 1.1
PASP <55 mmHg	PASP >55 mmHg
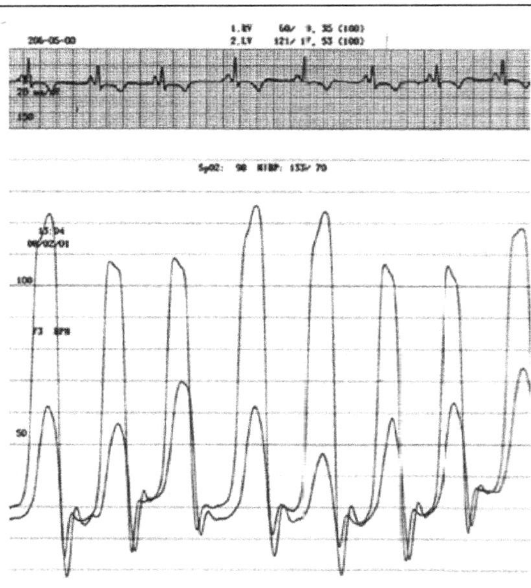	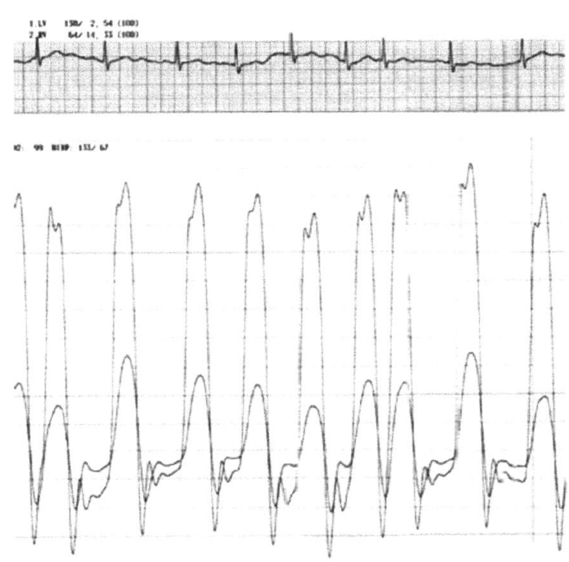

13. Acute Rheumatic Fever

- An autoimmune response to group A b-hemolytic streptococcus (GAS) infection
- Although rare in developed countries, ARF remains a major health problem in developing countries.

Cardinal clinical features

> - Carditis has significant long-term consequences
> - Arthritis usually resolves without residual deformity
>
> **ARF licks the joints, but bites the heart**

Carditis

- The most common major manifestation during the first episode of ARF is (50%-70% of the cases).
- Endocarditis with valvular involvement is most common. Pericarditis and myocarditis are also seen (Pancarditis).
- The most common valvular lesion is mitral regurgitation (MR), characterised by an apical systolic murmur and a transient apical mid-diastolic murmur.
- About 10-30% develop severe MR, and 10% develop heart failure
- **Subclinical carditis-** defined as echocardiographic evidence of valvulitis in the absence of murmur. Before the routine use of echocardiography, these were underdiagnosed.

Arthritis

- Seen in 35- 66% of cases of ARF
- Characters
    - Asymmetric polyarthritis predominantly involving large joints (knee, ankle, elbow, wrist)
    - Migratory in nature
    - Dramatic response to salicylates
    - Usually self-limiting within 4 weeks and without residual deformity

Subcutaneous nodule

- Firm and painless nodules over the extensor surface

Erythema marginatum

- Evanescent, erythematous, serpiginous macular lesion with a pale centre, usually over the trunk

Chorea (Sydenham's chorea/St Vitus' dance)

- Involuntary, purposeless, non-stereotypical movement
- Usually affecting pre-pubertal females
- Very long latent period after GAS infection (1-7 months) and usually without other manifestations of AR

The revised criteria updated the following points

- Defining low-risk and moderate/high-risk populations based on prevalence
- Inclusion of subclinical carditis (echocardiography evidence) as a major manifestation in all populations
- Monoarthritis/polyarthralgia in moderate/high-risk population as a major criterion
- Fever and erythrocyte sedimentation rate (ESR) cut-offs in low-risk and moderate/severe risk populations

Presence of **Chorea** does not require other features/ Jones criteria for diagnosis

Revised Jones criteria (2015)

	Low risk population	Moderate/high risk population
Definition	Annual incidence of ARF ≤ 2 per 1,00,000 school aged children or all age prevalence of RHD ≤ 1 per 1000	Those not fulfilling criteria for the low risk
Major manifestations		
• Joint manifestation • Carditis	Polyarthritis only Clinical/**subclinical (echo)** Erythema marginatum Subcutaneous nodule chorea	Polyarthritis/**Polyarthralgia/ monoarthritis** Clinical/**subclinical (echo)** Erythema marginatum Subcutaneous nodule chorea
Minor manifestation		
• Arthralgia • PR prolongation • Fever • ESR, CRP	**Polyarthralgia** In absence of carditis **>38.50 C** **ESR >60mm** in 1hr CRP > 3 mg/dl	**Monoarthralgia** In absence of carditis **>380 C** **ESR >30mm in** 1hr CRP > 3 mg/dl
Supporting evidence of recent GAS infection- ASO titre/ streptococcal antibodies (anti DNAseB) Positive throat culture for GAS or positive rapid GAS carbohydrate antigen **First Episode of ARF**: 2 major or 1 major plus 2 minor plus evidence of recent GAS infection **Recurrence**: 2 major or 1 major plus 2 minor or 3 minors (later only in moderate/high risk population) plus evidence of recent GAS infection		

Management

- Treatment of GAS pharyngitis- Single dose IM Benzathine penicillin or 10 days oral penicillin. Cephalosporin, azithromycin and clarithromycin are alternatives in penicillin-allergic patients.
- Treatment of ARF manifestations
    - **Arthritis**- Aspirin 75-100mg/kg/day for 2 weeks
    - **Carditis**- steroid (prednisolone 2mg/kg/day for 3 weeks followed by tapering) in severe carditis with heart failure. Aspirin only in mild carditis
    - **Chorea**- symptomatic management with valproate/carbamazepine

Secondary prophylaxis

- For all patients after an episode of ARF, to prevent the recurrence and progression of chronic rheumatic heart disease

Drugs

- Long-acting Benzathine penicillin

1.2 MU (weight >27kg) or 0.6 MU (<27 kg) deep IM every 2-3 weeks

- Oral penicillin V- 250mg twice daily
- Penicillin allergy- Erythromycin, sulphadiazine

GOAL study

- Secondary antibiotic prophylaxis reduces disease progression in latent rheumatic heart disease

Duration (ACC/AHA 2013)

Rheumatic fever with carditis and residual heart disease	10 years or until 40 years of age (whichever is longer)
Rheumatic fever with carditis but no residual heart disease	10 years or until 21 years of age (Whichever is longer)
Rheumatic fever without carditis	5 years or until 21 years of age (Whichever is longer)

14. Mitral Stenosis and BMV

Normal Mitral Valve Area (MVA)- 4-6 cm2

Severe MS <1 cm2

Etiology

- Rheumatic heart disease (MC)
- Uncommon causes- congenital (part of Shone complex), SLE, RA severe mitral annular calcification, large LA myxoma, large mitral vegetation

Clinical features and natural course

- Progressive dyspnea, orthopnea and PND (paroxysmal nocturnal dyspnea) are characteristic of MS
- Disease may remain silent for a long time and manifest when there is tachycardia (secondary to AF, anaemia, pregnancy, fever, thyrotoxicosis)
- Pulmonary hypertension is mostly associated with a progressive increase in the severity of MS, leading to dilated RA, RV, tricuspid regurgitation and right heart failure
- Hemoptysis resulting from rupture of pulmonary-bronchial venous connections secondary to high PVH
- Atrial fibrillation and stroke are late complications of untreated MS
- Signs

  Loud S1

  Opening snap (A2-OS gap inversely correlates with the severity of MS). Presence of OS indicates mobile valve, and reduced intensity of OS suggests calcified valves

  MDM- best heard at apex and left lateral position with presystolic accentuation. Duration of murmur correlates with severity, not the loudness of the murmur.

  ECG

  - RAD, RVH
  - LA enlargement (P mitrale- Biphasic wide II, Predominant negative in V1)
  - Atrial fibrillation

Graham Steell murmurs

PR murmur due to PAH secondary to mitral valve disease

Austin Flint murmur

AR murmur in diastole mimics MS

Straightening of the left heart border

- Mitral stenosis
- CCTGA
- Absent pericardium

CXR

- LA enlargement (widening of carinal angle, double shadow)
- Straightening of the left heart border (due to dilated LA appendage and pulmonary trunk, underfilled aorta and LV)
- Pulmonary venous hypertension (cephalisation, Kerley A, B lines, pleural effusion)

> MVA assessed by pressure half-time (PHT)
>
> **MVA (cm2) = 220/PHT (in sec)**

Echocardiography

- Morphological features (2D)
  - Thickened and calcified mitral leaflets with restricted opening
  - Dilated left atrium
- Mitral valve area: assessed by 2 methods.
  - Planimetry
  - Pressure half time (PHT)
    - MVA = 220 / PHT
- Mean gradient between LA and LV using Doppler.
  - > 5 mmHg is significant.

> Components of the **Wilkins Echo score**
>
> - Leaflet thickening
> - Leaflet mobility
> - Leaflet calcification
> - Subvalvular thickening
>
> Score ranges from 4 to 16
>
> A score less than 8 is favourable for BMV

Management

i. **Medical management**

- Penicillin prophylaxis
- Heart rate control- Beta blockers (increase in diastolic time allows better mitral inflow_
- Diuretics
- VKA(Warfarin) -In atrial fibrillation (NOAC not indicated)

ii. **BMV (Balloon mitral valvotomy)**

- Should be considered as a first line for symptomatic MS
- Echo assessment remains crucial for better patient selection
- Good candidate- No commissural calcification
  No mitral regurgitation
  No LA thrombus
  mild subvalvular disease
- **Wilkin's echo score** assesses suitability for BMV (score 8 or less suggests a high chance of successful BMV)

> - Overall, LA thrombus is considered a contraindication for BMV
> - Manjunath's classification of LA clot suggests that modified BMV can be done with type I, IIa LA clot

- Usually performed by the femoral vein- transseptal puncture and balloon dilation across the mitral valve using the Inoue Balloon
- Preferred treatment modality during pregnancy (usually done during the second trimester)

iii. **Surgery**

- Considered when not suitable for BMV
- Closed mitral valvotomy
- Mitral valve replacement

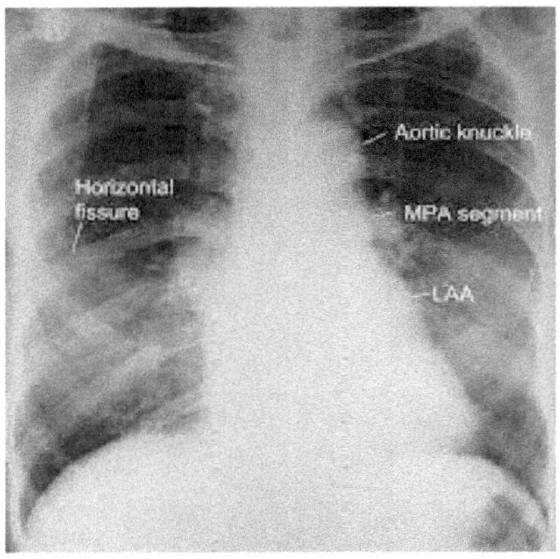

X-ray chest showing straight left heart border and pulmonary oedema

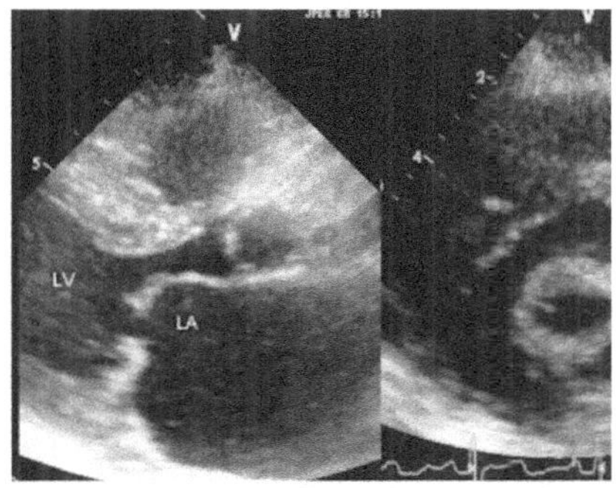

Echo images showing doming of mitral leaflets, fish-mouth appearance and increased gradient across the mitral valve

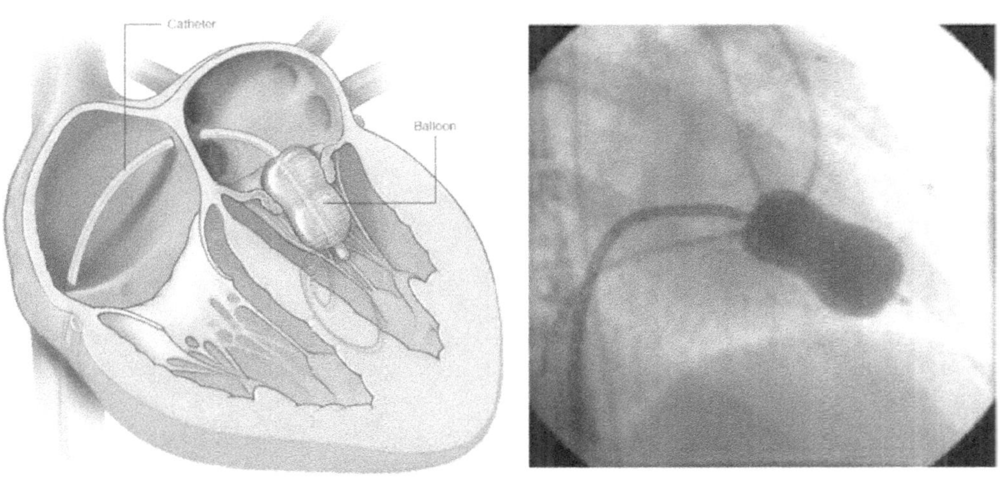

Balloon mitral valvotomy using the Inoue Balloon

Juvenile Mitral Stenosis

- Early onset of symptoms (before 20 years)
- Pulmonary oedema, PAH and right heart failure are common
- LA is usually not dilated much
- AF and thromboembolism are not common

Lutembacher syndrome

- Atrial septal defect (ASD), when associated with acquired mitral valve disease (mostly MS, sometimes MR)
- Elevated LA pressure decompressed via ASD and a very high left-to-right shunt
- Symptoms and signs of MS decreased due to less mitral flow
- soft S1, soft/absent MDM
- Signs of ASD (loud flow murmur and P2) due to increased shunt
- Right heart failure with peripheral oedema is more common

15. Mitral Regurgitation and TEER

> Posteromedial papillary muscle rupture is common due to its single blood supply

MR can result from a disease process affecting any of the components of the mitral valve apparatus, i.e, Leaflets, annulus, chordae, papillary muscle and myocardium

Etiology-

- **Primary MR** (primary disease of the valve leaflet/annulus)
    - Rheumatic heart disease
    - Mitral valve prolapse
    - Mitral annular calcification
    - Congenital anomaly (mitral cleft)
    - Infective endocarditis

> Progressive deterioration of MR secondary to dilated LA, LV and annulus
>
> **MR begets MR**

- **Secondary MR** (Myocardial disease leading to MR)
    - **Ischemic cardiomyopathy**
    - **Non-ischemic cardiomyopathy**

  Progressive dilation of the ventricle in cardiomyopathy causes displacement of the papillary muscle and tethering of the chordae, resulting in secondary MR

- Acute MR
    - Papillary muscle rupture in MI, trauma, endocarditis, and myomatous degeneration

> **Severe MR (Echo criteria)**
>
> - Effective regurgitant orifice area (EROA) >0.4 cm2
> - Regurgitant fraction >50%
> - Regurgitant volume >60 ml
> - Vena contracta >7 mm

- MR in HOCM occurs secondary to systolic anterior motion (SAM) of the anterior leaflet towards LVOT
- Symptoms
- Signs

  Management

    - **Medical management**
        - Diuretics
        - Vasodilators (ACE inhibitors, Nitroprusside in acute MR)
    - **Surgical management**
        - Surgical treatment is considered for all **symptomatic severe MR**

- Indications of surgery in **asymptomatic** severe MR
  - New onset AF
  - Pulmonary hypertension (PA pressure >50 at rest/ >60 with exercise)
  - Reduced LVEF <60 %
  - Increased LV end-systolic dimension > 40mm
- Repair vs replacement of the valve is decided based on anatomy
- Ischemic MR- Mitral valve replacement with CABG is preferred

- **Transcatheter intervention**

Transcatheter edge-to-edge repair of the mitral valve (m-TEER)

- Catheter-based therapy to appose part of the mitral leaflets, making a double orifice mitral valve
- Considered in selected patients with high surgical risk
- Mostly preferred in functional/secondary MR. Can be done in primary MR
- Approved TEER devices
  - **MitraClip**
  - **PASCAL**
  - **Myclip**
- Done via venous access and transeptal puncture

> - Alfieiri stitch- approximating mitral leaflets surgically (introduced by Prof Ottavio Alfieiri)
> - Mitra clip/TEER procedure is a transcatheter version of the Alfieri stitch

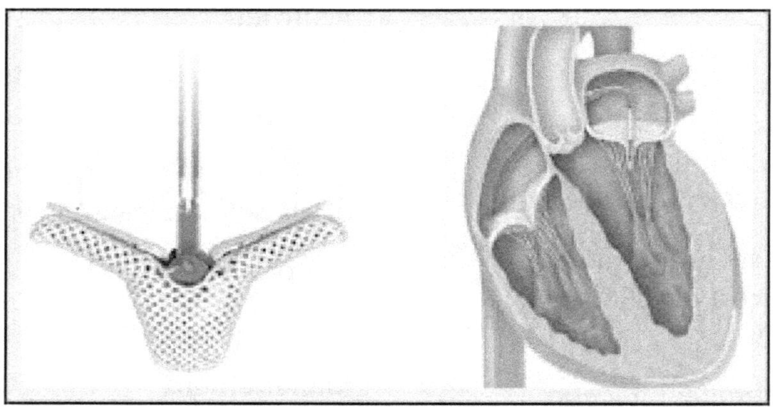

- Trial Evidence
  - **EVEREST II** – Safety and efficacy of the MitraClip procedure
  - **COAPT trial** - Reduced mortality and HF hospitalisation in selected patients of secondary MR
  - **MITRA FR** - No difference in mortality and heart failure hospitalisation with TEER vs medical therapy
  - **RESHAPE HF2** - reduced cardiovascular death and heart failure hospitalisations in patients with heart failure and moderate-to-severe functional MR.

Current guideline recommendation (AHA Valvular heart disease 2020)

Class IIa- severe secondary MR with suitable anatomy, LVEF 20- 50%, LV end systolic dimension <70 mm, PA systolic pressure <70 mmHg

Mitral valve prolapse (MVP)

- RHD is the commonest cause of primary MR in developing countries
- MVP is the most common cause in developed countries

- Also known as Barlow syndrome/Click-murmur syndrome
- Myxomatous degeneration with deposition of glycosaminoglycans and reduced type III collagen
- Irregularly thickened leaflets with increased mobility and prolapse
- Posterior mitral is more commonly affected
- Tricuspid and aortic valves can also be affected
- Common associations
  - Marfan syndrome
  - Ehlers-Danlos syndrome
  - Straight back syndrome
- Rupture of the chordae can lead to acute on chronic MR

- The posterior mitral leaflet and the posteromedial papillary muscle are commonly affected in MVP

Clinical features

- Young females are commonly affected
- Dyspnoea and palpitations with progressive deterioration of MR
- Chest pain resembling angina is common
- Arrhythmia- VPC, VT, AF and Sudden cardiac death reported with MVP
- Transient ischemic attack- embolism from the valve
- A midsystolic click followed by a murmur is characteristic
  - Click and murmur occur earlier with standing and Valsalva (reduced LV volume increase prolapse)
  - Squatting and isometric exercise increase LV volume and click-murmur, which may delay/ disappear

Management

- Beta blocker to relieve palpitations and chest pain
- ICD for secondary prevention after VT/aborted SCD
- Mitral valve repair/replacement when severe

Malignant MVP

- When MVP is associated with life-threatening ventricular arrhythmia and sudden death

Associated features-

- QT prolongation
- VPC
- Mitral annular disjunction
- **Picklehaube sign** in tissue Doppler

16. Aortic Stenosis and TAVI

Etiology

- Senile degeneration
- Bicuspid aortic valve or congenital abnormalities
- Rheumatic AS
- Rare causes
  - Familial hypercholesterolemia (valvular and supravalvular)
  - Rheumatoid arthritis
  - Ochronosis

> - ATTR amyloidosis has been attributed as a cause of AS in a few patients
> - Diagnosed by cMRI/Tc PyP nuclear scan

Cardinal symptoms of AS are

- **Dyspnea** – the commonest symptom, secondary to systolic and diastolic dysfunction
- **Angina** - imbalance between myocardial oxygen demand and decreased supply due to decreased capillary density of the hypertrophied ventricle.
- **Syncope** can be multifactorial.
  - Unable to increase cardiac output with exertion.
  - Malfunction of the baroreceptor mechanism
  - Transient AF
- **Natural course**
  - Usual presentation after the 6th decade and a rapid downhill course after symptom onset.
  - In untreated severe AS, the average life expectancy after the onset of angina, syncope and dyspnoea is 3 years, 2 years and 1 year, respectively
  - Bicuspid valve-related AS usually presents one decade earlier (50-60 yr
- **Echocardiographic Diagnosis of Severe AS**

  Valve area < 1 cm2

  Peak gradient >60 mmhg

  Mean gradient >40 mmhg

> **Hyede Syndrome**
>
> - Some patients with severe AS develop GI bleeding secondary to angiodysplasia of the colon.
> - Shear stress of AS leads to platelet aggregation and a reduction in high molecular weight VWF level.

- **Low flow, low gradient AS**
  - When a patient with AS develops ventricular dysfunction echocardiographically measured gradient across the aortic valve may be falsely low despite severe AS due to reduced flow.
  - Dobutamine stress echo helps to differentiate between true severe AS versus pseudo-severe AS.

Bicuspid Aortic Valve (BAV)

- Seen in 1 to 2% of the general population.
- NOTCH, eNOS, NKV 2.5 gene polymorphism
- Associated with aortopathy or aortic dilatation, which is not related to the severity of AS
- Associated with coarctation of the aorta / HLHS/Turner syndrome
- 3 types according to the fusion of leaflets
  - Right and left – **most common 70-80%**
  - Right and non-coronary – 20-30 %
  - Left and non-coronary – 5-10 %
- Clinical presentation
  - Most patients develop aortic stenosis
  - Aortic stenosis is usually present one decade earlier, at 50 to 60 years of age in compared to senile aortic stenosis (70 years)
  - Some patients develop aortic regurgitation (10 to 25%)

> - Aortopathy in BAV is not related to the severity of aortic stenosis

> In contrast to previous beliefs, antihypertensives can be safely given to patients with severe AS and have symptomatic benefit

Management of aortic stenosis

Indications of AVR (aortic valve replacement)

- Symptomatic severe AS
- Asymptomatic severe AS with
  - LVEF less than 50%
  - very severe AS (Vmax > 5 m/s)
  - Planning for other cardiac surgery
  - BNP level is more than 3 times normal
  - rapid progression of disease
- The aortic valve can be replaced in two ways
  - Surgically (Surgical AVR/**SAVR**)
  - Percutaneously (**TAVI/TAVR**)

> - The STS score (Society of Thoracic Surgeons) assesses surgical risk for major thoracic surgery and predicts 30-day mortality after surgery.
> - It takes into account
>   - Age
>   - Gender
>   - Comorbidity
>   - Pre-op condition (CHF/shock)

- Recent advancements in the transcatheter aortic valve implantation (TAVI) have led to a suitable alternative for surgical AVR
- Surgical AVR can be done with a mechanical(metallic) or bioprosthetic valve. However, TAVI always involves a bioprosthetic valve

The following factors should be considered while choosing SAVR Vs TAVI, Mechanical Vs bioprosthetic

- Age
- Surgical risk (STS score
- The need for anticoagulation use and patient preference

Management algorithm of AS

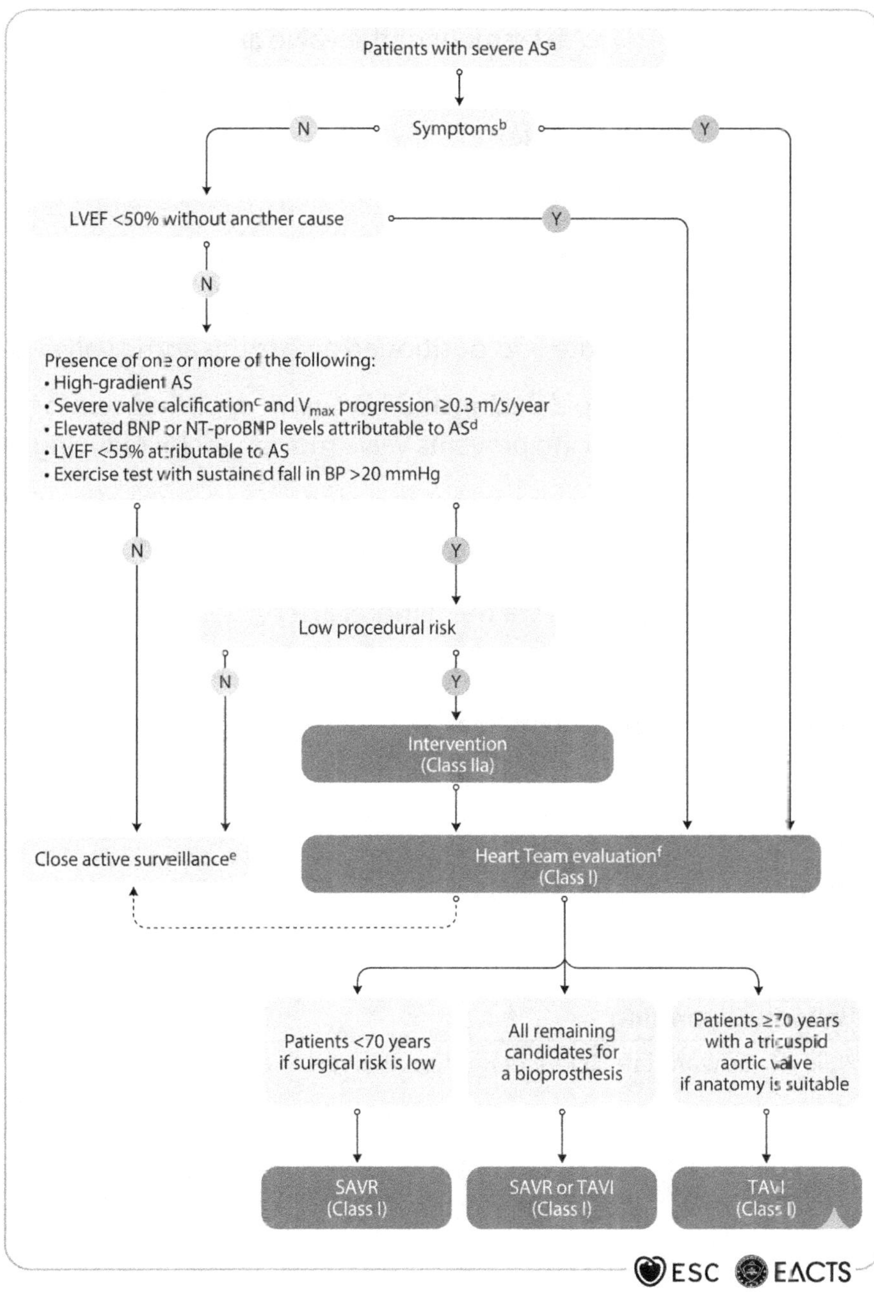

TAVI/TAVR (Transcatheter Aortic Valve Implantation)

First performed by **Alain Cribier** (France) in 2002 via trans septal approach in a patient with severe AS with Cardiogenic Shock.

- Now, the number of TAVIs has surpassed the number of surgical aortic valve replacements (SAVR)

CT Assessment before TAVI

- CT assessment is most crucial before TAVI

- MDCT plays a crucial role in the assessment of suitability and pre-procedure planning before TAVI
- Important parameters assessed are
  - Vascular access (diameter, calcification and tortuosity of ilio-femoral)
  - Assessment of the valve and annulus (size, calcification)
  - Height of the coronary origin from the valve annulus (>10 mm is safe)

TAVI Procedure

- TAVI is not recommended in patients with BAV and aortic regurgitation, used off-label
- However, various studies have shown good outcomes

- Large-bore femoral arterial access
- The valve delivery system is advanced retrogradely via the arterial route and positioned across the aortic valve
- Rapid pacing and TAVI valve deployed across the native valve (rapid pacing prevents valve movement by reducing cardiac output
- Vascular access is closed by a vascular closure device

Complications

- Vascular complications (12-14F sheath via the femoral artery)
- CHB / Permanent Pacemakers requirement (around 5%, more compared to SAVR)
- AKI and new-onset AF are more common in SAVR
- Endocarditis, the reintervention rate is similar.
- Rupture of the annulus
- Coronary occlusion

Valve types

Balloon Expanding	Self-Expanding
SAPIEN, SAPIEN XT (Edward Life Sciences) MyVal (Meril)	Core Valve Hydra Valve
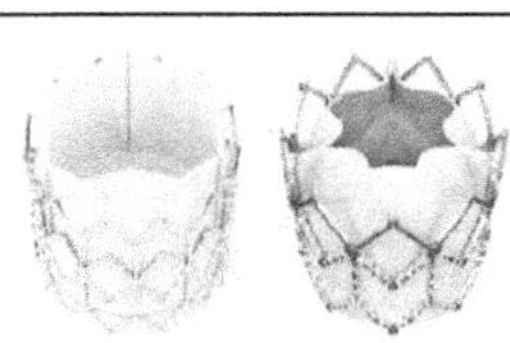 SAPIEN SAPIEN XT	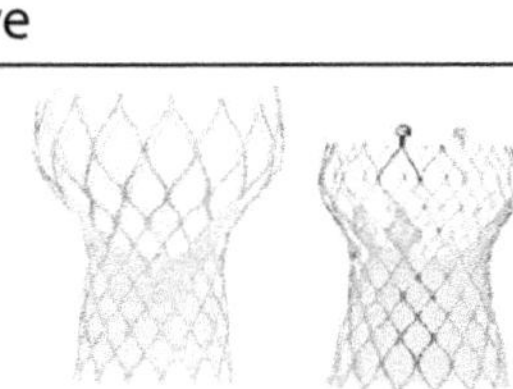 CoreValve Evolut R

- The overall outcome of both types of TAVI valves is the same. Self-expanding valve preferred in a small aortic annulus

Evidence

- The STS (Society of Thoracic Surgery) Score predicts 30-day mortality following major thoracic surgery
- Outcome of TAVI compared with SAVR in various populations according to surgical risk (STS Score)

Risk	Trial	Conclusion
Prohibitive Risk	**PARTNER 1B** (BE Sapiens Valve) Core valve Pivotal Study	Mortality benefit compared to standard medical therapy
High risk STS >8	**PARTNER 1A** Core valve high risk pivotal	TAVI non inferior to SAVR for mortality at 5 yrs.
Intrmediate Risk STS 4-8	**PARTNER 2** SURTAVI	TAVI non inferior to SAVR for Mortality and Stroke
Low Risk STS < 4	**PARTNER 3**	TAVI superior to SAVR for Death, Stroke, and hospitalization at 2 yrs.

17. Aortic Regurgitation

Peripheral signs of AR

- **Hill sign**

  Popliteal BP>Brachial BP

  Difference >60 mmHg most specific clinical sign
- **De Musset sign**

  Head nodding with heartbeat
- **Corrigan's/water hammer pulse**
- **Muller sign**

  Uvula pulsation
- **Quinke sign**

  Nailbed capillary pulsation
- **Traube sign**

  Pistol shot sound over femoral artery
- **Durozeiz mulmur**

  Diastolic bruit over femoral artery when compressed
- **Landolfi sign**

  Alternate constriction and dilation of the pupil

Etiology

- Degenerated tricuspid valve
- Bicuspid aortic valve
- Infective endocarditis
- Rheumatic heart disease
- Aortic root pathology
  - Hypertension
  - Root dilation (Marfan, Syphilis, Takayasu)
  - Aortic dissection

Key clinical findings

- Progressive volume overload leads to eccentric hypertrophy and subsequently LV dysfunction
- Exertional palpitation and dyspnea are prominent
- Signs
  - Wide pulse pressure
  - Bounding and high-volume pulse
  - High-pitched early diastolic murmur
  - Austin Flint murmur- functional MS/MDM murmur due to regurgitant jet hitting the anterior mitral leaflet, leading to inadequate opening
- Classical clinical findings of severe AR may not be there in acute severe AR

Management

- Medical management
  - Vasodilators (ACE inhibitors) reduce regurgitant volume
  - Diuretics for congestion
- Surgery (aortic valve replacement)
  - For all symptomatic severe AR

- **Asymptomatic severe AR with LVEF <50%**

  OR LV end systolic dimension **(LVESD) >50mm**
- Undergoing CABG

- **Bentall surgery**
  - Composite aortic root and valve graft when a dilated aortic root is associated with valve involvement
- **TAVI**
  - Off-label as of now. Done in selected patients at high risk for surgery

18. Prosthetic Heart Valves

Types of bioprosthesis

- **Xenograft**

  Animal tissue (porcine/ bovine)

- **Homograft**

  Human donor valve (cadaveric)

- **Autograft**

  Patient's own valve in a different position

TAVI valves are bioprosthetic in nature

VKA (warfarin) is the anticoagulant of choice. **NOACs are contraindicated** after a prosthetic valve

Broadly, 2 Types of prosthetic valves

Mechanical valve

- Made up of metal/pyrolytic carbon
- Durable (20-30 yrs)
- Requires lifelong anticoagulation with VKA (Warfarin)
- High risk for thromboembolism
- Preferred in young individuals with high life expectancy

  Available mechanical valves

  - Caged ball (star Edwards)- obsolete now
  - Tilting disc (Björk-Shiley)
  - Bileaflet (St Jude)- commonly used now
  - Chitra valve

Bioprosthetic valve (tissue valve)

- Made up of bovine/porcine pericardium
- Less durable (8-10 years)
- No need for lifelong anticoagulation (initial 3 months only)
- Preferred in older individuals or high-risk of bleeding or planning for pregnancy

  Available bioprosthetic valves

  - Carpentier, Perimount, Hancock, Mosaic

  Ross procedure

  - Pulmonary valve (autograft) placed at the aortic position, and pulmona dividuals with aortic valve disease for a better physiological outcome

Anticoagulation after valve replacement

	Duration	Target INR
Mechanical MVR	lifelong	2.5-3.5
Mechanical AVR	lifelong	2-3
Bioprosthetic valve	3 months	2-3
TAVI	**Lifelong single antiplatelet (Aspirin)**	

19. Supraventricular Tachycardia (SVT)

Tachyarrhythmia is classified based on QRS duration as it has diagnostic and management implications-

1. **Narrow QRS tachycardia (QRS duration <120ms)**
   a. Regular
      i. Sinus tachycardia
      ii. Sinus nodal reentrant tachycardia
      iii. Ectopic atrial tachycardia (focal AT)
      iv. AVNRT
      v. Orthodromic AVRT
      vi. JET
      vii. Atrial flutter with fixed AV block
      viii. Idiopathic VT (high septal)
   b. Irregular
      i. AF
      ii. MAT
      iii. Atrial flutter with variable block
2. **Wide QRS tachycardia (QRS duration > 120ms)**
   a. Regular
      i. VT
      ii. SVT with aberrancy (underlying BBB/rate related)
      iii. Antidromic AVRT
      iv. AT/junctional tachycardia with preexcitation
      v. Paced tachycardia
   b. Irregular
      i. AF with aberrancy
      ii. Preexcited AF
      iii. Antidromic AVRT with variable AV conduction
      iv. Polymorphic VT/Torsades
      v. VF

Supraventricular tachycardia (SVT)

Refers to tachycardia (atrial rate >100/min) with an arrhythmic substrate at the level of the His bundle or above

- In general, all arrhythmias except VT and AF are included under SVT
- Overall, AVNRT is more common than other SVTs
- AVRT (WPW syndrome) is common in the pediatric age group
- AVNRT is more common in women, and AVRT is common in men

Approach to narrow complex tachycardia

- Baseline ECG and ECG during tachycardia are crucial for correct diagnosis
- The presence of preexcitation in the baseline ECG in a patient with a history of regular paroxysmal palpitations is generally suggestive of AVRT.
- absence of apparent pre-excitation does not rule out the diagnosis of AVRT, as it may be due to a concealed accessory pathway (AP) that conducts only retrogradely or to an atypical (Mahaim) pathway, which is latent at sinus rhythm
- focal ATs are characterised by gradual acceleration of rate at start of tachycardia (warm-up phenomenon) and gradual deceleration (cool-down phenomenon) at termination

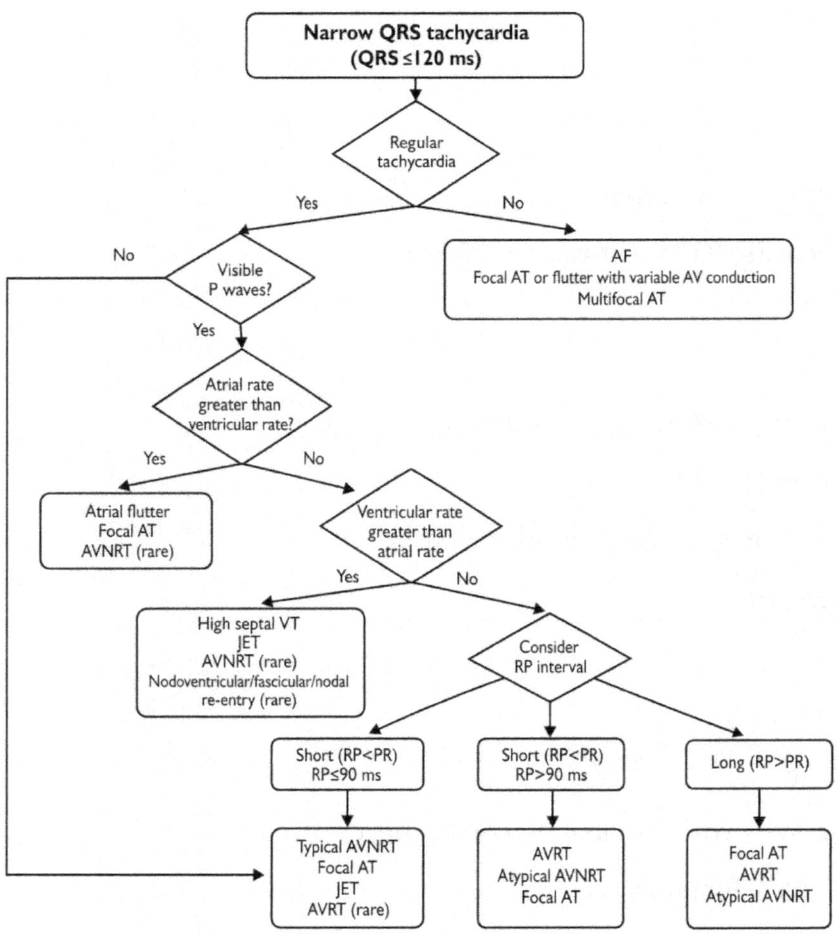

AVNRT (Atrioventricular nodal re-entrant tachycardia)

- A common paroxysmal supraventricular tachycardia (PSVT) caused by a reentrant circuit within or around the AV node using dual AV nodal pathways (slow and fast).
- Dual AV nodal pathways:
    - Fast pathway: fast conduction, long refractory period.
    - Slow pathway: slow conduction, short refractory period
- A premature atrial beat blocks the fast pathway (still refractory) and conducts down the slow pathway.
    - Retrograde conduction up the fast pathway → reentrant circuit → sustained tachycardia.
- Types of AVNRT
    - Typical (Slow-Fast) – 90% cases
        - Antegrade: Slow pathway and Retrograde: Fast pathway
        - Short RP tachycardia on ECG
    - Atypical (Fast-Slow / Slow-Slow) – less common
        - Longer RP intervals
        - P wave is often seen in the late ST segment or the early T wave
- Sudden onset and termination of palpitations. Often, young people with a normal heart
- ECG-Regular narrow QRS tachycardia (150–250 bpm)
    - P wave absent, or manifest as pseudo r′ in V1 or pseudo-S in inferior leads (II, III, aVF)
    - RP < PR in typical AVNRT
- Acute Termination:
    - Vagal manoeuvres (e.g., Valsalva, carotid massage)
    - IV Adenosine – first-line drug (6–12 mg bolus)
    - Alternatives: Verapamil, diltiazem, beta-blockers
- Long-term Management: Catheter ablation of the slow pathway (curative in >95%)

AVRT (Atrioventricular re-entrant tachycardia) (WPW syndrome)

- Conditions commonly associated with bypass tract- HCM, CCTGA, Ebstein anomaly
- Atrioventricular Reentrant Tachycardia (AVRT) is a type of paroxysmal supraventricular tachycardia (PSVT) that involves a macro-reentrant circuit using the AV node and an accessory pathway (bypass tract).
- Types
    - Orthodromic AVRT (95% cases):
        - Antegrade conduction through AV node and retrograde through accessory pathway

    - Regular narrow QRS tachycardia (150–250 bpm)
    - retrograde P waves after QRS
  - Antidromic AVRT:
    - Antegrade conduction through the accessory pathway and retrograde through AV node
    - Wide QRS tachycardia
- Acute Termination:
  - Vagal manoeuvres
  - IV Adenosine (avoid in manifest WPW with atrial fibrillation)
  - Alternatives:beta-blockers, or calcium channel blockers
- Long-term Management:
  - Catheter ablation of accessory pathway (curative in >95%)

Asymptomatic WPW pattern

- WPW pattern without any arrhythmia
- Needs risk stratification for further management- catheter ablation considered if high-risk bypass tract. Ablation is considered in high-risk profession (pilot)
- Risk stratification methods
  - Exercise ECG- Loss of preexcitation at higher heart rates indicates low risk
  - Holter monitoring- intermittent preexcitation indicates low risk
  - EP study- Accessory pathway refractory period of more than 250 ms suggests low risk
  - SPERRI (Shortest pre-excited RR interval) during AF, less than 250 ms, suggest a high-risk pathway

Preexcited Atrial Fibrillation

- Atrial fibrillation conducted via an accessory pathway (e.g., in WPW syndrome), leading to very rapid ventricular rates
- It can cause a wide QRS irregular tachycardia and risk of ventricular fibrillation.
- Dangerous arrhythmia with high risk for sudden death
- Management
  - AV nodal blockers (Beta blockers, CCB and amiodarone) are contraindicated as they promote conduction via the accessory pathway
  - Urgent cardioversion mostly for unstable patients
  - Procainamide or Ibutilide in stable patients
  - RF ablation of the accessory tract is a definitive treatment

Mahaim Tachycardia

- Mahaim tachycardia is a rare form of **antidromic AV reentrant tachycardia (AVRT)** involving a **Mahaim fibre**—an accessory pathway that conducts **only in the anterograde direction** and has **decremental conduction**, similar to the AV node.

Atrial tachycardia

- Tachycardia focus lies in the atrium and is classified into 3 types
  - Focal AT
  - Multifocal AT
  - Macro re-entrant atrial tachycardia (Atrial flutter)

Focal AT

- **Ectopic atrial focus** outside the sinoatrial (SA) node, leading to **regular atrial rates between 100–250 bpm**.
- **Regular rhythm** with **abnormal P-wave morphology** (depends on focus location)
- **Ventricular rate** may be variable, depending on AV conduction

Multifocal atrial tachycardia (MAT):

- Irregular rhythm with ≥3 distinct P-wave morphologies
- Common causes are
  - Structural heart disease
  - Digoxin toxicity
  - Hypoxia, COPD (especially in MAT)
  - Post-cardiac surgery
- **Management:**
  - **Rate control:** Beta-blockers or calcium channel blockers
  - **Antiarrhythmic therapy:** Class IC or III agents in selected cases
  - **Catheter ablation** for symptomatic or recurrent focal AT
  - **Avoid AV nodal blockers** in MAT unless necessary (especially if digoxin-related)

Atrial flutter

- A macro re-entrant atrial tachycardia, usually with atrial rate ~300 bpm and ventricular rate ~150 bpm (2:1 block).
- The classic type is counterclockwise flutter in the right atrium, showing sawtooth flutter waves in inferior leads on ECG.
- Common in structural heart disease and post-surgery

- **Management:**
  - Rate control: Beta-blockers or calcium channel blockers
  - Rhythm control: Electrical or pharmacologic cardioversion
  - Definitive: Cavotricuspid isthmus ablation for typical flutter

20. Ventricular Tachycardia (VT)

Etiology

- 2 Broad etiologies underlie the origin of VT.
- Need to be differentiated correctly, and it has management and prognostic implications.

VT associated with structural heart disease	Idiopathic VT
• VT secondary to myocardial scar	mostly enhanced automaticity/triggered activity
• poor prognosis	good prognosis
• high chance of sudden cardiac death	low chance of sudden cardiac death
• low success rate of catheter ablation	high success rate of catheter ablation
• ICD usually indicated for secondary prevention	ICD not indicated for all
• different morphologies of VT can be seen	usually single morphology of QRS complex during VT

- Common causes of VT associated with structural heart disease: CAD-ICMP, DCMP, HCM, ARVC, Congenital heart disease, Inflammatory cardiomyopathy (myocarditis, sarcoidosis)

Idiopathic VT

- monomorphic VT in the absence of structural heart disease/myocardial scar (assessed by ECHO/MRI)
- Several types are named according to the focus of origin
    - Outflow VT(RVOT/LVOT VT)
    - Fascicular VT
    - Annular VT
    - Papillary muscle VT
    - Crux VT

Outflow VT

- RVOT & LVOT are the most common sites of idiopathic VT origin.
- Triggered activity underlies the VT origin
- Can be paroxysmal/exercise induced/stress induced
- ECG-
    - RVOT VT-LBBB with inferior axis
    - LVOT VT-RBBB with inferior axis.
- Responsive to vagal manoeuvre, beta blockers, verapamil, diltiazem

Fascicular VT

- Usually exercise-induced
- VT originates from either the fascicle (left anterior or left posterior) of the left bundle.
- ECG
    - Left posterior fascicle commonly involved-RBBB with superior axis
    - Anterior fascicle-RBBB With inferior axis
- Respond well to IV verapamil (verapamil-sensitive VT)
- Relatively narrow QRS mimics SVT

Bundle branch re-entry VT (Not an idiopathic VT)

- Usually associated with significant structural heart disease and myocardial scar
- VT re-entry involves antegrade through the right bundle and retrograde through the left bundle branch
- Predominantly LBBB morphology of VT
- Catheter ablation of the right bundle is the treatment of choice

Antiarrhythmic Drug (AAD) therapy for VT

- Considered to prevent recurrence of VT even after ICD
- **Cardiac Arrhythmia Suppression Trial (CAST)**
    - Sodium channel blockers (e.g., ecainide, Flecainide) increase mortality in patients after MI
    - Subsequently, Sodium channel blockers (Class I) drugs were contraindicated in ICMP/Structural heart disease
    - This increased mortality is likely secondary to pro-arrhythmic effects
- **Choice of AAD**
    - With structural heart disease,- Amiodarone, Sotalol
    - Amiodarone- consider long-term adverse events (lung, eye, thyroid)
    - Idiopathic VT- Beta blocker, CCB, Flecainide, Propafenone
    - Brugada/early repolarisation- Quinidine
    - LQT syndrome- Beta blockers (Propranolol/Nadolol)
    - Idiopathic VF- Quinidine
- Class Ic (Flecainide) and class III (Dofetilide, Ibutilide, sotalol) have maximum pro-arrhythmic potential

Management Algorithm

Episode of VT

ACUTE MANAGEMENT

- According to ACLS protocol
- DCCV if hemodynamically unstable
  With cardiac resuscitation
- Drug therapy can be tried if stable

LONG-TERM MANAGEMENT

- Rule out structural heart disease by echo and cardiac MRI
- Look for ventricular function and scar

STRUCTURAL HEART DISEASE

- Secondary prevention AICD
- Treatment of underlying heart disease
- Drug therapy: amiodarone and sotalol
- Catheter ablation

NO STRUCTURAL HEART DISEASE

Likely idiopathic VT

Consider Drug therapy-

- beta blockers
- calcium channel blocker
- Flecanide
- Propafenone

Catheter ablation is curative

ICD usually not indicated

ICD Therapy

- An implantable device that terminates VT/VF by delivering a DC shock and prevents sudden cardiac death
- It aims to prevent SCD and does not prevent the recurrence of VT
- The device is implanted in the left prepectoral area in a subcutaneous pocket, and the defibrillator lead is inserted transvenously into the RV apex.
- Indications
  - Secondary prevention
    - After an episode of aborted SCD/ hemodynamically unstable sustained VT/VF
    - Unstable VT/VF documented 48 hours after MI without evidence of active ischemia
  - Primary prevention
    - ICMP with LVEF <30 % assessed 40days after MI (Class I)
    - DCMP with LVEF < 30 % , NYHA I, 3months after OMT (Class IIa)
    - HCM with high risk of SCD
    - Inherited arrhythmia syndromes in selected patients
- Previous trials for primary prevention ICD in HFrEF showed mortality benefit in ICMP as well as DCMP (CAT, AMIOVIRT, DEFINITE, COMPANION, and SCD-HeFT).
- Recent DANISH trial- No mortality benefit with primary prevention ICD in non-ischemic cardiomyopathy. This trial downgraded the role of primary prevention ICD in DCMP.
- Idiopathic VT- Catheter ablation usually prevents recurrence, and ICD therapy is not indicated

Sub-cutaneous ICD

- The defibrillator lead is placed underneath the skin over the precordium without entering the heart (PIC)
- Avoid lead-related vascular complications/infection
- However, it cannot have a pacing function

Wearable ICD

- Temporary ICD device to prevent SCD when an implantable ICD is not indicated
- Mostly used early after MI/revascularisation with reduced ejection fraction
- VEST trial - Among patients with a recent myocardial infarction and an ejection fraction of 35% or less, the wearable cardioverter–defibrillator did not lead to a significantly lower rate of the primary outcome of arrhythmic death than control

Polymorphic VT

- Rapidly changing QRS morphology during VT
- Torsades De pointes is a specific type of polymorphic VT that has waxing and waning QRS amplitude and is associated with a prolonged QT interval.

Common Causes

Structural Heart Disease

- Acute ischemia
- DCM
- Myocardial scar.

Structurally normal heart

- Inherited arrhythmia syndrome
    - LQT
    - SQT
    - Brugada
    - CPVT
    - Early Repolarisation Syndrome.
- Digoxin Toxicity
- Acquired Long QT (Hypokalemia, Hypocalcemia)

Management

- Mostly unstable vitals requiring defibrillation
- IV magnesium sulphate
- Beta blocker for long QT syndrome
- Temporary pacing if bradycardia
- Correct underlying causes-
    - Revascularisation if on-going ischemia
    - Correct electrolyte imbalance.

VT storm/electrical storm

- 3 or more episodes of VT within 24 hours

Management options:

- Correct electrolyte imbalance/ischemia
- Beta blockers, nonselective (Propranolol is more effective than selective beta blockers)
- General anaesthesia
- Percutaneous stellate ganglion block
- High thoracic epidural anaesthesia
- Emergency catheter ablation.

Bidirectional VT

- Rare variant of VT characterised by beat-to-beat alteration of frontal QRS axis
- Etiology
    - Digoxin toxicity
    - CPVT (Catecholinergic polymorphic VT)
    - Aconite poisoning

VT and SVT with aberrancy

- Regular wide complex tachycardia can be VT or SVT with aberrancy. This needs to be differentiated as the prognosis and management differ between the two.
- The following factors need to be considered while differentiating -

  Clinical background/history:-

  - Known structural heart disease/prior MI/CAD-more likely VT
  - History of ICD implant-likely VT
  - Young age is more likely to have SVT
  - Symptoms usually do not differentiate.
  - Hemodynamically unstable- more chance of VT.

ECG Characteristics

	VT	SVT with Abberancy
• QRS duration	more wide QRS RBBB>140ms LBBB>160ms	less wide QRS <140-150ms
• QRS axis	northwest axis(-90 to 180 degree) RBBB with QRS axis left of -30 degree(LAD) LBBB with QRS axis Right of +90 degree(RAD)	Usually normal axis
• AV dissociation	Present there is 2 separate foci controlling atrium (SA node) and ventricle VT focus	Absent
• concordance	positive or negative QRS complex (concordant) in all chest lead suggest VT	No concordance
• fusion and capture beat	considered most specific/diagnostic of VT	absent

- Prolonged initial part of QRS complex manifested by RS interval (> 100 milliseconds) suggests VT as there is myocardial conduction in VT
- On the contrary, there is rapid initial conduction in SVT, as there is impulse transmission via the conduction system
- Various algorithms have been proposed to differentiate VT Vs SVT with aberrancy, including the above parameters-

  VERECKEI approach

  BRUGADA Criteria

21. Inherited Arrhythmia Syndrome

LQTS (Long QT syndrome)

- One of the common causes of sudden cardiac death (20% of SCD in young)
- Prolonged QTc leads to classical Torsades, causing syncope/SCD. Torsades events are mostly self-limited and sometimes fatal.

M -FACT risk stratification score used for assessing risk of arrhythmia in LQTS

Genetic mutations

The following 3 mutations account for 75% of LQTs

- **KCNQ1** (Loss of function of K+ channel)- **LQT1**
- **KCNH2** (Loss of function of K+ channel)- **LQT2**
- **SCN5A** (Gain of function of Na Channel)- **LQT3**

Other minor mutations – CACNA1, CALM1, CALM2, CALM3, SCN4B **Associated syndromes**

- Jarvel Lange Nielson- sensorineural hearing loss
- Anderson-Tawil Syndrome-
- Timothy syndrome
- Ankyrin B syndrome

- Genetic testing to identify the type of LQT syndrome is useful in choosing appropriate management
- There are specific identified triggers for each type of LQTs to provoke syncope/SCD

	LQT1	LQT2	LQT3
Trigger	Swimming exercise	Auditory stimuli Post-partum	Sleep Rest
ECG pattern	Broad based T	Low amplitude notched T	Long ST segment and narrow based T
Therapy Beta blocker	Very useful	Less protective	Less protective
Na Channel blocker (Mexilitine Flecainide Ranolazine)	Not useful	Not useful	Useful (as there is gain of function mutation of Na channel)

Management

- Avoid triggers
- Beta blocker
  - The first line of therapy in symptomatic patients
  - Propranolol and nadolol are useful (membrane-stabilising property)
  - LQT1 and LQT2 respond well to exercise-induced sympathetic drive, which provokes syncope
- Left cervical sympathetic denervation (LCSD)
  - Consider when recurrent syncope occurs despite maximal beta-blocker
- AICD
  - Syncope despite the drug and LCSD
  - SCD survivor
  - Very high QTc (>550) with signs of electrical instability on ECG (T alternans)

J Wave Syndrome

Repolarisation abnormality leading to VF/SCD

- ER Syndrome
- Brugada Syndrome

SQTS (Short QT syndrome)

- Defined as QTc < 340-360 ms
- Predisposed to **polymorphic VT and atrial fibrillation**
- Secondary to a loss-of-function mutation of the L-type Ca channel or a gain-of-function mutation of the K+ channel
- SCD is the initial manifestation in 40% patients, and a family h/o SCD is common
- ICD insertion in symptomatic patients
- Quinidine may be helpful

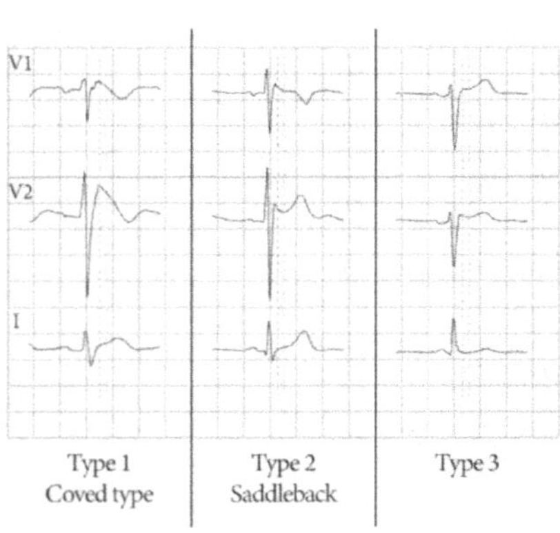

Brugada Syndrome

- Genetically inherited arrhythmia syndrome characterised by a specific ECG abnormality
- Autosomal dominant and SCNSA mutation (Na channel)
- SCD (sudden cardiac death), usually secondary to polymorphic VT/VF, happen **during rest, sleep or febrile illness,** commonly involving young males
- Structural abnormality involving the RVOT epicardium as the source of arrhythmia (focal epicardial arrhythmogenic cardiomyopathy)

ECG- Transient or persistent coved ST elevations (J point elevation followed by down-sloping ST) in precordial leads are characteristic

- Mimic RBBB and STEMI/AWMI
- ECG can be normal and Brugada pattern and induced with enhanced vagal tone, fever and drugs (Na channel blocker, psychotropic drugs)

Diagnosis

- Typical clinical history + type I Brugada pattern on ECG (spontaneous/provoked by Na+ channel blockade)

Management

- AICD to prevent SCD for patients who had aborted SCD/ syncope
- Quinidine / Hydroquinidine (DOC)
- Catheter ablation of epicardial RVOT (arrhythmia focus)

ERS (Early repolarisation syndrome)

- When a patient with an early repolarisation pattern on ECG, with a history of VF/aborted SCD, called ER Syndrome
- ECG-J point elevation > 1 mm in two contiguous inferior or lateral leads and QRS duration <120 ms in leads without J point elevation
- ER pattern on ECG is seen in 1% to 24% of the general population, but the rate of SCD is very low
- Heterogeneity of transmural voltage gradient across the ventricular wall is considered an arrhythmogenic mechanism
- VF is usually initiated by Purkinje cells and myocardial cells
- Currently, no risk stratification tool is available for the asymptomatic ER pattern to predict high risk

Management

- ICD who sustained VF/aborted SCD and ER pattern
- Quinidine for recurrent episodes
- Catheter ablation of the target epicardial substrate

CPVT (catecholaminergic polymorphic VT)

- Characterised by exercise-induced ventricular arrhythmia (VPC, bidirectional VT, polymorphic VT/ VF)
- Bidirectional VT is not very common but pathognomonic
- Mutation of the **ryanodine receptor (RYR2)** leading to abnormal calcium handling underlies arrhythmogenicity
- Other mutations, such as calsequestrin, calmodulin, Kin 2.1 and triadin, are also responsible in a few cases
- Resting ECG is nearly normal, and a structurally normal heart
- Exercise stress testing (TMT) can be done for diagnosis

Management

- Avoidance of exercise
- beta blocker-1st line treatment
- Persistent episodes- Flecanide, propafenone, verapamil
- Left cervical sympathectomy

ICD is usually avoided, as inappropriate shock may precipitate sympathetic activity leading to VT storm

Causes of bidirectional VT

- Anderson–Tawil Syndrome
- CPVT
- Aconite poisoning
- Myocarditis
- Digoxin toxicity

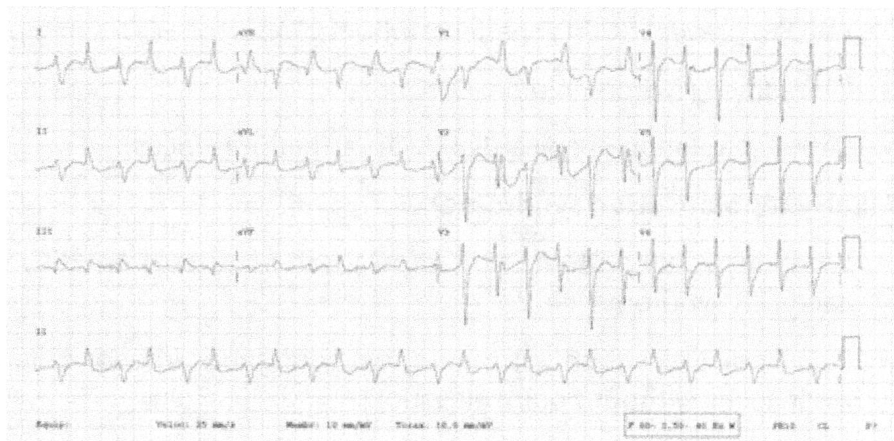

Bidirectional VT in CPVT

Causes of exercise-induced VT

- CPVT
- ARVC
- RVOT VT
- LQT
- CAD

ARVC (Arrhythmic Right Ventricular Cardiomyopathy)

- Fibrofatty replacement of myocardium -predominantly involves RV, biventricular/isolated LV involvement is less common
- Defective cell adhesion molecule-Desmosome
- Clinically progresses in 3 stages
- long subclinical stage → symptomatic ventricular arrhythmia → dilated RV with RV failure
- Exercise precipitates arrhythmia
- Cardiomyopathy predominantly involves the RV outflow tract

ECG - T inv in v1-3 (repolarisation abnormality)

- **Epsilon waves** (delayed depolarisation of dilated/dysplastic RVOT)
- **VT (LBBB with superior axis**)

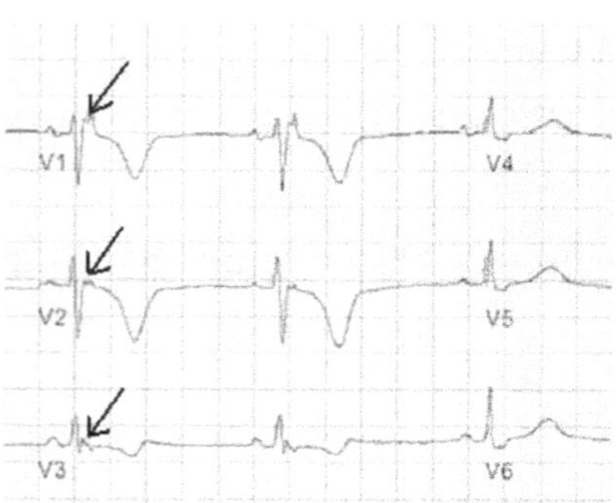

Diagnosis-

- Task Force Criteria 2010 diagnoses ARVC, including clinical, ECG, imaging (ECHO, MRI) and genetic study
- MRI plays an important role in assessing RVOT dilation, fatty infiltration of the myocardium

- **Management**
  - Avoid heavy exertion
  - Beta blocker
  - AICD for secondary prevention
  - Catheter ablation

Cardio cutaneous syndrome

ARVC is associated with skin manifestations

NAXOS syndrome	Carvajal syndrome
Plakoglobin Mutation	Desmoplakin Mutation
Hyperkeratosis of Palms and sole with wooly hair	Epidermolytic Keratoderma (like pemphigus)
ARVC	ARVC

22. Management of Atrial Fibrillation (AF)

Management of AF aims at following the 3 important aspects

1. Stroke risk assessment and anticoagulation
2. Symptom control (rate and rhythm control)
3. Risk factor management

Initial management of new-onset AF

- Spontaneous restoration of sinus rhythm is commonly seen in new-onset AF in the majority of patients within 48 hours.

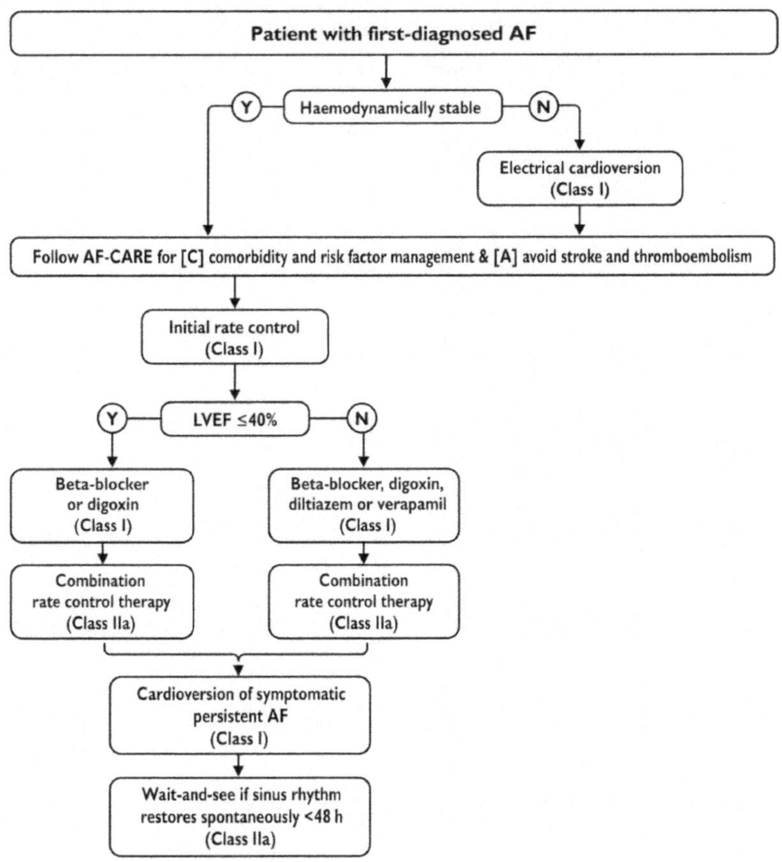

- Long-term, according to the CHADS2 VASC Score
- Anticoagulation for 4 weeks for all AF patients who persisted for more than 48 hours, even if sinus rhythm is achieved (risk of thromboembolism due to atrial stunning)

Wait and watch strategy in new onset AF

- Spontaneous restoration of sinus rhythm is seen in 55 to 60% of patients with new-onset AF within 24 hours and in 69% of patients within 48 hours. **(RACE 7ACWAS trial)**

So, a wait-and-watch strategy may be appropriate if the patient is asymptomatic or with minimal symptoms

Symptom control (Rate versus Rhythm Control)

- Decided based on the following factors.
  - Age and duration of AF
  - LA size
  - Symptom burden
  - Heart failure or LV dysfunction
  - Prior recurrence
  - Reversible cause

Example – A patient with advanced age with long-standing AF, mitral stenosis with large LA size, recurrence rate will be very high with rhythm control, so rate control strategy would be appropriate.

On the contrary, a recent onset of AF with no structural heart disease should go for a rhythm control strategy.

Rhythm control strategy in AF

- AF can be reverted to sinus rhythm in the following ways
  - Electrical cardioversion
  - Antiarrhythmic drugs (AAD)
  - AF ablation
    - Percutaneous catheter ablation
    - Endoscopic and hybrid ablation
    - Surgical ablation
- Older studies of a rhythm control strategy using AADs compared to rate control only do not reduce mortality and morbidity, and may increase hospitalisation (AFFIRM)
- However, recent studies using catheter ablation showed a favourable outcome with rhythm control strategy (CASTLE AF, EAST-AFNET, CABANA)

Pill in pocket approach

- In patients with infrequent AF episodes and a structurally normal heart, patients can take AAD during episodes of AF to restore rhythm
- **Flecainide** (100-200 mg) or **propafenone** (300-600 mg) is the preferred drug for this approach.

> - Flecainide and propafenone are preferred as Pill in pocket approach

- Beta blockers should be taken one hour before Flecainide is administered.

Antiarrhythmic Drugs

- Choice of AAD for chronic suppression of AF depends upon the underlying heart disease, efficacy and side effects.

- Class I drugs (flecainide, propafenone) have better cardioversion property, but have shown increased mortality in CAD/Heart failure patients
- Amiodarone is the drug of choice in HF/CAD patients, with monitoring of adverse effects

- Class Ic drugs (flecainide, propafenone) increase mortality in CAD patients. (CAST trial)
- **Pro-arrhythmic risk**
  - Class Ia (quinidine, procainamide) & class III (Sotalol, amiodarone, dronedarone) are associated with increased QTc and polymorphic VT
  - Class Ic drugs (flecainide, propafenone) are associated with QRS widening and monomorphic VT (not QT prolongation)
- **Choice of AAD**
  - Structurally normal heart (No LV dysfunction/LVH/CAD)- Flecainide, Propafenone
  - Heart failure/CAD- Amiodarone, Dronedarone

Catheter Ablation in AF

Indications:

  - Paroxysmal/persistent AF non-responsive/intolerant to antiarrhythmic drugs
  - AF with HFrEF to reverse LV dysfunction secondary to tachycardiomyopathy
  - AF related bradycardia and pauses to reduce symptoms and avoid a pacemaker
- Catheter ablation predominantly involves **pulmonary vein isolation,** which is ablation around the ostium of the pulmonary vein, as pulmonary veins are considered major foci for AF.
- **AV node ablation along with a permanent pacemaker** is considered in patients with AF unresponsive to rate/rhythm control strategies to reduce symptoms

Rate control strategy

- Agents -beta blockers, CCB, digoxin
- Choice of drugs
  - Beta blockers and CCB preferred.
  - CCB should be avoided in case of LVEF less than 40%

  Digoxin reduces the resting heart rate, making it less useful in exercise-induced tachycardia. Useful in patients with heart failure
- No difference between **strict heart rate control** (resting heart rate less than 80 beats per minute and exercise heart rate less than 110 beats per minute) versus **lenient heart rate control** (resting heart rate less than 110 beats per minute)
- So lenient heart rate control is also acceptable.

Stroke risk and anticoagulation

- The CHADS2VASC2 score is used for risk stratification for stroke in patients with AF who require long-term oral anticoagulant

NOAC preferred over VKA for stroke prevention in all except in severe MS and mechanical heart valves.

Score >2 OAC recommended (class I)

Score 1 OAC should be considered after shared decision making with the patient (Class IIa)

- The need for anticoagulation should not be based on paroxysmal or persistent AF
- NOACs are preferred over VKAs for stroke prevention except in certain scenarios

LAA device closure

- Left atrial appendage is a common site of thrombus formation in patients with Airtel fibrillation leading to stroke.
- Percutaneous devices have been developed to occlude the LAA.
  - FDA-approved are WATCHMAN and WATCHMAN FLEX
  - PROTECT AF and PREVAIL AF trials showed that watchman devices were inferior to VKA in stroke prevention. However, the quality of evidence is not robust as of now.
- Percutaneous LAA Occlusion devices may be considered in patients with AF with contraindication to anticoagulation. (class II b)

Antiplatelet therapy (aspirin/ clopidogrel) is not useful for stroke prevention in AF

NOAC/DOAC

- DOACs have demonstrated non-inferior benefit for stroke prevention compared to warfarin and an added benefit of 50% more reduction in ICH
- Advantages of NOAC over VKA
  - The lack of INR monitoring
  - Fewer drug and food interactions
- All NOAC excretion is dependent on the Pgp protein. Rivaroxaban and apixaban metabolism are CYP3A4 dependent. Enzyme inducer (e.g. Rifampicin) decreases the plasma level and effectiveness
- Contraindicated in
  - Mechanical heart valve
  - Severe MS

	dose	Inhibit	Monitoring	Other remarks
Apixaban	5mg BD 2.5 mg BD if age >80, wt <60	Factor Xa	Anti Xa level	Lowest bleeding risk Safe in elderly Better tolerated in CKD
Rivaroxaban	20mg OD 15 md OD	Factor Xa	Anti Xa level	Significant hepatic clearance

	dose	Inhibit	Monitoring	Other remarks
Dabigatran	150mg BD 110MG BD	Factor IIa	apTT	Higher GI bleeding Maximal hepatic clearance Contraindicated in CKD
Edoxaban	60mg OD 30 mg OD	Factor Xa	Anti Xa level	

Antidote for DOAC

- Factor Xa inhibitors (Apixaban, Rivaroxaban)- **Andexanet alpha**
- Dabigatran- **Idarucizumab**
- **Ciraparantag**- a newer universal antidote for both heparin and NOAC

23. Left-to-right shunts

- Sinus venosus ASD is usually associated with anomalous pulmonary venous drainage (PAPVC)

Atrial septal defect (ASD)

1. **OS (Ostium secundum ASD) is the** most common type (50-70 %)
   - The inferior or mitral rim is preserved
2. **OP (Ostium primum ASD)** - 30 %
   - Also known as a partial endocardial cushion defect
   - Absent mitral rim of ASD
   - Associated with a cleft mitral valve and MR
3. **Sinus venosus defect** (10%)
   - Defect located at the entry of SVC or IVC into the RA
   - Associated with anomalous pulmonary venous drainage (PAPVC)
4. **Unroofed coronary sinus**
   - Not a true ASD
   - A defect in the roof of the CS leads to shunting of blood from LA to RA through the coronary sinus, behaving like an ASD

Clinical features

- Usually asymptomatic in childhood, and develops progressive dyspnea around 20 to 30 years of age
- Characteristic auscultatory findings
  - Wide and fixed S2
  - secondary to dilated and compliant pulmonary artery (it may persist after ASD closure)
  - Loud P2 even without PAH
  - Flow murmur across the pulmonary valve
- Eisenmenger in ASD is very rare (less than 10%) as it has only volume overload. It develops in the 3rd to 4th decade.
- Cardiomegaly may be present even with ES. There is a high chance of right heart failure.

ECG changes

- ostium secundum ASD

  RV volume overload leads to RVH, RAD, RBBB (RsR′)

  Crochetase sign – notching in QRS in inferior leads
- Ostium primum ASD

  Left axis deviation.

ECG in ASD

- **OS-ASD** – RAD, RBBB
- **OP-ASD** – LAD
- **SV ASD**- Negative P inferior leads

- Sinus venosus ASD

  Negative P wave in II, III and avF (Low-lying ectopic pacemaker)

Management of ASD

- ASD closure is indicated when there is a significant shunt (QP: QS more than 1.5) and evidence of RV volume overload (RV enlargement in ECHO)

A. Device closure

- Currently, it is most preferred, and it is the standard of care for **ostium secundum ASD.**
- Devices - AMPLATZER septal occluder

  Helix septal occluder

- Defects up to 38-40 mm can be closed with the device

ASD Eisenmanger

- very rare (less than 10%)
- Cardiomegaly may be present
- (cardiomegaly disappears in VSD/PDA Eisenmenger)

B. Surgical closure

- It is done when anatomy is not suitable for device closure, like a large defect and no adequate rim
- A pericardial or Teflon patch is used

Asymptomatic child	Elective closure between **2-5 years** to prevent RV dilation and arrhythmias later.
Symptomatic infant	Rare, but if heart failure due to ASD alone → consider early closure.
Older children & adults	Closure recommended regardless of age if significant shunt and RV volume overload before pulmonary hypertension develops.

Partial anomalous pulmonary venous return (PAPVC)

- One or more (but not all) pulmonary veins drain into the systemic venous circulation (e.g. SVC, IVC, RA) instead of the left atrium.
- **The right upper pulmonary veins to the SVC** (most common)
- Frequently associated with **sinus venosus type ASD**
- Clinical features similar to ASD

Scimitar syndrome

- A rare form of **partial anomalous pulmonary venous connection (PAPVC)** where the **right pulmonary veins drain into the IVC**
- Often associated with **right lung hypoplasia**

- Warden procedure for Sinus venosus ASD

- May have systemic arterial supply to the right lower lung (from the aorta)
- The anomalous vein on chest X-ray resembles a **Turkish curved sword (scimitar)** along the right heart border

VSD (Ventricular septal defect)

An abnormal communication between the right and left ventricles due to failure of the interventricular septum closure.

Types (by location)

1. **Perimembranous (most common)** – near the membranous septum.
2. **Muscular (trabecular)** – anywhere in the muscular septum, often multiple ("Swiss cheese" septum).
3. **Outlet (supracristal / subarterial / infundibular/conal septal)** – beneath aortic and pulmonary valves; more common in Asians.
4. **Inlet (AV canal type)** – near tricuspid and mitral valves; associated with AV septal defects.

Pathophysiology

- **Left-to-right shunt** → increased pulmonary blood flow → volume overload of pulmonary circulation, LA, and LV.
- **Pulmonary hypertension** may develop with large VSDs.
- **Eisenmenger's syndrome**: reversal to right-to-left shunt due to severe pulmonary hypertension leading to cyanosis.

Clinical Features

- **Small VSD (restrictive)**: often asymptomatic; loud, harsh pansystolic murmur at LLSB with normal growth.
- **Moderate/large VSD (non-restrictive)**:
  - Symptoms of heart failure: tachypnea, feeding difficulty, poor weight gain, and sweating.
  - Frequent respiratory infections.
  - **Murmur:** loud pansystolic murmur at LLSB
  - **Large VSD** may have a softer murmur if pulmonary pressures equal systemic (low gradient).

> **Katz Wachtel phenomena**
>
> - Large biphasic QRS complex V2-V5 suggestive of biventricular hypertrophy in large VSD

Investigations

- **ECG**: LVH or biventricular hypertrophy depending on defect size.
- **Chest X-ray**: Cardiomegaly, increased pulmonary vascular markings in large VSD.
- **Echocardiography (Gold standard)**:

- Defines size, location, and hemodynamic significance.
- Assesses pulmonary pressures and associated lesions.

Management

- **Small VSD**:
  - Usually close spontaneously (esp. muscular type).
  - Monitor for infective endocarditis risk.
- **Moderate to large VSD**:
  - **Medical:** manage heart failure (diuretics, ACE inhibitors, nutrition support).
  - **Surgical:**
    - Indicated if failure to thrive despite optimal therapy, persistent pulmonary hypertension, or large defects.
    - Best done **before irreversible pulmonary vascular disease develops (preferably <1 year of age for large VSD)**.
  - Device closure: for selected muscular/perimembranous VSDs in suitable anatomy.

Gerbode defect

- Communication between the LV and the right atrium
- High-pressure left-to-right shunt

Complications

- Eisenmenger's syndrome.
- Aortic regurgitation (esp. in outlet VSD).
- Acquired right ventricular outflow tract obstruction (infundibular hypertrophy). **(Gasul phenomena)**
- Infective endocarditis.

PDA (Patent Ductus Arteriosus)

Persistent patency of the ductus arteriosus connecting the pulmonary artery to the descending aorta distal to the left subclavian artery beyond the neonatal period.

Aetiology / Risk Factors

- Prematurity (most common)
- Congenital rubella infection
- High altitude
- Hypoxia, respiratory distress
- Female sex (2:1)

Pathophysiology

- **Left-to-right shunt (aorta → PA)** → ↑ pulmonary blood flow → pulmonary congestion → volume overload of **LA and LV** → heart failure if significant.
- **Eisenmenger PDA**: Long-standing large PDA → pulmonary vascular disease → shunt reversal (**right-to-left**) → **differential cyanosis (cyanosis of lower limb**

Clinical Features

Small PDA	Large PDA
Asymptomatic	Heart failure signs (tachypnea, poor feeding, FTT)
Incidental murmur	Recurrent respiratory infections

- **Pulse**: Bounding pulses, wide pulse pressure
- **Murmur**: Continuous **"machinery murmur"** at **left infraclavicular area**, +/- mid-diastolic flow murmur at apex (↑ MV flow).

> - Device closure is the first line in ASD and PDA
> - Surgical closure is the first line in VSD

Investigations

- **ECG**: LVH ± LAE; biventricular hypertrophy if pulmonary hypertension.
- **CXR**: Cardiomegaly, ↑ pulmonary vascularity.
- **Echo (Gold standard)**: Defines PDA size, flow, and LV volume overload

Management

Preterm PDA

- **Indomethacin/Ibuprofen (NSAIDs)** – inhibit prostaglandin synthesis → closure
- **Paracetamol**: Alternative

Term infants & older children

- **Device closure (preferred)**: Coil or Amplatzer occluder
- **Surgical ligation**: If device closure is unsuitable or fails

Operability in left-to-right shunt

- The natural course of left-to-right shunt (ASD, VSD, PDA) play an important role in management.
- Shunt lesions, when left untreated, lead to irreversible pulmonary vascular changes secondary to increased pulmonary blood flow.

The ideal age for closure of

- VSD - <1 year
- PDA
- ASD

Untreated shunt lesion (ASD, VSD, PDA)

↓

Irreversible pulmonary vascular changes

↓

Obstructive PAH

↓

Reversal of shunt and cyanosis

[Eisenmenger syndrome]

Age of development of Eisenmenger syndrome

- VSD <10 years
- PDA <10 years
- ASD 30-40 years

Hyperkinetic Vs obstructive PAH

- In the presence of ASD/VSD/PDA, there is increased pulmonary blood flow, and there is pulmonary hypertension secondary to high flow (Hyperkinetic PAH)
- With the development of irreversible pulmonary vascular changes(Eisenmengerization), there is increased pulmonary vascular resistance and high PA pressure (obstructive PAH). Shunt flow is usually very low or reversal of shunt at this stage. Shunt should not be closed at this stage (inoperable)

Assessment of operability

- The development of irreversible pulmonary vascular changes takes years to develop
- When a patient comes for the first time beyond the ideal age of shunt closure, they need to be assessed for operability to rule out obstructive PAH
- If the shunt is closed after the setting of obstructive PAH, there will be right heart failure as the RV cannot pump against high PA pressure, and there is no shunt to decompress

Comprehensive assessment done, including clinical features and investigation (ECG, CXR, echo and cath study)

Operable	inoperable
Clinical features	• Silent chest
• Hyperdynamic cardiac impulse, Cardiomegaly, loud shunt murmur, flow murmur across PV and flow murmur across the mitral valve, suggesting active shunt and operability	• No shunt murmur • Loud S2
CXR	
Cardiomegally, e/o increased PBF	No cardiomegaly
Echo	normal or reduced vascularity
Significant left to right shunt, dilated LA, LV	mild left to right shunt/right to left shunt dliated RA, Rv only (except ASD)
ECG	
Evidence of LVH or biventricular enlargement (watz kachtel sign)	Evidence of RVH only (qR pattern in V1)
Cath study	
• Qp/Qs>1.5-2	• Qp/Qs<1.5
• PVRI <4	• PVRI 4-8 borderline, >8 inoperable

Anomalous left coronary artery from pulmonary artery (ALCAPA)

- Anomalous origin of the left coronary artery from PA rather than the aorta
- Also known as Bland -White-Garland syndrome
- Reversal of blood flow towards the PA (low pressure) leads to myocardial ischemia
- Manifest as heart failure in infancy (LV dysfunction, Mitral regurgitation)
- Deep Q waves I,avL, V5-6 characteristic
- Management
- Reimplantation to the aorta
- Tekeuchi repair (intrapulmonary tunnel)

24. Eisenmenger Syndrome

Definition-irreversible pulmonary vascular changes with severe PAH in patients with unrepaired left-to-right shunt.

- Common in post-tricuspid shunts (VSD, PDA, AVSD, AP window) due to both volume and pressure transmission in the pulmonary circulation.
- Eisenmengerization develops in the first few years (2-3 years) if a shunt is not closed, although clinical manifestations start in the 2nd-3rd decade.
- less common in pre-tricuspid shunts (ASD), seen in <10% patients.

Clinical features

- Cyanosis is a late manifestation and is usually mild.
- Markedly reduced exercise capacity
- Haematological manifestations- polycythemia, thrombocytopenia, leucopenia
- Coagulation disturbances, both thrombotic and bleeding complications seen
- Rheumatological complications- gout, arthritis, myalgia.
- Infections-brain abscess, endocarditis

> Eisenmengerization develops in the first few years (2-3 years), although clinical manifestations start in the 2nd-3rd decade.

Cardiovascular examination

- Prominent a wave in JVP, precordium usually silent, rt parasternal heave, shunt murmur usually absent.
- S2 loud, no flow murmur across the pulmonary valve,
- High-pitched diastolic murmur of PR+

CXR

- normal heart size, (cardiomegaly of VSD & PDA regresses once obstructive PAH develops; however, cardiomegaly persists in ASD even after severe PAH)
- Normal to decreased pulmonary blood flow.
- Dilated central PA, with peripheral pruning.

> - No cardiomegaly with VSD/PDA Eisenmenger
> - Cardiomegaly persists with ASD Eisenmanger

Echocardiography

- Dilated RA, RV, with TR.
- Poor shunt flow, bidirectional/right-to-left shunt, dilated pulmonary arteries

Management considerations

Non-estrogen-containing contraceptives are preferred as estrogen increases thromboembolic events

- Adequate hydration
- Pregnancy contraindicated (very high mortality, 30%)
    - Choice of contraception: Non-estrogen-containing contraceptives are preferred as estrogen increases thromboembolic events
- Very high risk for non-cardiac surgery and should be avoided (high intra op mortality),
- Manage iron deficiency

- Hyperviscosity symptoms-
    - hydration, correct iron deficiency,
    - Therapeutic phlebotomy is recommended if symptomatic after volume and iron repletion.
    - Routine phlebotomy is not recommended as it increases stroke risk
- Pulmonary vasodilator-
    - Endothelin antagonist (bosentan) and PDE4 inhibitors (sildenafil) are beneficial in improving exercise capacity
    - BREATHE 5 trial-bosentan
- Transplantation options-
    - combined heart and lung transplantations
    - Lung transplantation with repair of shunt

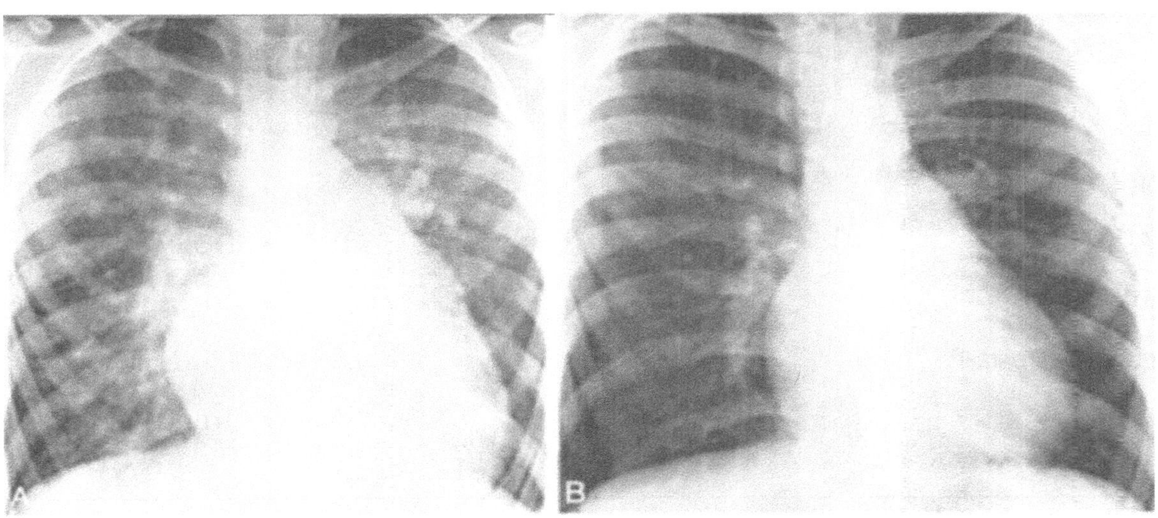

Chest X-ray depicting cardiomegaly with increased pulmonary vascularity during active VSD shunt (left) and oligemic lung fields with resolution of cardiomegaly with development of Eisenmenger

25. Cyanotic Congenital Heart Disease

Broadly divided into 3 types of physiology

TOF Physiology

- There is a large non-restrictive VSD and severe pulmonary stenosis
- R-> L shunt at VSD and cyanosis depend on the pulmonary blood flow
- PBF reduced (decreased Qp)
- PaO2 <SpO2

Include

- TOF
- DORV-VSD-PS
- TGA-VSD-PS
- Single ventricle-PS
- Tricuspid atresia-PS

TGA Physiology

- Ventriculo-arterial discordance (PA connected to LV and Aorta to RV)
- Systemic and pulmonary circulation in parallel connection
- ASD/VSD/PDA shunting between these two circulations is a must for survival.
- Severe desaturation and early presentation
- PBF increased (Increased Qp)
- PaO2> SpO2

Include

- dTGA

Admixture physiology

- There is an admixture of systemic and pulmonary venous return at the level of the atria, ventricles or great vessels
- No RVOT obstruction/PS
- Cyanosis is usually mild and due to admixture of right and left-sided blood
- PBF increased (Increased Qp)
- PaO2 = SpO2

Include

- TAPVC
- Common atrium
- DORV
- Tricuspod atresia
- Mitral atresia
- Truncus arteriosus

Predominant clinical presentation		
Cyanosis	**CHF**	**Shock**
TOF TGA-PS	TGA TAPVC	Hypoplastic left heart syndrome (HLHS) Severe coarctation/AS

I. Tetralogy of Fallot (TOF)

- The most common CCHD in children and adults.
- Comprise of
  - Large subaortic VSD
  - Severe RVOT obstruction (valvular/subvalvular)
  - RV hypertrophy
  - Overriding of the aorta
- Other associations
  - Right-sided aortic arch (25%)
  - Coronary anomaly (5%)

    (LAD from RCA and crossing over RVOT- the most common coronary anomaly in TOF)
- **Clinical signs**
  - Central cyanosis
  - Single S2 (because of soft/faint P2)
  - Ejection systolic murmur

    Murmur loudness is inversely proportional to the severity of cyanosis

    (In isolated PS without VSD, murmur increases with increased PS severity. If PS is associated with VSD, there is increased right-to-left shunt with an increase in the severity of PS, reducing RVOT outflow and a decrease in the loudness of the murmur.
- **ECG**
  - RVH and Right axis deviation
  - Sudden transition from dominant R to S in V2/V3

    Lead V2 lies just over the large VSD, recording a negative voltage of the posterior wall
- **CXR**
  - Boot-shaped heart (due to RV hypertrophy with upturned apex)
  - Pulmonary oligemia
  - Small PA segment
- **Echocardiography**
  - Large VSD
  - Small PA annulus with severe pulmonary stenosis
  - RVH
  - Large aortic root and overriding of the aorta towards the RV
  - Asses

Management/surgical correction

- Complete repair /intracardiac repair is the surgery of choice (VSD patch closure, RVOT muscle band resection, pulmonary valvotomy, transannular RVOT patch when PV annulus is very small)
- Ideal timing of surgery is around 3-4 months, but may be delayed up to 1 year if acyanotic or minimally cyanotic.
- Procedure performed via right atrium(transatrial) or pulmonary artery(transpulmonary) and rt ventricular(transventricular) is least preferred to avoid the ventricular scar site for VT afterwards.
- Use of a transannular patch leads to severe free PR and needs PV replacement in the long term.
- In case of a coronary anomaly (LAD crossing over RVOT), primary repair may lead to LAD injury. In such cases, a conduit is placed between the RV and PA(Rastelli). In such cases, surgery is usually delayed till 1yr age.
- The need for palliative shunt-direct surgical repair is done in most cases

Surgical shunts for palliation

- classic BT shunt-end to side anastomoses of the subclavian artery and ipsilateral PA
- Modified BT shunt-Side-to-side Gore-Tex shunt between the subclavian artery and the PA
- Waterson shunt-ascending aorta to RPA
- Pott shunt-descending aorta to LPA

- Indications
    - TOF with pulmonary atresia and severe cyanosis
    - Infants <3-4 months with severe cyanosis/cyanotic spells are not fit for corrective surgery
    - Hypoplastic PA, annulus

Hypoxic spell/Cyanotic spell/Tet spell

- Paroxysms of respiratory distress, irritability and worsening of cyanosis
- Various triggers set a vicious cycle, as in the flow diagram
- Murmur becomes soft during the spell, indicating reduced pulmonary blood flow

Management

- Target the underlying pathogenesis and block the vicious cycle
- Knee-chest position- Increase SVR and decrease venous return
- Morphine(0.2mg/kg)- suppresses the respiratory centre and controls tachypnoea
- Inhaled O2
- Beta blocker (Propranolol 0.05mg/kg IV bolus) to reduce RVOT spasm and heart rate
- Ketamine- Increase SVR and sedation
- Sodium bicarbonate to correct acidosis

Transcatheter Pulmonary Valve Replacement (TPVR)

- Severe PR in patients with prior transannular patch for TOF surgery is detrimental and leads to right heart failure
- TPVR is an alternative to surgery in such patients
- Valves- Melody valve (made of bovine jugular valve, for a smaller annulus)

  TAVI valves (Sapien, venous P valve, MyVal - for larger annuli)

TOF with absent pulmonary valve

- Mild to moderate PS and severe PR
- Grossly dilated pulmonary arteries, contrary to small PAs in classic TOF
- Airway obstruction by dilated PA and recurrent LRTI

Hoffman variant TOF

- VSD is restrictive

Pink TOF

- Large VSD with mild pulmonary stenosis
- The shunt is predominantly left to right
- Cyanosis is absent or minimal

II. TGA (Transposition of the Great Arteries)

- Normal relation of great arteries- the aorta is posterior and right of the pulmonary artery
- Transposition – when the aorta is anterior to the pulmonary artery
  - d-TGA- Aorta is **right** and anterior to PA
  - l-TGA/CCTGA- Aorta is **left** and anterior to PA

d-TGA

- The aorta arises from the RV, and the PA arise from the LV (VA discordance). The aorta is right and anterior to the PA
- Systemic and pulmonary circulation are in parallel connection (normally in series connection).

There has to be a shunt (ASD/VSD/PDA) for survival

- Usually symptomatic with cyanosis and heart failure at birth/early neonatal period
- CXR- Egg on side appearance

Surgical correction

- **Arterial switch operation (ASO)-** Surgery of choice (anatomic correction)
- Aorta and PA resected above the level of the coronaries and anastomosed to the correct ventricle, and transfer of the coronaries.

- Ideal age- usually done within 4-8 weeks of age.
- When the patient presents late, after 4-8 weeks, LV usually becomes hypoplastic as it faces pulmonary circulation. In such cases, a transient palliative procedure (PA banding, PDA stenting) is usually done, and ASO is done in a staged manner.
- Atrial switch when ASO cannot be done due to a difficult coronary anomaly. (physiologic correction).

- TGA VSD PS- LV routed to the aorta via VSD and RV to PA with conduit

III. l-TGA/CCTGA (congenitally corrected TGA)

- RA drains into the anatomic LV on the right side, which drains to PA, and LA drains to the anatomic RV on the left side, which drains to the aorta
- Physiologically, circulation is maintained (congenitally corrected), and there is ventricular inversion only
- However, anatomic RV is facing high-pressure systemic circulation, which eventually fails with tricuspid regurgitation

  CCTGA is usually associated with other anomalies
  - VSD (80%)
  - PS (50%)
  - Congenital CHB
  - SVT
- Isolated CCTGA is usually asymptomatic in childhood and presents with heart failure in adulthood, mimicking DCMP
- When associated with VSD/PS, present with cyanosis/CHF in early childhood

ECG- Absence of q wave in V5-6 and presence of q wave in V1 (septal depolarisation right to left)

Evidence of AV block/preexcitation

CXR- Egg on a string appearance (due to narrow upper mediastinum)

Straight up left heart border (due to L positioned ascending aorta)

Management

- Double switch operation (DSO) - involves an atrial switch (Mustard/Senning procedure) where RA is connected to RV and LA connected to LV, plus arterial switch (ASO).
- In case of associated VSD-PS-Atrial switch plus Rastelli.

IV. TAPVC (Total Anomalous Pulmonary Venous Connection)

- Pulmonary venous drainage to the right atrium rather than the left atrium
- Usually associated with ASD to allow right-to-left shunt (obligatory shunt for survival)
- There is an admixture of pulmonary and systemic venous return in RA. After this admixture, same blood is circulated to both the pulmonary and systemic circulations
- Similar Sp02 in all cardiac chambers

4 types depending upon the drainage pattern

i. **Supracardiac** (most common type, 50%)
   - All pulmonary veins connect to the left vertical vein, → left innominate vein →SVC→ RA
   - Figure of 8/ Snowman sign on chest X-ray (secondary to dilated vertical, innominate and SVC)

ii. **Cardiac**
   - Pulmonary veins drain directly to the RA or via the coronary sinus

iii. **Infracardiac**
   - Pulmonary veins drain to the portal vein, or hepatic vein, or the IVC
   - Infracardiac types are usually associated with obstruction (obstructive TAPVC)

iv. **Mixed**
   - A combination of either of the above

TAPVC can clinically be

- **Obstructive**- obstruction at the site of anomalous pulmonary drainage usually present as pulmonary oedema/CHF
- **Non-obstructive**- No obstruction/pulmonary oedema. Usually present with cyanosis

Management

Surgical correction with reimplantation of pulmonary veins to the left atrium

V. Ebstein anomaly

- Apical displacement of the septal and sometimes the posterior leaflet of the tricuspid valve
- (insertion of septal TV leaflet >8mm/m2 of BSA towards apex than mitral leaflet insertion)
- Part of the RV cavity is incorporated inside RA (atrialized RV), leading to a small functional RV and a large RA
- Abnormal tricuspid valve leads to TR (low-pressure TR), dilating RA further
- Almost all patients have ASD/PFO, causing cyanosis with right-to-left shunt secondary to elevated RA pressure

Clinical features

- Can present from neonatal age to adulthood, depending upon severity
- Common presentations are
  - Cyanosis
  - Right heart failure
  - SVT/WPW syndrome
- Triple/quadruple rhythm on auscultation characteristics

  split S1, split S2, S3, S4

ECG- tall and broad P waves (Himalayan P waves), increased PR interval, RBBB

preexcitation/WPW pattern (15-20% patients)

Management

- Surgery is usually avoided if the patient is asymptomatic or minimally symptomatic.
- indications of surgery-
    - CHF: NYHA >III,
    - Cyanosis, spo2<80,
    - life-threatening arrhythmia with WPW,
    - paradoxical embolism,
    - RVOT obstruction by the tricuspid valve.
- Surgical options-choice of surgery depends on the severity of TV displacement/amount of functional RV available.
- Biventricular repair- when adequate functional RV, TV repair, plus ASD closure
    - Carpentier technique
    - Danielson technique.
- Single ventricular repair-when RV is inadequate for biventricular repair. (Fontan surgery)

VI. Single ventricle palliation (Glen and Fontan)

- Biventricular repair (RV connected to PA, LV connected to aorta) is the most physiological and has the best long-term outcome in any CHD.
- However, in certain situations, biventricular repair cannot be done for several reasons. (absence of one AV valve, single ventricle or when great arteries cannot be connected to the respective ventricle/non-routable)
- In such cases, univentricular palliation (not correction) is done.
    - Systemic venous return (SVC and IVC) is directly connected to the pulmonary artery

Common Indications

- Tricuspid atresia, mitral atresia
- single ventricle,
- DORV with non-routable VSD
- This can be done in a staged manner (Glenn at an early age and Fontan later), or the Fontan procedure can be done directly.

Glen procedure

- End-to-side anastomoses to the SVC to the right pulmonary artery (half of venous return connected to the PA)
- Usually performed at 2-3 months of age.

Fontan procedure

- SVC to PA anastomoses and IVC connected to PA by artificial graft
- 3 types - cardiac, lateral tunnel, total extra-cardiac.

Suitability for Fontan procedure

- There should be minimal resistance in the pulmonary circulation to accept systemic venous return without a ventricle. (low PVR)
- There should not be any left heart disease (normal ventricular function and competent valves)

Long-term complications-

As there is direct drainage of venous return to the PA, there is elevated venous pressure for a long time, leading to the following complications.

- Low cardiac output, pleural effusion, peripheral oedema, hepatomegaly, ascites, protein-losing enteropathy, thromboembolism, supraventricular arrhythmia.

Adequacy of pulmonary artery size

Pulmonary artery size should be adequate for a better outcome after TOF surgery /Fontan surgery

The following tools assess the adequacy of PA size

McGoon's ratio-

- diameter of RPA+LPA/diameter of DTA just above the diaphragm
- Normal 2-2.5,
- for TOF surgery at least > 1
- for Fontan at least> 1.8

Nakata index-

- Cross-sectional area of RPA+LPA/BSA
- Normal 330+-30mm2/BSA

  For TOF >100

  Fontan >250

PA banding

- Surgically ligate the pulmonary artery to create pulmonary stenosis.
- Usually done in the setting of congenital heart disease to protect pulmonary circulation from increased flow.
- A palliative procedure is used when corrective surgery is delayed for some reason.

Example

In a patient with tricuspid atresia with a large VSD and no VS. Definitive surgery is a Fontan once the child grows for more than 6 months to 1 year. However, by this time, pulmonary vascular damage will have occurred secondary to increased flow. Palliative PA banding will protect pulmonary circulation.

Common indications

- large VSD, multiple VSDs with failure.
- Any complex congenital heart disease with VSD without PS where definite surgery was delayed.
- D-TGA presents late to train the hypoplastic LV before the arterial switch operation.
- L-TGA to reduce TR and reduce the septal bulge to the right
- Sometimes in DCMP to induce PS and make the IVS bulge towards LV, reducing further LV dilation

Balloon atrial septostomy (Rashkind procedure)

- Usually done via IVC using Rashkind balloon/ Fogarty catheter
- Atrial septal defect created percutaneously to decompress the LA / RA in the following situations.
  - TGA with restrictive ASD/No ASD to allow adequate admixture before going for surgery
  - TAPVS with restrictive ASD
  - Tricuspid atresia with restrictive ASD
  - Pulmonary atresia with intact IVS
  - Failing Fontan circulation to decompress the RA
  - Post-operative RV failure
  - End-stage idiopathic PAH before lung transplantation

Condition	Surgery
Sinus venosus ASD with PAPVC	Warden procedure
ALCAPA	Tekeuchi repair
Ebstein	Carpentia repair/Danielson repair
HLHS	Norwood procedure
DTGA	Arterial switch operation (ASO)
CCTGA	Double switch operation
SV with interrupted IVC	Kawasima procedure
DTGA VSD PS	NIKAIDOH procedure, REV procedure
DTGA VSD subaortic stenosis	Damns kays stansel
TOF with Pulmonary atresia	Rastelli procedure

26. Echocardiography Basics

Basic Principle

Current generation echocardiography comprises the assessment of the heart in two ways

2D Echo	Doppler
Assessment of structure/morphology	**Assessment of function** (such as pressure gradient between chambers)
e.g., Chamber dimension, valve opening and closing, vegetation/clot, RWMA	**e.g.:** Stenosis/ regurgitation of the Valve VSD Gradient, PAH assessment

Combining information from 2D Echo and Doppler findings leads to the final diagnosis of any cardiac condition

Example 2D echo → Calcified mitral valve, which is not Opening normally + Doppler → increased gradient (> 5 mmHg) between LA and LV

= **Mitral Stenosis**

Standard Views of 2D Echocardiography

As a three-dimensional structure, the heart is imaged in multiple views for complete assessment

Apical	**Short Axis (PSAX)**	**Long Axis (PLAX)**
Apical 4 chamber (A4C)	Basal Short Axis	
Apical 3 Chamber (A3C)	Mid	
Apical 2 Chamber (A2C)	Apical	

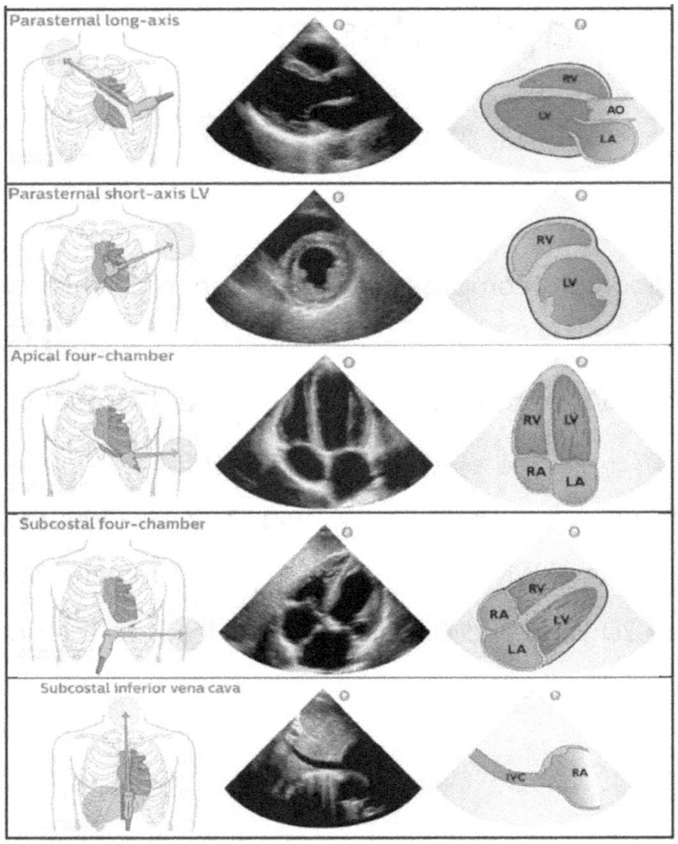

Principles of Doppler Echocardiography

- Ultrasonic waves are emitted from the echo probe at a certain frequency.
- These waves hit the moving RBCs and reflect back to the probe.
- The velocity of RBCs changes the frequency of an ultrasonic wave.
- Based on the change in frequency of ultrasonic waves (frequency shift), the velocity of RBCs (velocity of blood) at that point is measured.

Fd= Ft (V/C), where:

Fd: frequency of reverted sound (Doppler shift)

Ft: frequency of transmitted sound

V: Velocity of blood

C: speed of sound in tissue

After measuring velocity, the gradient between chambers is calculated using the derivative of the **Bernoulli equation**

Pressure Gradient (ΔP) = 4V2

where V is the velocity of blood

E.g. Doppler velocity across the aortic valve = 4 m/s

Gradient = 4 X 42 = 64 mmHg, Suggestive of severe AS

Types of Doppler

Pulse Wave Doppler (PW)	Continuous wave Doppler (CW)
Discrete pulses of waves emitted targeting a specific location	Ultrasound waves emitted continuously across a line
Measures velocity of exact location / sample volume	Measures velocity of all points in the line and maximum velocity record
Can be used only for low velocity lesions (<1.5 m/s). e.g.: mitral valve, tricuspid valve	Can be used for high velocity lesion (>1.5 m/s) e.g.: Aortic valve

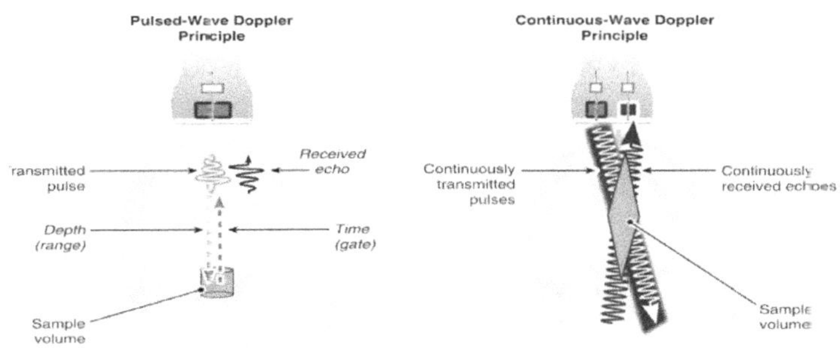

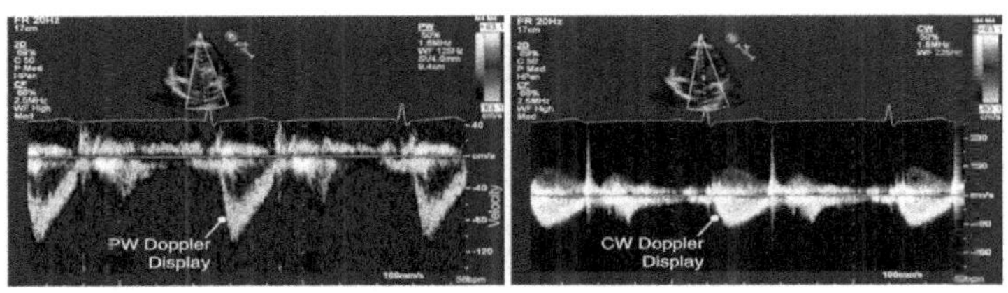

Colour Doppler

- Type of PW with colour representation of the velocity of blood
- Blood coming toward the probe appears red, and blood away from the probe appears blue.
- Turbulent blood appears mosaic pattern.
- Help in qualitative assessment of stenotic, regurgitant and shunt lesions.

Ventricular contractility/systolic function

- Ejection fraction of LV is assessed by the following methods:
  - Visual / Eye balling (VEF)
  - Simpson method
  - M Mode
- Other echo parameters to assess LV function are
  - Tissue Doppler velocity of the mitral annulus
  - EPSS
  - MPI (myocardial performance index / Tei Index)

When there is left ventricular systolic dysfunction, we need to assess whether it is a global hypokinesia (likely non-ischemic aetiology/DCMP) or regional ventricular dysfunction (ischemia likely/ICMP)

- The function of RV is assessed by
  - TAPSE (Tricuspid annular plane systolic excursion)

RWMA (regional wall motion abnormality)

- Part of the left ventricle is dysfunctional (RWMA), which indirectly suggests stenosis of the supplying artery (CAD)
- Assessed in all views to detect any hypokinetic/akinetic segment of LV suggestive of Ischemia / Scar.
- The whole of LV is divided into 16 segments to report RWMA uniformly

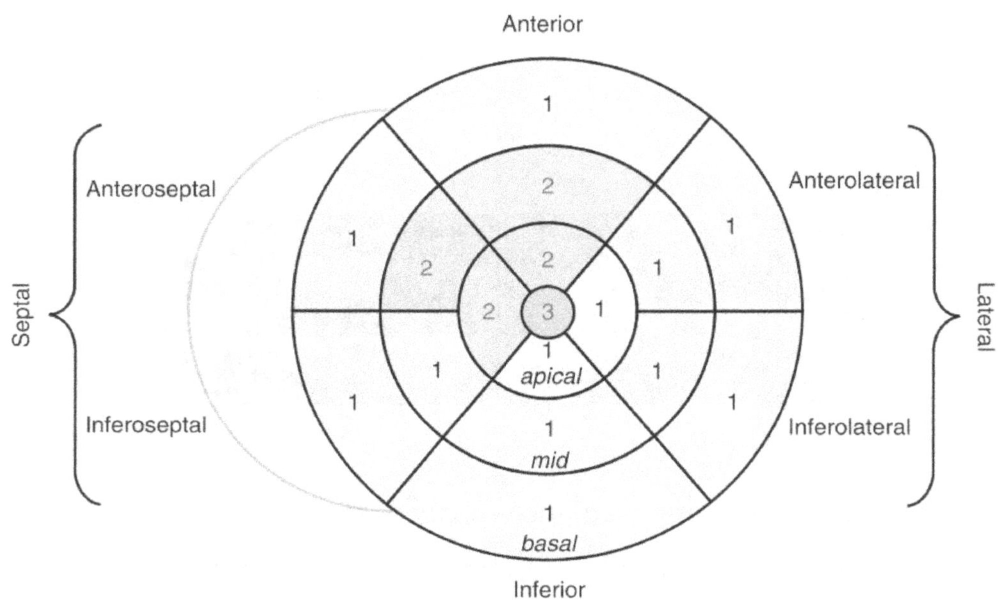

ASE Wall motion score index (WMSI) = Σ17 scores/17 segments

For this case: WMSI = 23/17 = 1.35

Points:	1 = normal 2 = hypokinetic (reduced wall thickening) 3 = akinetic (absent or negligible wall thickening, i.e., scar) 4 = dyskinetic (systolic thinning or stretching, i.e., aneurysm)

- E.g. Basal, mid-anterior and anteroseptal hypokinesia suggestive of LAD territory ischemia

Diastolic dysfunction

Various ways to assess diastolic dysfunction

Mitral Inflow Doppler

- Early and late LV filling (LA contraction) produce two waves, i.e. E and A, respectively.
- Normally, early filling (E) is more than late filling (A)

- With mild diastolic dysfunction, early filling remains the same, but atria contract more to maintain LV filling (So A > E)
- With the worsening of diastolic dysfunction, LA pressure increases more, leading to high velocity of early filling (E >> A)

Tissue Doppler

- Tissue Doppler assesses the velocity of the mitral annulus.
- Normally mitral annulus moves towards the apex with ventricular relaxation.
- Normal velocities are :
  - Peak velocity of the lateral mitral annulus during systole (Lateral E') > 10 cm/s
  - Peak velocity of the lateral mitral annulus during systole (Medial E') > 7 cm/s
- With diastolic dysfunction, the velocities decrease
- The ratio of E/E' suggests the filling pressure of the ventricle
  - E/E' > 10 suggests elevated filling pressure
- Other evidence of Diastolic dysfunction is:
  - Dilated LA
  - Change in pulmonary vein Doppler
  - PAH (Increased TR gradient)

	Normal	Grade I	Grade II	Grade III
Mitral E/A	> 0.8	< 0.8	0.8- 2	> 2
E/e'	< 10	< 10	10-14	> 14
Peak TR velocity m/s	< 2.8	< 2.8	> 2.8	> 2.8
LA Volume ml/m2	< 34	< 34	> 34	> 34

Valvular Heart Disease

1. Mitral stenosis

- Morphological features (2D)
  - Thickened and calcified mitral leaflets with restricted opening
  - Dilated left atrium
- Mitral valve area: assessed by 2 methods
  - Planimetry
  - Pressure half time (PHT)

    The time it takes for the pressure gradient across the mitral valve to decrease to half its initial value.

    - **MVA = 220 / PHT in msec**

- Mean gradient between LA and LV using Doppler
  - > 5 mmHg is significant.

Echo severity of MS

	Mild	Moderate	Severe
Mean gradient (MDG)	< 5 mmHg	5-10 mmHg	>10 mmHg
Mitral valve area (MVA)	> 1.5 cm2	1-1.5 cm2	<1 cm2

Wilkins Score- to assess suitability for balloon mitral valvotomy (BMV)

Components of the Wilkins Echo score

- Leaflet thickening
- Leaflet mobility
- Leaflet calcification
- Subvalvular thickening

Score ranges from 4 to 16. A score less than 8 is favourable for BMV

2. Mitral regurgitation

- Morphological features :
  - Mom coaptation/prolapse of leaflets towards LA.
  - Dilated LA / LV.
- Doppler: colour doppler jet into L
  - Vena contracta, area of the colour jet
  - Access EORA, Regurgitant fraction, Regurgitant volume (PISA Method)

Severe MR-

- vena contracta >7 mm
- Regurgitant volume > 60 ml
- Regurgitant fraction >50%
- Effective regurgitant orifice area(EROA) > 0.4 cm2

3. Aortic Stenosis

- Morphological features (2D)
  - thickened aortic valve with restricted mobility,
  - bicuspid/tricuspid valve
  - hypertrophied LV
- Doppler: increased gradient across the aortic valve. Peak and mean gradient measured.

- Aortic valve area (AVA): calculated using the continuity equation
  - LVOT area X Velocity LVOT = AVA X Velocity Aortic Valve

Severity of AS

	Mild	Moderate	Severe
Peak gradient	< 40 mmHg	40-60 mmHg	> 60 mmHg
Mean gradient	< 20 mmHg	20-40 mmHg	> 40 mmHg
Aortic valve area (AVA)	> 1.5 cm2	1-1.5 cm2	<1 cm2

4. Aortic Regurgitation

- Morphology (2D) :
  - Dilated aorta and LV
  - Non-coaptating / Abnormal Leaflets
- Doppler
  - Regurgitant jet into LV
  - EORV, Regurgitant Fraction and Regurgitant Volume calculated
  - PHT (pressure half time)
  - Flow reversal in DTA

Severe AR-

- vena contracta >6 mm
- Regurgitant volume > 50 ml
- Regurgitant fraction >50%
- Effective regurgitant orifice area(EROA) > 0.3 cm2
- PHT < 200 ms
- Holodiastolic flow reversal in DTA

Pulmonary hypertension

- Morphological features (2D) – dilated and hypertrophied RV and D-shaped LV cavity, Dilated RA, dilated pulmonary artery
- RV systolic pressure equals PA systolic pressure when there is no RV outflow obstruction / PS
- PA systolic pressure is indirectly estimated from the TR gradient.
  - PASP = RVSP = TR Gradient + RA pressure
  - RA pressure estimated using IVC diameter
- Diastolic PA pressure is estimated using the PR gradient if present
  - MPAP: PR peak gradient + RAP
  - DPAP = end diastolic gradient

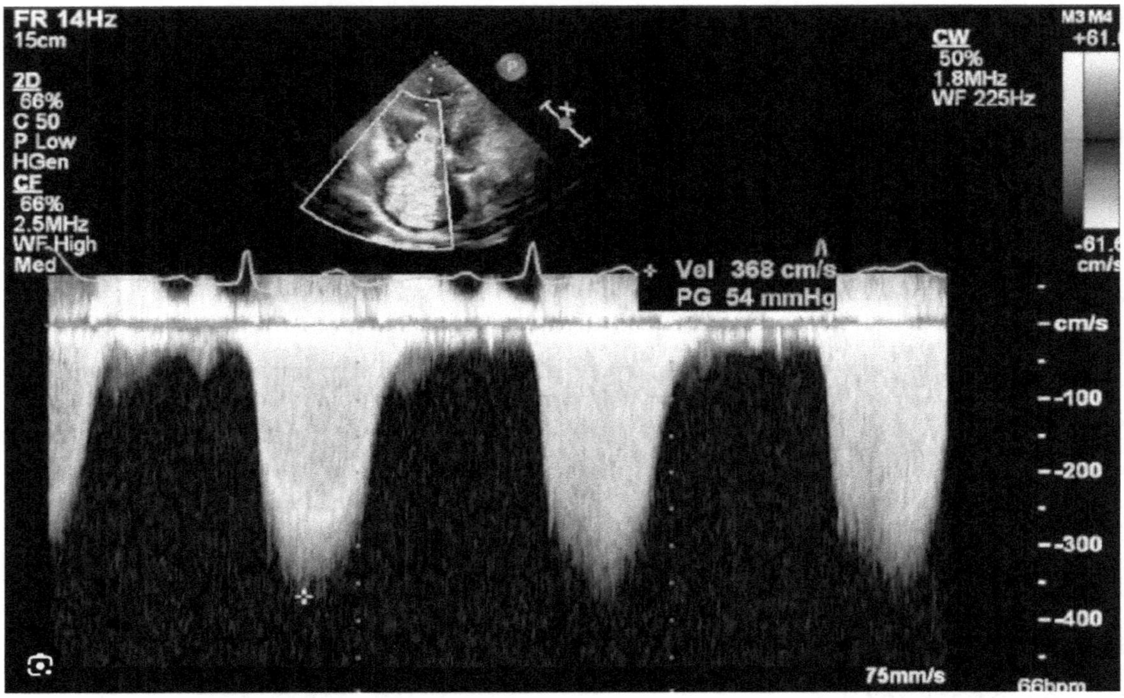

Severity of pulmonary hypertension

PAH	MPAP (mmHg)
Mild	20-29
Moderate	30-39
severe	≥40

Dobutamine Stress Echo

- Dobutamine is a selective β1 agonist, which increases cardiac contractility and HR.
- Echocardiography done during dobutamine infusion (start with 5 μg/kg/min, increase up to 20-40 μg/kg/min)
- Uses:
    - CAD: used as a non-invasive stress test, the appearance of new RWMA suggests underlying CAD
    - Low flow, Low Gradient AS: to differentiate true AS from pseudo-severe AS

M Mode Echocardiography

- M-mode echo was used before this real-time 2D Echo (B Mode)
- Images are created linearly with time. It is a one-dimensional echo
- Uses:
    - Assessment of LV ejection fraction
    - Accurate measurement of the dimensions of LV, LA.
    - EPSS: Measure of LV function
    - SAM (Systolic anterior Motion) of the mitral leaflet, characteristic of HO

27. Cardiac CT and MRI

ECG gating during cardiac CT is useful to reduce motion artefact of beating heart

CAC scoring involves non-contrast low dose cardiac CT

ECG Gating:

- The heart is a moving structure, and it poses a challenge in image acquisition.
- ECG gating synchronises image acquisition with the heart's electrical activity, to acquire images during a relatively motionless period of the cardiac cycle, minimising motion artefact.
  - **Prospective Gating:** Scans during a specific phase of the cardiac cycle (usually diastole for coronary arteries), reducing radiation dose but requiring a stable, low heart rate.
  - **Retrospective Gating:** Acquires data throughout the cardiac cycle, allowing for functional assessment (e.g., ventricular volumes, ejection fraction) but with higher radiation
- **Contrast Enhancement:** Iodinated contrast material is typically injected intravenously to visualise blood vessels and cardiac chambers.

Types of Cardiac CT

- **Coronary Artery Calcium (CAC) Scoring (Non-contrast CT)**
  - Low-dose, non-contrast CT.
  - Quantifies calcified plaque burden in the coronary arteries (Agatston score).
  - Used for cardiovascular risk stratification in asymptomatic or low-to-intermediate risk patients.
- **Coronary CT Angiography (CCTA)**
  - Contrast-enhanced, ECG-gated CT.
  - Primary application: visualisation of coronary arteries to detect and characterise atherosclerotic plaque (calcified, non-calcified, mixed), assess stenosis severity, and evaluate bypass grafts and stents

Cardiac MDCT remains the most useful tool for planning before TAVI

- **CT for Structural Heart Disease:**

  Detailed anatomical assessment for pre-procedural planning (e.g., TAVI, LAA occlusion, congenital heart disease).

- **Congenital Heart Disease:** Delineating complex anatomy, surgical planning, and follow-up
- **Pericardial Disease:** Pericardial effusions, constrictive pericarditis
- **Cardiac Masses:** Characterisation of tumours or thrombi.

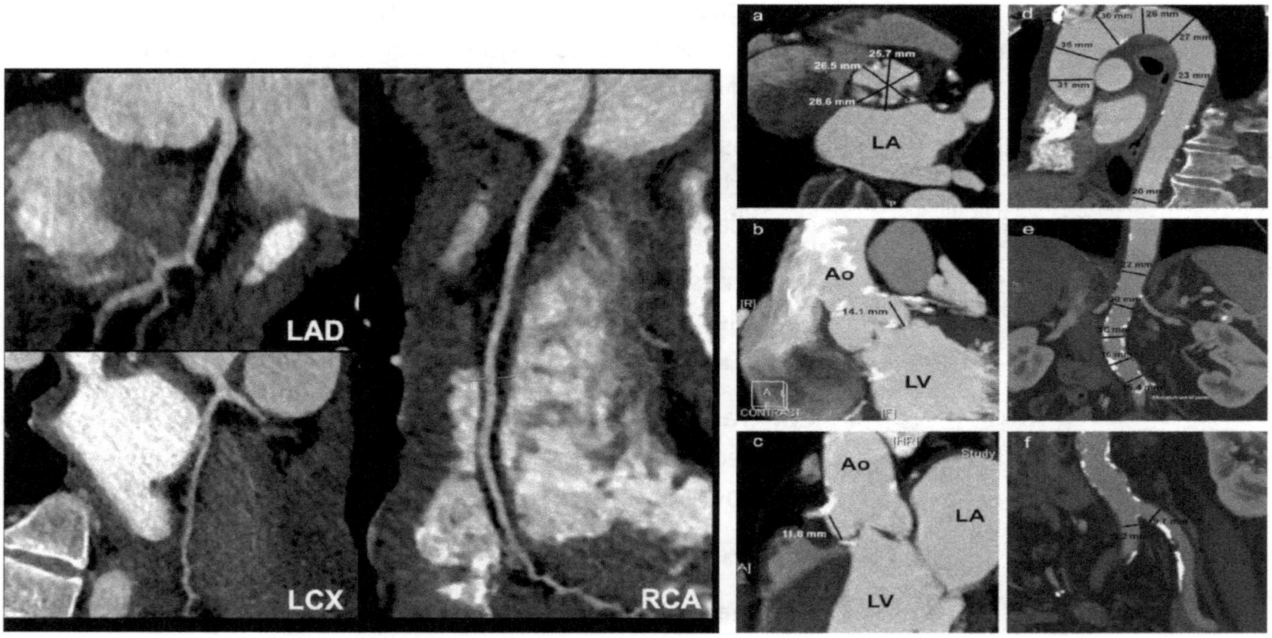

Cardiac CT for planning for TAVI

Cardiac MRI

T1 weighted -Morphology of cardiac chambers.

T2 weighted -for myocardial oedema.

LGE (Late gadolinium enhancement)

- A type of T1-weighted image acquired 5-15mm after (late) gadolinium injection.
- Normally, gadolinium should wash out by this time.
- Late persistent gadolinium in the interstitial space suggests fibrosis, infarction, or infiltration.

T1 mapping - quantitative assessment of extracellular space/volume [ECV] to better assess fibrosis or infiltration.

T2 mapping - quantitative assessment of myocardial oedema.

T2 star - for assessment of myocardial iron deposition.

Current indications of Cardiac MRI-

- Better characterisation of myocardial disease (cardiomyopathy/Infiltrative cardiomyopathy)
- Coronary artery disease-
    - myocardial viability after MI
    - Stress perfusion imaging for stable CAD.
- rarely indicated for valvular, pericardial, congenital, and cardiac tumours.

Myocardial disease with specific CMR findings described as follows:

Cardiac amyloidosis

- Diffuse subendocardial LGE in the ventricle.
- High ECV (Extracellular volume) quantification in T1 mapping to suggest amyloid protein deposition.

Cardiac sarcoidosis

- Patchy multifocal LGE involving the septum, basal anterior RV, and RV insertion points.
- Evidence of oedema (in T2 weighted sequence) in acute phases of disease.

Idiopathic DCM

- Linear mid-septal LGE is characteristic

Iron overload cardiomyopathy/hemochromatosis

- Quantitative T2 star sequence is useful.
- T2* value< 20msec suggests significant iron overload.
- Used to guide iron chelation therapy in thalassemia.

ARVC

Fibrofatty infiltration of myocardium.

MRI features consistent with ARVC are

- Regional RV Akinesia/dyskinesia/ dyssynchronous contraction/RV dysfunction/ dilation of RVOT
- LGE involving RV/LV
- ARVC involves predominantly
    - RV-41%
    - Biventricular- 37%
    - predominantly LV-12%

Dallas criteria for histological diagnosis of myocarditis

Myocarditis

Lake Louise Criteria (diagnostic of myocarditis)

- T2 (myocardial oedema)

- EGE (capillary leak)
- LGE (necrosis and fibrosis)

T1 & T2 mapping is more diagnostic for myocarditis than this criterion

HCM

- For the diagnosis of HCM
- Burden of LGE – extent of fibrosis

A high LGE burden (>10%) predicts a high risk for SCD and an indication for AICD.

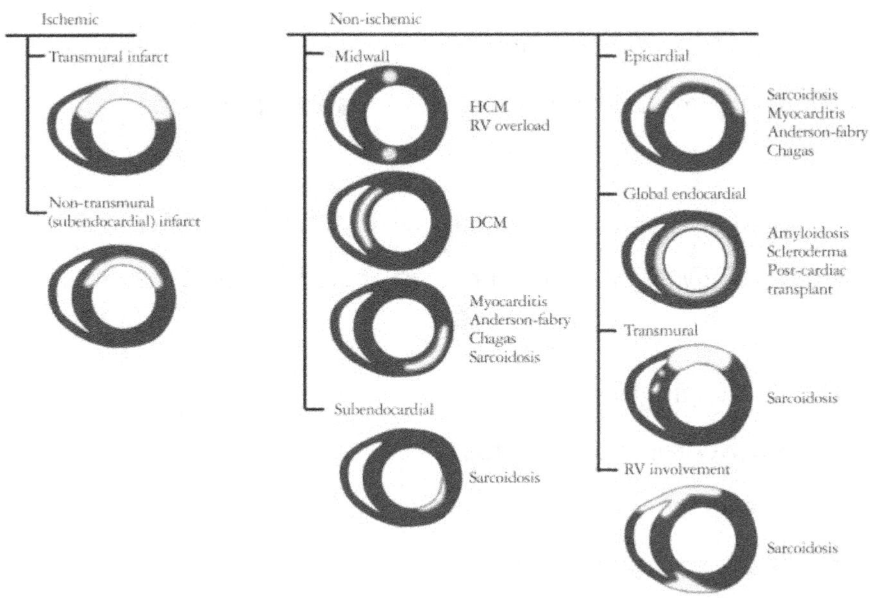

Stress MRI in CAD

- To assess myocardial ischemia in stable CAD.
- MRI performed using pharmacological stress (Adenosine/sometimes dobutamine) to assess reversible perfusion defect or regional wall motion abnormality.
- Comparable diagnostic accuracy with SPECT.

MRI for myocardial viability-

To predict recovery of myocardium after revascularisation in patients with significant ventricular dysfunction.

Differentiate viable tissue from dead myocardium by better tissue characterisation and contrast enhance

28. Nuclear Cardiology

Indications of Nuclear Scan in Cardiology

A. Coronary artery disease (CAD)

a. To assess stress-induced Ischemia in stable CAD (SPECT MPI)

b. To assess myocardial viability after MI (Cardiac PET)

Helps in decision-making for coronary revascularisation

B. Inflammatory cardiomyopathy / Sarcoidosis

a. To detect focal myocardial Inflammation (Cardiac PET)

C. Infective Endocarditis

a. Mostly in Prosthetic valve endocarditis and infection of the implanted device/lead (Cardiac PET)

D. Accurate assessment of ventricular function (MUGA Scan)

E. Amylodosis

a. ATTR amyloidosis can be imaged with 99Tc PYP (PYP scan)

Nuclear scan in CAD

Perfusion Scan (usually SPECT, can be done with PET)

- Radioactive tracers injected intravenously and distributed in the myocardium if the blood supply is intact (Perfusion)
- Images acquired during rest and stress are compared.
- Reduced perfusion to a part of the myocardium (perfusion defect) during stress suggests significant stenosis in the supplying artery.
- Mostly useful in stable CAD/chronic coronary syndrome: - Indicate severe Ischemia by obstructive CAD

Metabolism Scan (PET)

- Specific radioactive racers (FDG) injected intravenously will be taken up only by viable myocardium.
- Useful after ACS/MI to look for Hibernating / Viable Myocardium, which is expected to recover after coronary artery revascularisation.

In cardiac PET

- **Perfusion and metabolism match suggest an infarct**

  In an infarct, both blood flow (perfusion) and metabolic activity are reduced in the affected area. This indicates irreversible cell death due to prolonged ischemia.

- **Perfusion and metabolism mismatch suggest Hibernating Myocardium**

  In hibernating myocardium, the blood supply to the tissue is reduced, but the cells are still alive and can utilise glucose for energy. This mismatch between reduced blood flow and preserved or even increased glucose metabolism is a hallmark of hibernating myocardium.

Cardiac SPECT	Cardiac PET
• Access Myocardial perfusion	• Access myocardial perfusion and metabolism.
• Commonly used tracers:	• 2 types of PET tracers
• ^{201}Thallium	**Perfusion** **Metabolism**
• ^{99}Tc Sestamabi	^{82}Rb ^{18}F-FDG
• ^{99}Tc Tetrofosmin	^{13}N – Ammonia ^{11}C- Glucose
Thallium can be used for viability if no PET available.	^{15}O- Water
• Less spatial / temporal resolution	^{18}Flurpiridaz
• Assess relative perfusion defect compared to normal area i.e. qualitative assessment. (Less helpful in diffuse TVD)	• More resolution
• More radiation	• Quantitative assessment of coronary flow can be assessed in each coronary artery.
• High risk features suggesting significant CAD:	• Less radiation
○ Large perfusion defect (>15% of LV myocardium)	• Perfusion and metabolism scan done with different tracers and compared as seen in figure.
○ Transient Ischemic Dilation of LV	• **Perfusion metabolism**
○ Transient drop in LVEF	**Match- suggestive of infarct**
○ Increased lung uptake of tracers.	**Mismatch- suggestive of hibernating myocardium**

29. Hypertension

- Prevalence of hypertension worldwide: 20-35 %
- **ESC 2024 Guideline provides the latest classification of Blood pressure**

> Hypertension has the **highest attributable risk** for cardiovascular disease amongst CV risk factor

Non elevated blood pressure	Office BP <120/70 mmHg	No pharmacotherapy
Elevated Blood pressure	Office BP 120-139/70-89	Pharmacotherapy in high CV risk individuals
Hypertension	Office BP > 140/90	Pharmacotherapy useful in all

> **Out-of-office BP** measurement (ABPM/HBPM) has been given more importance in new guidelines for confirming hypertension

- **Office BP** is considered a **screening method** and diagnosis of hypertension/elevated BP confirmed using ABPM (Ambulatory BP monitoring) OR HBPM (Home BP monitoring)
- Several new studies supported the "Lower the better" approach for BP control, leading to a change in the new guidelines. A few landmark trials are highlighted here

SPRINT Trial

> **Out-of-office BP** measurement (ABPM/HBPM) has been given more importance in new guidelines for confirming hypertension

- RCT to assess Intensive BP control (SBP <120 mmHg) Vs standard BP control (<140 mmHg) in patients with high CV risk and without diabetes.
- Intensive BP control had a significantly lower primary composite outcome (myocardial infarction, other acute coronary syndromes, stroke, heart failure, or death from cardiovascular causes).
- Adverse events (hypotension, syncope, non-fatal falls, AKI, electrolyte disturbance) were higher with the intensive arm.

> **Diagnosis of Hypertension**
>
> - **office BP** >140/90
> - **Avg HBPM** >135/85
> - **ABPM**
>
>   24 hr. Avg >130/85
>
>   Daytime avg ≥135/80
>
>   Night time avg ≥120/70

ACCORD BP Trial

- In patients with type 2 diabetes at high cardiovascular risk, intensive blood pressure control (target systolic blood pressure <120 mmHg) compared to standard control (<140 mmHg) **did not** reduce the risk of major cardiovascular events

When to start antihypertensives?

- Pharmacotherapy, along with lifestyle modification, for all patients with confirmed hypertension **(BP>140/90 mmHg)**
- Patients with DM pharmacotherapy should be started if BP remains >130/80 after 3 months of lifestyle modification

Antihypertensive with established CVD prevention

- ACEI/ARB
- DHP-CCB
- Thiazide/thiazide like diuretics
- Beta blockers

Antihypertensive with NO established CVD prevention

- MRAs
- Clonidine
- Hydralazine
- Prazosin

Antihypertensive causing erectile dysfunction

- Beta blocker
- Diuretics
- Central sympatholytic

ARBs improve erectile dysfunction

- In patients with moderate to severe CKD (GFR >30), pharmacotherapy is started if BP>130/80

Highlights of Antihypertensive Drugs

- Antihypertensive agents should have BP BP-lowering effect as well as CVD prevention potential
- Drug classes that have shown CVD prevention are ACEI/ARB, Thiazide /thiazide-like diuretics, and Dihydropyridine CCB, and are considered as first-line antihypertensives
- RAS blockers are less effective antihypertensives in the **black population** compared to CCB/diuretics
- Recent guidelines omitted beta-blockers as the first-line antihypertensive list because of
    - It is a less potent antihypertensive compared to CCB/ACEI/ARB
    - More adverse effects and metabolic derangements (new onset DM)
    - Worsening in isolated systolic hypertension with stiff arteries, where bradycardia increases cardiac output
- Beta blockers are antihypertensives of choice in patients with angina, heart failure and after MI. Vasodilating beta blockers (Carvedilol, nebivolol and labetalol) are preferred in such situations
- **ALLHAT Trial**
    - RCT to determine the superiority of newer antihypertensives (ACEII, CCB and alpha blocker) over thiazide-like diuretic (Chlorthalidone)
    - **No significant difference** between the two arms for the primary endpoint
    - Chlorthalidone is superior in reducing stroke and heart failure
    - Alpha blocker (Doxazocin) arm was terminated early due to increased congestive heart failure
    - Overall, chlorthalidone is suggested as a first-line antihypertensive agent with low cost.
- However, **irrespective of the drug used,** if BP lowering is achieved, reduction in BP corresponds to a decrease in CV events

ACCOMPLISH trial

- ACEI-CCB combination (Benzapril and amlodipine) is superior to the ACEI-diuretic combination with similar BP reduction

In general, the recommended SBP **target for treatment is 120-129 mmHg**

TOPSPIN study

- Indian patients single-pill combination of Perindopril-amlodipine, perindopril-indapamide and amlodipine-indapamide for BP control
- All combinations are equally well tolerated with equal efficacy in 24 hr BP control

Newer antihypertensive agents

The following drugs are in the pipeline for primary use as antihypertensives

- ARNI (Sacubitril/valsartan)
- SGLT2 inhibitors
- Finerenone (Non-steroidal MRA)
- Aprocitentan (dual endothelin receptor A and B antagonist)
- Zilebesiran (experimental RNAi agent, inhibits hepatic angiotensinogen synthesis, administered 6 monthly SC inj)

Osler phenomena

Pseudohypertension in the elderly due to severe calcific arteries.

Falsely labelled as resistant HTN.

Treatment target

- In general, on treatment, the SBP target should be 120-129 mmHg
- A higher target (SBP <140 mmHg) may be kept for
    - severe frailty
    - age >85 yrs
    - pre-treatment orthostatic hypotension
- After achieving target systolic BP (120-129 mmHg), enhancing drug therapy to lower diastolic BP to below 70 mmHg has not shown a CV advantage

Upfront Monotherapy Vs Combination Therapy

- Low-dose combination therapy (preferably a single pill) should be considered for the initial treatment of hypertension. (Class IIa)
- It helps to target two different physiological pathways, and low doses of individual drugs can be used to reduce adverse reactions
- However, there is a poor level of evidence for this (observational studies only)
- In elderly/frail individuals who are at risk of orthostatic hypotension, monotherapy can be considered.

Resistant Hypertension

- BP target not achieved despite maximally tolerated combination of 3 drugs (ACEI/ARB, CCB and diuretics)

Spironolactone is the **drug of choice** for resistant hypertension

- Spironolactone is considered the preferred 2nd line agent for resistant hypertension (PATHWAY 2 study)
- Other 2nd line drugs are beta blockers, prazosin, hydralazine, and clonidine

Hypertension in pregnancy

- Hypertension in pregnancy – BP>140/90 mmHg, Severe HTN- BP>160/110 mmHg
- Drug therapy for all pregnant females with confirmed BP > 140/90
- Safe Drugs: Beta blocker (Most evidence for Labetalol, Metoprolol, bisoprolol also safe), DHP CCB (Most evidence for Nifedipine, Amlodipine, Felodipine, nicardipine also used) and Methyl dopa
- Severe HTN (BP>160/110) should be hospitalised

  IV Labetalol DOC, Other drugs- IV Nicardipine, IV Hydralazine (2nd line)
- Safety data of thiazide diuretics is not clear.
- RAASi contraindicated (Foetal RAAS inhibition causing renal failure, renal agenesis, Oligohydramnios, Lung hypoplasia, Potter syndrome)
- Atenolol should be avoided- foetal growth retardation
- Methyldopa is associated with post-partum depression

Drug-induced hypertension

- NSAID
- Corticosteroid
- Cyclosporine
- Estrogen OC Pills
- Antidepressants
- Anticold drugs
- amphetamine

Secondary hypertension

Overall prevalence is 10-35 % and up to 50 % in the resistant hypertension population

Common causes of secondary HTN are highlighted here

1. Primary aldosteronism (Conn's Syndrome)

- The most common cause of secondary hypertension
- Clinical clues- **Hypokalemia with resistant HTN**, severe hypokalemia after low-dose diuretic therapy, muscle weakness/tetany
- HMOD (stroke and MI) and AF are more common
- Adrenal adenoma is more common than bilateral adrenal hyperplasia
- **Diagnosis**

  Screening- ARR (Aldosterone Renin Ratio)

  Drugs affecting ARR (RAASi, Beta blocker, clonidine, spironolactone) should be stopped before testing. CCB can be continued.

  Confirmatory- Saline suppression test/oral salt loading/ captopril challenge

  Adrenal venous sampling

  Adrenal imaging

- **Treatment**

  Surgery for adenoma/unilateral causes

  Drug therapy for hyperplasia

  MRA- spironolactone, eplerenone, Finerenone

  Aldosterone synthase inhibitor- Baxdrostat

2. Renovascular hypertension

- Aetiology- Atherosclerosis (MC), Fibromuscular dysplasia, Neurofibromatosis, Takayasu arteritis, aortic dissection, thromboembolism, retroperitoneal fibrosis
- Clinical clues- unexplained unilateral small kidney, bruit, multisite atherosclerosis, aortic dissection, young female with migraine and pulsatile tinnitus (FMD)
- Recurrent flash pulmonary oedema (Pickering syndrome)
- **Management**

  Drug therapy- ACEI/ARB is the first-line agent

  Contraindicated in severe b/l renal artery stenosis and

  Single kidney with renal artery stenosis

  PTRA (Percutaneous transluminal renal angioplasty) without stenting for fibromuscular dysplasia and with stenting in atherosclerosis

Interventions for hypertension

1. Renal denervation therapy

- Catheter-based RF ablation of the sympathetic nervous system in renal artery adventitia.
- It may be considered in patients with resistant HTN or uncontrolled HTN with high CVD risk after risk-benefit discussion (Class IIb)
- Not a first-line treatment modality as of now (class III)
- Modest BP reduction (4-6mmHg) and no large RCT evidence to suggest long-term safety and CVD prevention.
- Trials- RADIANCE HTN, SIMPLYCITY HTN3, SPYRAL Off MED

2. Device-based therapy

- Baroreceptor activation therapy
- Endovascular baroreflex amplification therapy
- Carotid body ablation

30. Bradyarrhythmia

A heart rate less than 50 per minute in the resting state is considered bradycardia; it can be physiological or pathological.

SA NODAL DISORDERS

Sinus bradycardia

- ECG - heart rate less than 50, normal P wave morphology, positive P wave in II, III, avF, P wave preceding each

  QRS with a constant PR interval

- Causes- physiological in healthy young and athletes, drug-induced (beta blocker, calcium channel blocker,

  Clonidine, ivabradine, lithium, amiodarone, raised ICT, myxedema, gram-negative sepsis

Sinus Arrhythmia

- Phasic variation of P-P interval with respiration
- increased heart rate during inspiration and decreased heart rate during expiration
- Lack of sinus arrhythmia is considered a risk factor for sudden cardiac death
- Non-respiratory sinus arrhythmia, phasic variation in pp interval seen in digitalis toxicity.

Ventricular phasic sinus arrhythmia

Seen in complete AV block and low ventricular rate, where the PP interval containing the QRS interval is shorter than without the QRS. Caused by an alteration in autonomic tone secondary to changes in stroke volume.

Sinus pause/arrest

- Absence of the P wave transiently
- No SA nodal impulse formation
- The duration of the pause is not equal to a multiple of the PP interval

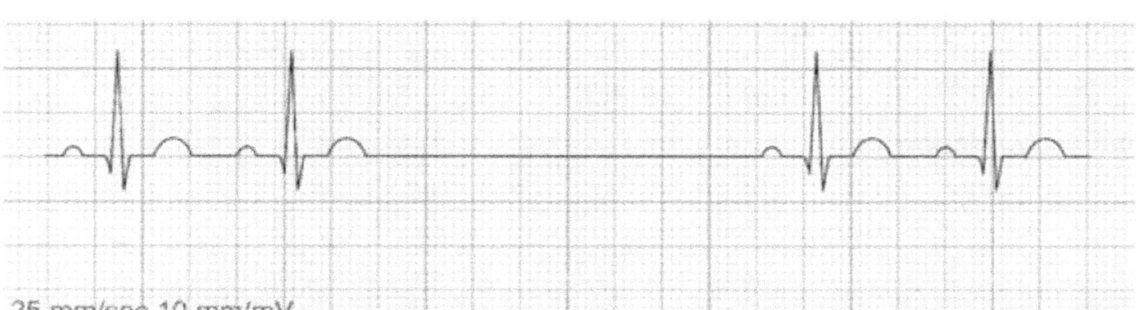

SA nodal exit block

- Impulse formed in the SA node failed to conduct to the atria
- Duration of pause is a multiple of the preceding pp interval

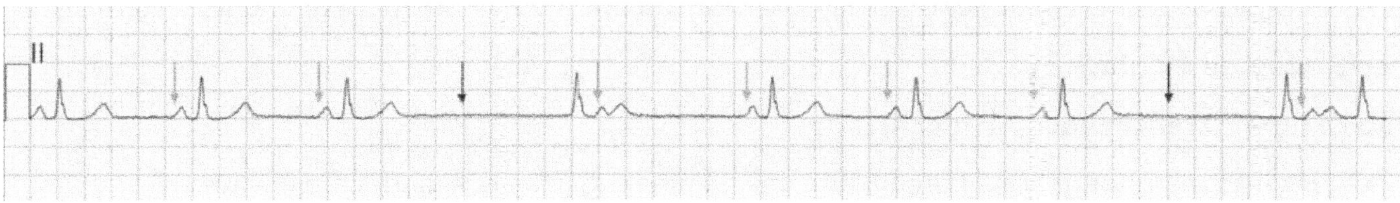

Sick sinus syndrome

Syndrome comprising several SA nodal abnormalities

i. Persistent sinus bradycardia (inappropriate for the physiological state)
ii. Sinus arrest or sinus exit block
iii. A combination of the SA node and AV nodal block
iv. Tachy-Brady syndrome (episodes of bradycardia and regular or irregular supraventricular tachycardia)

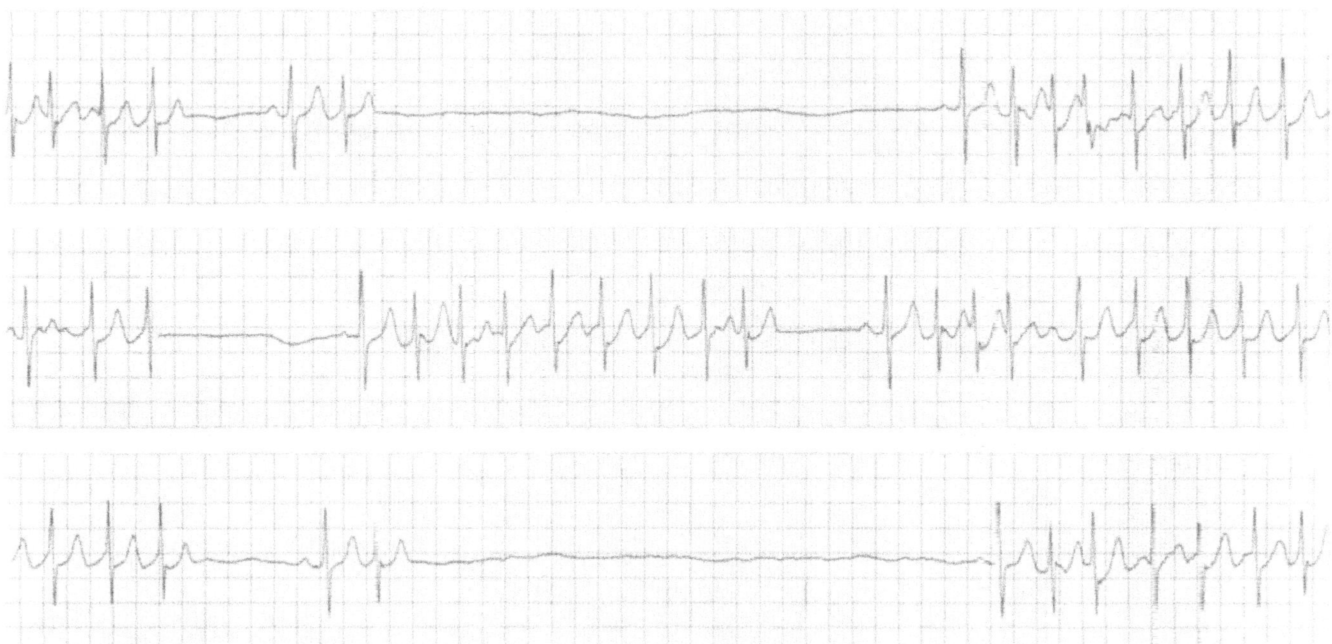

- Various combinations of the above abnormalities can present in the same patient
- Unpredictable disease course, and can be intermittent
- Permanent pacing is considered if symptomatic

Chronotropic incompetence

- Failure to increase heart rate appropriate to physiological demand

  (Less than 80 to 85% of the maximum expected heart rate, MPHR = 220-age)

AV NODAL DISORDERS

First-degree AV block

- Each atrial impulse is conducted with a prolonged PR interval of more than 200 ms
- PR prolongation can be due to a delay in conduction of the AV node or His-Purkinje system

Second-degree AV block

Mobitz Type I (Wenckebach AV block)

- Progressive prolongation of the PR interval culminating in a non-conducted P wave
- PR interval is the longest immediately before the dropped beat and is the shortest immediately after the dropped beat
- Can be physiological

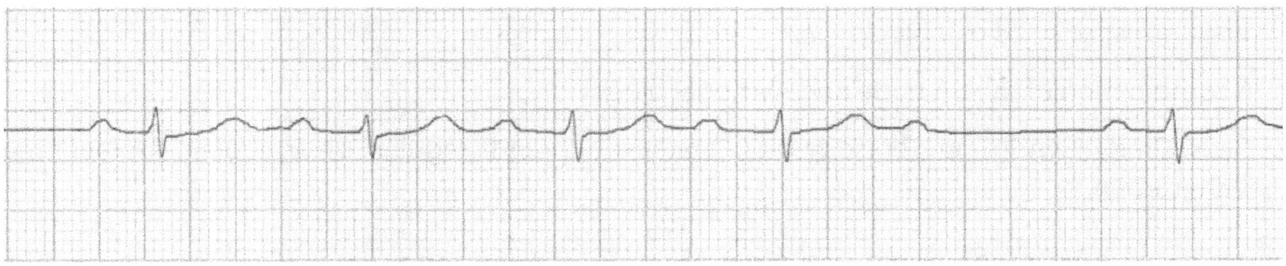

Mobitz Type II

- Intermittent non-conducted P waves without progressive prolongation of the PR interval
- PR interval in the conducted beats remains constant.
- The RR interval surrounding the dropped beat(s) is an exact multiple of the preceding RR interval
- Usually suggests conduction system disease and infra-nodal involvement

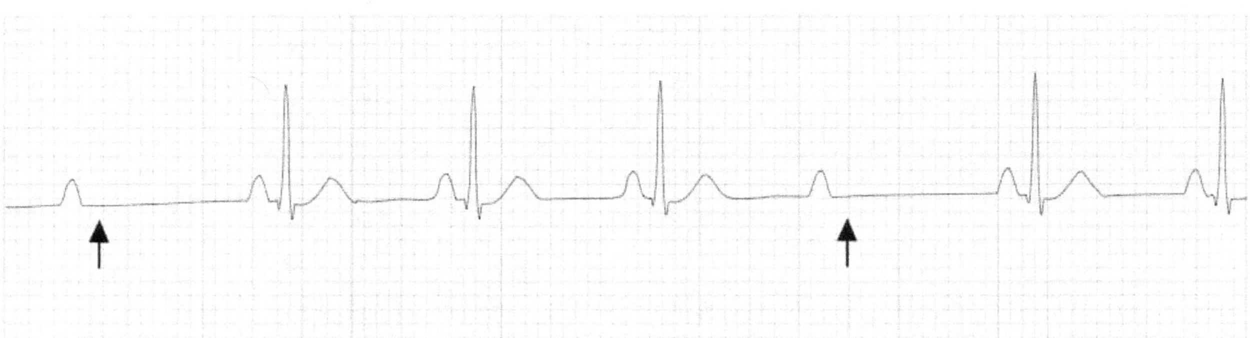

High-grade AV block

- **Second-degree heart block** with a **P: QRS ratio of 3:1 or higher**. That means two or more consecutive P waves are not conducted.

Third-degree AV block/Complete AV block

- The ECG demonstrates complete **AV dissociation**, with independent atrial and ventricular rates
- There is a fixed P-P and R-R interval with a variable PR interval, suggestive of AV dissociation

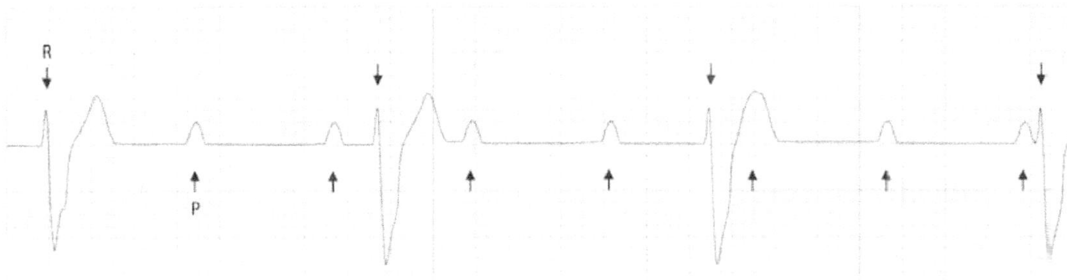

Nodal and infranodal conduction system disease

- The level of conduction system disease should be determined for appropriate management
- EP study is confirmatory
  - AH interval
  - HV interval

	Nodal	**Infranodal**
• Site of disease	• AV node	• His-purkinjee system
• ECG clues	• Mobitz type I	• Mobitz type II
• Escape rhythm	Narrow QRS escape	wide QRS escape
• Response to atropine/ isoproterenol	• Junctional, stable (40-60 bpm)	• Ventricular, unstable (20-40 bpm)
	• Improves conduction	• No response/worsening
• EP study	Prolonged	Normal
AH interval	Normal (35-55ms)	prolonged (>55ms)
HV interval • Prognosis	• Usually benign. Require pacemaker only if symptomatic	• High risk of sudden death. Pacemaker strongly indicated

Bundle branch block

- Conduction system disease can affect one of the bundle branches

LBBB	RBBB
Causes	Causes
• Less common in normal population	• Common in general population
• Usually suggest underlying CAD, cardiomyopathy	• RV strain, pulmonary embolism, ASD
Increased risk of mortality	Not increased
Deep S in v1 and broad R in v5-6 with discordant T	rsR', RsR' iv V1 and broad S in v5-6 with discordant T

Fascicular block

- Conduction disturbance in one of the fascicles of the left bundle manifests as axis deviation

LAFB	LPFB
• Left axis deviation • qR inl, avL • rS in II, III, avF	• Right axis deviation • qR II, III, avF • rS in I, avL

Rate-dependent conduction block

- Tachycardia or bradycardia can induce abnormal conduction

Tachycardia dependent block	Bradycardia dependent block
• Phase 3 block • It is more common • it can be seen in normal heart • Mechanism- post repolarization refractoriness i.e. conduction system fails to recover in first rate	• Pause dependent/phase 4 block • It is less common • Suggest advanced conduction system disease • Mechanissm- after a pause/brady, there is abnormal phase 4 depolarization causing conduction tissue inexcitable for next beat

- Bundle branch block can develop during tachycardia, known as rate-related aberrancy/phase 3 block
- RBBB is more common in this scenario due to the long refractory period of the right bundle than the left

Congenital CHB

- The most common cause of AV block in children
- Causes
  - Maternal autoimmune disease (SLE/Sjogren). Maternal antibodies crossing the placenta, destroying the conduction system
  - Associated congenital disease (CCTGA, AVSD, DILV)
- Maternal screening of antibodies (Ro/La, dsDNA) is done if the baby has congenital CHB without any structural abnormalities
- Children are mostly asymptomatic, with a good escape rate
- Indications of a permanent pacemaker
  - Symptomatic- syncope, heart failure, chronotropic incompletence
  - Asymptomatic
    - Average daytime HR <50
    - Pause for more than 3 cycle lengths of escape rhythm

- Wide QRS escape
- Prolonged QT interval
- Complex VPC

Ashman Phenomena

- A type of aberrant ventricular conduction mimicking VPC
- After a long-short cycle in atrial fibrillation, the next beat is conducted with aberrancy mimicking a VPC
- Usually, RBBB morphology (the right bundle has a longer refractory period than the left)

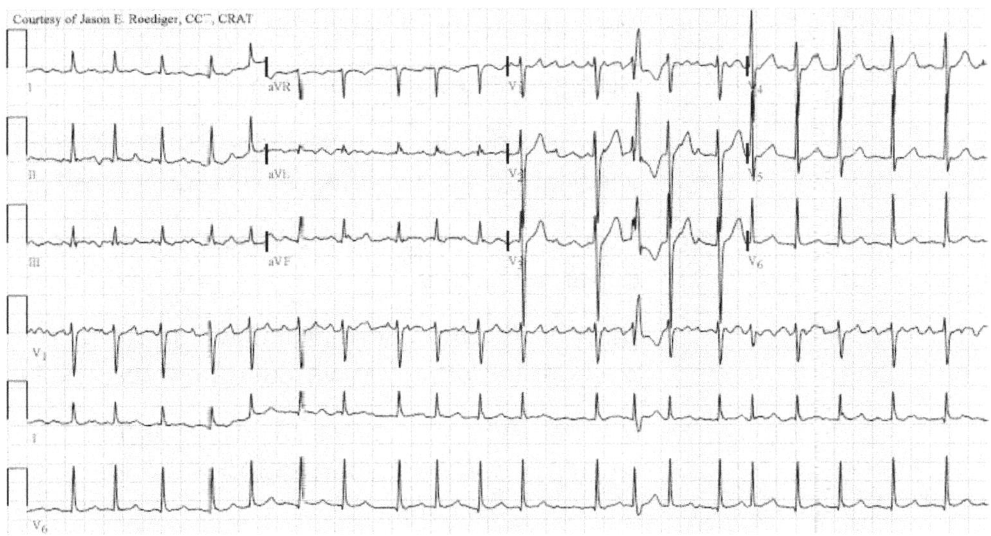

31. Pulmonary Hypertension

- Normal mean PA pressure is 10-15 mmHg
- Normal PVR- less than 2 wood units

Definition- Elevated mean pulmonary artery pressure (**mPAP > 20 mmHg**) at rest/exercise

- PA pressure measured by invasive right heart catheterisation (RHC). Echocardiography can provide an estimation of PA pressure.
- **Pulmonary vascular resistance**
  - Resistance to blood flow through the pulmonary circulation
  - Measured by right heart catheterisation (RHC).
  - Objective assessment of primary
  - PVR is affected by vascular tone, structural changes in vasculature, lung volume, and blood viscosity
  - Normal PVR- less than **2 Wood** units (between 30 and 180 dynes/sec/cm−5)
  - High PVR with normal PCWP suggest primary structural changes in pulmonary vasculature (pre-capillary)
  - Normal PVR with elevated PCWP suggest left heart disease with pulmonary hypertension secondary to back pressure change (post-capillary)

Chest X-ray features of PAH

- Dilated pulmonary trunk
- Prominent hilar shadow
- Pruning of peripheral PA
- Peripheral oligemia of the lung parenchyma

Pre-Capillary PH (Suggestive of pulmonary vascular change)	mPAP > 20mm Hg PVR > 2 Wood PCWP <15 mm Hg
Post-Capillary PH (Suggestive of left heart disease)	mPAP > 20mm Hg PVR < 2 Wood PCWP > 15 mm Hg

Primary /Idiopathic Pulmonary Arterial Hypertension (PAH)

- Primary changes involving the pulmonary vasculature
- Female preponderance
- Familial in up to 20 % of iPAH (autosomal dominant)
- Mutation of **BMPR II** (bone morphogenic protein receptor) and **TGF beta** (transforming growth factor)
- Very poor prognosis (mean survival 2-3 years from diagnosis without therapy)

- **PH** denotes an increase in mean PA pressure irrespective of aetiology
- **PAH** denotes only Group 1.

Clinical classification of PH

Classified into 5 groups according to their pathophysiology, clinical presentation, haemodynamics and management.

Group 1: pulmonary arterial hypertension (PAH)

- Idiopathic (sporadic/familial)
- Connective tissue disease
- Congenital left-to-right shunts (Eisenmenger)
- Drugs and toxins
- Portal hypertension
- HIV
- PPHN of newborn
- Pulmonary capillary hemangiomatosis (PCH)
- Pulmonary venoocclusive disease (PVOD)

PCH and PVOD

- Rare cause of PAH
- PCH denotes abnormal proliferation of capillaries
- PVOD involves venules
- Overlap clinical feature
- **EIF2AK4** Mutation
- Reduced DLCO
- Lung biopsy is diagnostic
- Ground glass opacity in HRCT
- Worsening symptoms with PAH therapy

Group 2: pulmonary hypertension due to left heart disease

- HFpEF/HPrEF
- Valvular heart disease
- Congenital left heart disease

Group 3: pulmonary hypertension due to lung diseases and/or hypoxia

- Obstructive/restrictive lung disease
- Hypoventilation/hypoxia

Group 4: pulmonary hypertension due to chronic thromboembolic disease

- CTEPH

Group 5: pulmonary hypertension with unclear, multifactorial mechanisms

- Haematological disorders (chronic anaemia)
- CKD
- Fibrosing mediastinitis
- Pulmonary tumour thrombotic microangiopathy

Management of idiopathic PAH

A) supportive therapy

- REVEAL 2 Score

  Risk stratification of PAH

- Loop diuretics and mineralocorticoid receptor antagonist.
- Supplemental O2 reduces hypoxic pulmonary vasoconstriction.

- Digoxin improves RV cardiac output.
- vaccination (influenza and pneumococcal)
- Routine anticoagulation is not recommended.

- Pulmonary vasodilators are useful in Category 1 (PAH) and Category 4 (CTEPH)
- Contraindicated in PH with left heart disease (Category 2)

B) Specific therapy/pulmonary vasodilators

I. NO pathway

- PDE5 inhibitors- Sildenafil, Tadalafil
- Soluble Guanylyl Cyclase stimulator- Riociguat

II. Endothelin pathway

- Endothelin receptor antagonist- Bosentan, Macitentan, Ambrisentan

III. Prostacyclin pathway

- Epoprostenol, treprostinil, Iloprost (parenteral route)
- Selexipag -Newer oral prostacyclin receptor agonist
- Choice of therapy depends on the WHO functional class (severity)
- Current evidence suggests that starting **upfront combination therapy (ambrisentan + tadalafil)** is superior to either monotherapy **(AMBITION TRIAL)**
- Continuous parenteral prostacyclin in patients with end-stage disease.
- Lung transplantation/heart-lung transplantation last resort
- Palliation during the waitlist for transplantation to decompress the right heart pressure and increase cardiac output
    - **Balloon atrial septostomy**
    - **Percutaneous Pott shunt**

Selexipag

- **Oral** Prostacyclin IP receptor agonist
- Dose-200-1600mcg six to nine times daily
- **GRIPHON** trial showed a favourable result in idiopathic PAH

Vasoreactive PAH

- All patients with PAH should be tested for vasoreactivity (change in PA pressure to inhaled NO)
- **Positive test** defined by a fall in mean PAP ≥ 10mm of Hg with mPAP < 40 mmHg with increase or no change in cardiac output
- **High-dose Calcium Channel Blocker**(Nifedipine 20-80 TDS, Diltiazem 60-240 TDS, Amlodipine 10mg) is treatment of choice for vasoreactive PAH

Sotatercept

An activin signalling inhibitor improves clinical outcome in Group I/PAH

CTEPH (Chronic Thromboembolic PAH)

- Inadequate treatment/impaired natural thrombolysis after an episode of pulmonary thromboembolism leads to chronic obstruction of the pulmonary vasculature
- Primary PTE episode may go unnoticed and present directly as CTEPH
- The incidence of CTEPH after an episode of PTE is 0.1 to 4.8% in various follow-up studies
- A CT pulmonary angiogram/ Lung perfusion scan is diagnostic

Management

Lifelong anticoagulation for all patients (VKA/NOAC)

- 3 other modalities depending on suitability

A) Pulmonary thromboendarterectomy

- Suitable for patients with a clot in the proximal large pulmonary artery that is accessible surgically.
- An experienced surgical team is required.

B) Balloon pulmonary angioplasty

- Balloon dilation of occluded segmental/subsegmental arteries, which are surgically not accessible.
- done in multiple stages.

Pulmonary endarterectomy is the treatment of choice in CTEPH

C) Drug therapy

- Riociguat(soluble guanylate cyclase stimulator) has shown favourable benefits.
- Sildenafil, macitentan can also be used

Riociguat

- Soluble guanylate cyclase (sGC) stimulator
- Increase cGMP level, causing vasodilation (independent from NO)
- Route of administration: oral (0.5 -2.5mg TDS)
- Improve functional capacity (6MWD) and pulmonary vascular resistance in PAH and CTEPH
- Trials

  CHEST1 (CTEPH inoperable/persistent symptom after endarterectomy)

  PATENT1 (PAH)

32. Lipids and Dyslipidemia

> - During routine lipid profile testing, the LDL level is usually not measured directly
> - It is estimated using the **Friedewald Formula**
>
> **LDL Ch = Total Ch – (TG/5) – HDL.**

Lipid profile testing

- Lipid profile screening should be done at age 10 years and repeated every 5 years.
- If family history of hypercholesterolemia / premature CAD, cholesterol screening should be done at 2 years and repeated every 3-5 years.
- CV risk estimation (ASCVD Score) includes total cholesterol and HDL Cholesterol level.
- LDL level used to guide statin initiation, monitoring and intensification.
- Standard lipid profile testing measures total cholesterol, HDL and TG levels.
    - LDL level is estimated using the Friedewald Formula

      LDL Ch = Total Ch – (TG/5) – HDL.
- Fasting and non-fasting lipid profile measurement have similar clinical implications (ASCOT LLA trial)
- In patients with High TG levels, LDL estimation may be inaccurate. Non-HDL Ch (Total Ch- HDL Ch) and apo B levels were measured in such patients.

LDL Cholesterol

- Causal risk factor for CV disease.
- Lowering LDL level by 1 % corresponds to 1% decrease in CV events.
- LDL level and percentage reduction guide statin therapy.

HDL Cholesterol

- Epidemiological studies suggest an inverse relationship of HDL level and CV disease.
- Each 1 mg/dl higher HDL is associated with a 2%-3% lower CV disease.
- However, drugs that increase HDL levels have not shown cardiovascular benefit.

Triglyceride

- TG levels also increase CV risk.
- Fasting/non-fasting TG level >175 mg/dl is considered a risk enhancer and should be considered for statin therapy beyond this.
- Dietary and lifestyle modification (decreased calorie intake, decreased alcohol intake, exercise, weight reduction) should be the first measure to reduce TG levels.

- Drugs to reduce TG level in Severe Hypertriglyceridemia (>500), are used to reduce the incidence of pancreatitis.

Apo B

- Major structural protein of VLDL, IDL, LDL, Lp(a).
- Each particle has one Apo B molecule. → Apo B reflects the total number of atherogenic particles
- Better marker of **atherogenic particle burden** than LDL-C alone, especially when LDL particle size is small.
- Normal value **<90 mg/dL**

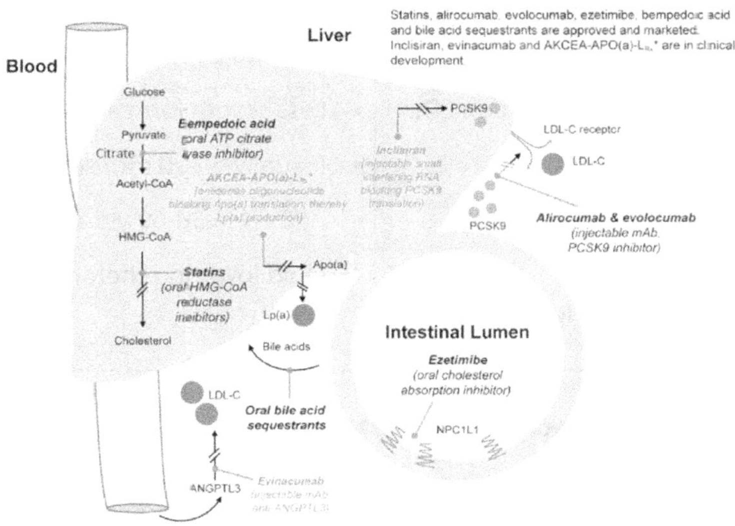

Lipoprotein (a)

- LDL-like particle with Apo B + Apo(a) attached.
- Atherogenic & prothrombotic:
  - Apo(a) is structurally similar to plasminogen → promotes thrombosis.
- High Lp(a) is an independent risk factor for ASCVD and aortic stenosis.
- Genetically determined. Not significantly modified by lifestyle.
- Screening is recommended in patients with premature CAD, family history of early CAD, or unexplained high LDL-C.
- Normal value <30 mg/dL. Levels >50 mg/dL (125 nmol/L) associated with increased risk.
- Treatment- No approved specific therapies yet.

Statins do not lower Lpa level. There may be a modest

increase in the level

PCSK9 inhibitors modestly reduce Lp(a).

Pelacarsen (antisense oligonucleotide) Lp(a)

LIPID DISORDERS/DYSLIPIDEMIA

FAMILIAL HYPERCHOLESTEROLEMIA (FH)

- Autosomal dominant. Can be homozygous/heterozygous
- The following are 3 underlying mutations responsible for FH
- LDL receptor (most common)
- Gain of function of PCSK9
- Apo B100 mutation

Homozygous FH	Heterozygous FH
• 1 in every 1 million people • Severe form with very high LDL • (often >500 mg/dl) • Early onset xanthoma and ASCVD (<10 yrs) • Response to lipid lowering therapy is poor	• 1 in 500 people • Less severe form and high LDL • (usually > 190 mg/dl) • ASCVD in 30-60 yrs age • Lipid lowering therapy usually effective

Diagnosis of Homozygous FH

- Elevated LDL level (> 190 mg/dl)
- Family history
- Clinical signs (tendon xanthoma, corneal arcus)

  Premature ASCVD
- Genetic testing is mostly confirmatory- LDLR, PCSK9, Apo B100

  Several diagnostic criteria have been proposed, comprising the above parameters
  - Dutch Lipid Clinic Network Criteria
  - Simon Broome Criteria

> Deposition of lipid in the aortic root may cause valvular or supravalvular aortic stenosis in FH

Treatment options

- Drugs
  - High-intensity statin is the mainstay of therapy
  - Other drugs- Ezetimibe, Mipomersan, Lomitapide
  - PCSK9 inhibitors – Evolocumab, Alirocumab, Inciseran

    Effective in heterozygous FH.

    Variable effect in homozygous FH depending upon receptor activity. No effect in receptor-negative FH. Useful if there is residual LDL receptor activity

- Evinacumab- Inhibits the **NPC1L1 transporter** in the **intestinal brush border**, thereby reducing cholesterol absorption.
- LDL apheresis
- Liver transplantation

TANGIER'S DISEASE

HDL deficiency and Orange Tonsil characteristic of Tangier disease

Familial HDL deficiency (ABCA1 gene mutation)

- Increased risk of premature CAD
- Orange tonsil is characteristic

SITOSTEROLEMIA

- A mutation in the ABC transporter, which helps in the biliary excretion of plant sterols (plant sterols are absorbed only in small amounts).
- Increased sitosterol suppresses the LDL receptor, resulting in elevated LDL-C levels.
- Clinical presentation and lab findings similar to familial hypercholesterolemia (atherosclerosis in young, xanthomas, very high level of LDL-C).
- Additional characteristic findings-
  - Joint pain and arthritis
  - Hematological findings
    - RBC anisopoikilocytosis
    - Mega thrombocytes/platelets
    - Episodic hemolysis & splenomegaly

Haematological manifestation and non-response to statin differentiate Sitosterolemia from FH

Treatment:

- No response to statins
- Dietary restriction of plant sterol-containing food
- Ezetimibe
- Bile acid sequestrant

LIPID LOWERING DRUGS

Statins

- Inhibits HMG CoA reductase, a crucial step in cholesterol synthesis
- Also has anti-inflammatory properties/pleotropic effects other than lipid-lowering, targeting atherosclerosis

LDL reduction

- High intensity statin 50%
- Ezetimibe 20%
- PCSK9 inhibitors 60%
- Statin + ezetimibe 65 %
- Statin + ezetimibe + PCSK9 inhibitors 85%

- CV benefit (Cholesterol Treatment Trialist meta-analysis)
- Overall, 1 % decrease in LDL-C is associated with 1 % lower CV risk
- LDL lowering by 1 mmol (39mg/dl) reduced 21% MACE, 10 % all-cause mortality and 24 % coronary revascularisation
- Similar benefits in both primary and secondary prevention of ASCVD

Facts to note about statins

- Adverse effects
    - New onset diabetes (1 in 100 patient years)
    - Hemorrhagic stroke (rare)
    - Muscle symptoms- myalgia, myositis, rhabdomyolysis
- Statins do not affect cognitive function
- No effect on cancer mortality
- No effect on heart failure mortality in ICMP/DCM
- Lovastatin, simvastatin, and atorvastatin are metabolised by CYP 450 enzymes and have drug interactions with enzyme inhibitors
- CYP does not metabolise Rosuvastatin and pravastatin, and does not have drug interactions with enzyme inhibitors
- Dose-dependent LDL reduction

High intensity	Moderate intensity	Low intensity
LDL reduction >50 %	30-50%	<30 %
Atorvastatin 40-80mg Rosuvastatin 20-40 mg	Atorvastatin 10-20 mg Rosuvastatin 5-10 mg Simvastatin 40 mg Pravastatin 40-80 mg	Simvastatin 10mg Pravastatin 10-20mg

Ezetimibe

IMPROVE-IT trial
showed adding ezetimibe to simvastatin reduced cardiovascular events post-ACS compared to statin alone

- Inhibits the **NPC1L1 transporter** in the **intestinal brush border**, thereby reducing cholesterol absorption.
- Leads to the upregulation of hepatic LDL receptors, resulting in increased clearance of LDL-C.
- **10 mg once daily** (standard dose). Lowers **LDL-C by 15-20%**
- Mostly combined with statin when LDL target is not achieved.

Adverse effects: Elevated liver enzymes (especially with statins), myalgias, diarrhoea.

PCSK9 inhibitors

- Monoclonal Ab against PCSK9- Evolocumab, Alirocumab
- PCSK9 binds LDL receptors and promotes their degradation.
- Inhibiting PCSK9 → increases LDL receptor activity → more LDL-C cleared from blood → LDL-C reduction.
- Lowers **LDL-C by 50-60%. along with high-intensity statin and ezetimibe 85 %**
- Mostly combined with high-intensity statin when LDL target is not achieved.
- **Subcutaneous injection** every 2-4 weeks

Adverse events- injection site reactions, nasopharyngitis, flu-like symptoms, neurocognitive events (rare)

> - **FOURIER trial (Evolocumab):** Reduced CV events in high-risk patients.
> - **ODYSSEY OUTCOMES trial (Alirocumab):** Reduced major CV events post-ACS

Incliseran

- siRNA inhibiting the synthesis of PCSK9, leading to increased LDL receptor activity
- Subcutaneous injection with a unique dosing schedule:

  Initial dose at Day 0, Second dose at 3 months and then every 6 months.
- **ORION-10 & ORION-11 trials:** Showed significant LDL-C reduction

> **Drugs targeting PCSK9**
> - Monoclonal Ab- **Evolocumab, Alirocumab**
> - siRNA inhibiting synthesis- **Incliseran**

Bempedoic acid

- Inhibits **ATP citrate lyase** in the liver → reduces cholesterol synthesis → upregulation of LDL receptors → **increased LDL-C clearance**
- Lowers LDL-C by ~15-20% alone. 35% reduction when combined with ezetimibe
- **Used in Statin-intolerant patients**

Adverse events- Increased uric acid levels → risk of gout, tendon rupture

> **CLEAR Outcomes trial** showed modest reduction in major CV events with Bempedoic acid in statin-intolerant patients.

Niacin

- **Also called:** Vitamin B3
- **Use: ↑ HDL (20–30%)**, ↓ LDL (10–20%), ↓ TG (20–35%)
- **Mechanism:** Inhibits **hepatic VLDL synthesis**
- **Side effects:** Flushing, hyperuricemia (gout), hyperglycemia, hepatotoxicity
- Limited current use due to **side effects and lack of CV outcome benefit**

> **NIACIN,** although it increases HDL level, does not improve CV outcome

Fibrates

- Examples: Fenofibrate, Gemfibrozil
- Use: ↓ Triglycerides (30–50%), ↑ HDL modestly
- Mechanism: Activate PPAR-α → ↑ lipoprotein lipase activity → TG breakdown
- Side effects: Myopathy (esp. with statins), gallstones
- First-line for severe hypertriglyceridemia to prevent pancreatitis

> **REDUCE-IT trial:**
> Icosapent ethyl (pure EPA) reduced CV events in high-risk patients with elevated TG despite statins.

Omega-3 fatty acid

- EPA & DHA from fish oil
- Decrease hepatic VLDL synthesis and lower TG by 20-50%. Minimal effect on LDL
- Dosing 2-4 gm/day
- **Side effects:** Fishy taste, GI upset, ↑ bleeding risk (high dose)

Bile acid sequestrants

- Cholestyramine, Colesevelam
- **Use: ↓ LDL (10–20%)**
- Bind bile acids in gut → ↑ hepatic cholesterol conversion to bile acids → ↑ LDL receptor activity
- **Safe in pregnancy**, used in children for familial hypercholesterolemia
- **Side effects:** GI upset, bloating, ↑ TG, interferes with the absorption of other drugs

Evinacumab

- Monoclonal antibody; angiopoietin-like protein 3 (ANGPTL3) inhibitor
- Inhibition of ANGPTL3 enhances lipolysis and clearance of triglyceride-rich lipoproteins → **reduces LDL-C, HDL-C, and triglycerides**, independent of LDL receptor activity
- Recommended in Familial Hypercholesterolemia- ELIPSE -HoFH trial

> **In pregnancy**
> - Bile acid sequestrants DOC
> - Statins, Ezetimibe, fibrate, PCSK9i, and niacin are contraindicated

CURRENT RECOMMENDATIONS (Cardiology Society of India clinical practice guideline for dyslipidemia management 2024)

- LDL and non-HDL cholesterol as treatment targets according to risk stratification
- High-intensity statin is first-line therapy in established ASCVD
- Upfront combination therapy Statin+ezetimibe in ACS patients (Hit hard and hit early)

- Subsequent addition of non-statins therapy (ezetimibe, Bempedoic acid and PCSK9 nhibitors) if LDL target not achieved

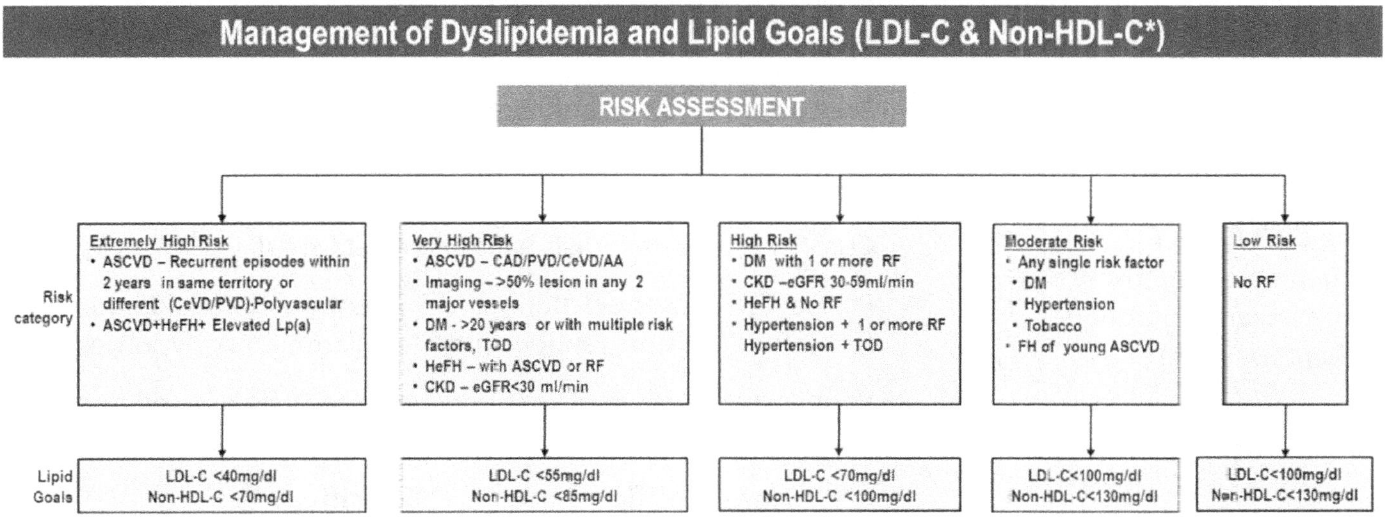

- In the absence of our own risk score calculator, only risk factors are used for risk assessment
- *Non-HDL-C as co primary Goal because of increase prevalence of atherogenic dyslipidemia in our country
- CeVD – Cerebrovascular disease, AA- aortic aneurysm, HeFH – Heterozygous Familial Hypercholesterolemia, TOD-Target organ damage, RF-Risk factor, CKD- Chronic kidney disease, DM- Diabetes mellitus, FH – Family history LDL-C – low density lipoprotein cholesterol, HDL-C – high density lipoprotein cholesterol, ASCVD – atherosclerotic cardiovascular disease, PVD- Peripheral vascular disease, CAD- Coronary artery disease

33. Antiinflammatory drugs for CAD

The **CRP-IL6-IL1** inflammatory pathway has been linked to coronary atherosclerosis.

- Even after the use of antiplatelets, statins, PCI/CABG, there is still a risk of recurrent MI/Death.
- The role of inflammation in the underlying progression of Coronary Atherosclerosis has been established.
- Raised CRP observed during ACS events and considered a risk factor for CV events (Supporting the inflammatory hypothesis)
- Various anti-inflammatory drugs have been developed targeting this pathway to reduce coronary events:

Non-Specific	**Specific**
Methotrexate	Canakinumab (IL-1β receptor antagonist)
Colchicine	Tocilizumab (IL-6 antagonist)

A. Methotrexate

- MTX has not shown CV benefit in various clinical trials (CIRT)

B. Colchicine

The following trials showed a favourable CV benefit of low-dose colchicine

i. **LODOCO:** phase II study

ii. **LODOCO 2**: In patients with stable CAD, low-dose colchicine reduced MACE (CV death, MI, stroke, and revascularisation) over a 2-year follow-up.

iii. **COLCOT**: Reduced ischemic events with colchicine after MI

ESC guidelines recommend the use of low-dose (0.5mg) colchicine for secondary prevention in patients with uncontrolled risk factors.

C. Canakinumab

- **CANTOS Trial:** Post MI patients with elevated CRP (>2), canakinumab reduced CV events and hs-CRP on 4 yrs follow-up.
- SC Injection (50-100 mg) given every 3 months
- Risk of serious infection and high cost

D. Tocilizumab

- **ASSAIL MI** trial showed increased myocardial salvage in patients after MI

34. Cardiac Embryology and Anatomy

Embryology of the Cardiovascular System

- Development of the cardiovascular system starts from the 10th day of fertilisation and at the 6th week, the first heartbeat can be recorded by USG.

Formation of the primitive heart tube

- In the cranial end of the mesodermal layer of the embryo, cardiac development starts in the form of two heart fields (cardiogenic field)
- Initially, they form two endocardial tubes, which subsequently merge to form a single primitive heart tube
- The primitive heart tube is further segmented into the following parts from cranial to caudal direction
  - truncus arteriosus
  - bulbus cordis
  - primitive ventricle
  - primitive atrium
  - sinus venosus

Derivatives of heart field

First heart field

- Atrium
- Ventricle
- Atrioventricular canal

Second heart field

- Aortopulmonary trunk
- Systemic and pulmonary vein
- Part of RV

Looping (around 23 days)

- Bulbus cordis (outflow part) moves ventrally, caudally and towards the right
- The inflow part moves dorsally, cranially and towards the left

Development of atrium

- **Right atrium-** develops mainly from the primitive atrium (trabeculated part) and partly from the sinus venosus (smooth part)
- **Left atrium-** develops mainly from the absorbed pulmonary veins (smooth part) and a small part from the primitive atrium

Interatrial septum

- A septum develops from the roof of the developing atrium towards the endocardial cushion, known as the septum primum
- The space between septum primum and endocardial cushion is known as ostium primum
- When the septum primum meets the endocardial cushion, a hole is formed in the midseptum, known as ostium secundum

- Subsequently, another septum develops right side of the septum primum, known as septum secundum, which closes ostium secundum

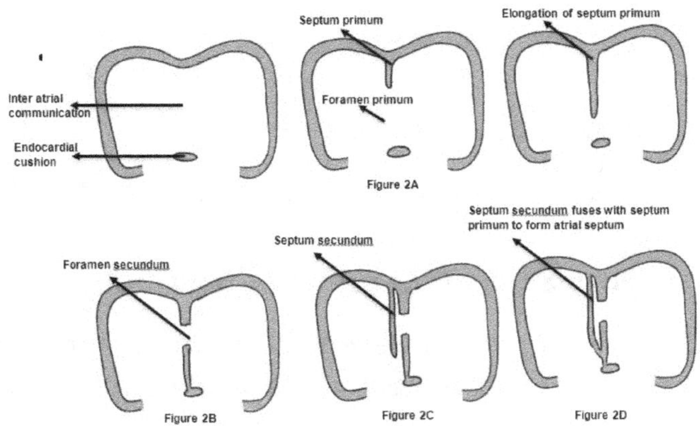

Figure 2. Formation of Atrial Septum

Ventricle and Interventricular Septum

- The muscular septum develops from the floor of the developing ventricle, and membranous septum develops from the endocardial cushion to meet the muscular part
- Left ventricle
- Right ventricle

> - Neural crest cells are responsible for the development of the spiral septum
> - **Abnormal neural crest cell migration** leads to anomaly of spiral septum/ conotruncal development, causing-
>   - **TOF**
>   - **DORV**
>   - **TGA**
>   - **Truncus arteriosus**

Outflow tract

- A spiral septum divides the truncus arteriosus and bulbus cordis, forming the aorta and pulmonary trunk, which subsequently meets the interventricular septum

Derivatives of the branchial arch vessels

- Branchial arch vessels from the cranial end of the primitive heart tube develop into the aortic arch with branches and the pulmonary artery

Arch vessel	Derivative
1st arch vessel	Maxillary artery
2nd arch vessel	Stapedial artery
3rd arch vessel	b/l common carotid and part of internal carotid
4th arch vessel	Left- arch of aorta Right- proximal rt subclavian artery Left subclavian from left segmental artery
5th arch vessel	disappear
6th arch vessel	Right and left pulmonary artery Ductus arteriosus on left side

> Common cardinal vein also known as **duct of Cuvier**

Development of the venous system

Three pairs of veins develop around 5th week and drain to the right and left horns of the sinus venosus

- Common cardinal vein- drains from the body of the embryo
- Umbilical vein- drains oxygenated blood from the placenta
- Vitelline vein- drains from the yolk sac

> **Valve of Vieussens** at the ostium of the great cardinal vein near CS

	derivative
Vitelline vein	• Portal vein, liver sinusoids and hepatic IVC
Umbilical vein	• Right vein disappear and proximal left disappear • Distal left vein persists and connect to IVC via ductus venosus
Cardinal vein	• Right anterior cardina +common cardinal --> SVC • Distal Rt anterior cardinal vein → Rt brachiocephalic vein • Anastomosis between Rt and Lt cardinal vein → left brachiocephalic vein • Distal anterior cardinal vein → IJV • Rt supracardinal vein → Azygous vein • Lt supracardinal vein → hemiazygous vein

- SVC develops from- Rt anterior cardinal vein, the Rt common cardinal vein and the Rt horn of sinus venosus
- IVC develops from- Rt common cardinal vein, vitelline vein, subcardinal vein, supracardinal vein and some part of posterior cardinal vein

LSVC (persistent left SVC)

- Persistent left anterior and left common cardinal vein → left SVC
- Mostly associated with absent Rt SVC
- Maybe with bilateral SVC

Oblique vein of LA/Vein of Marshall

- Persistent intracardiac portion of the left anterior cardiac vein
- Drains to the coronary sinus posterior to LA
- Vein of Marshall ablation has been tried as a treatment option for atrial fibrillation

Foetal circulation

- The umbilical vein carries oxygenated blood from the placenta to IVC
- The Umblical vein bypasses the liver by the ductus venosus to join the IVC

Umblical vein- the highest PO2 in foetal circulation

- There is preferential streaming of SVC and IVC blood in RA
- One-third of oxygenated blood is directed to LA via the foramen Ovale. This oxygenated blood reaches aorta via LV and supplies the coronary and cerebral circulation
- Deoxygenated blood from the SVC, two-thirds blood from the IVC, reaches to RV to PA and then to descending aorta via ductus arteriosus supplying abdominal viscera and lower limbs
- Two umblical arteries arising from the iliac artery carrying deoxygenated blood to the placenta for oxygenation

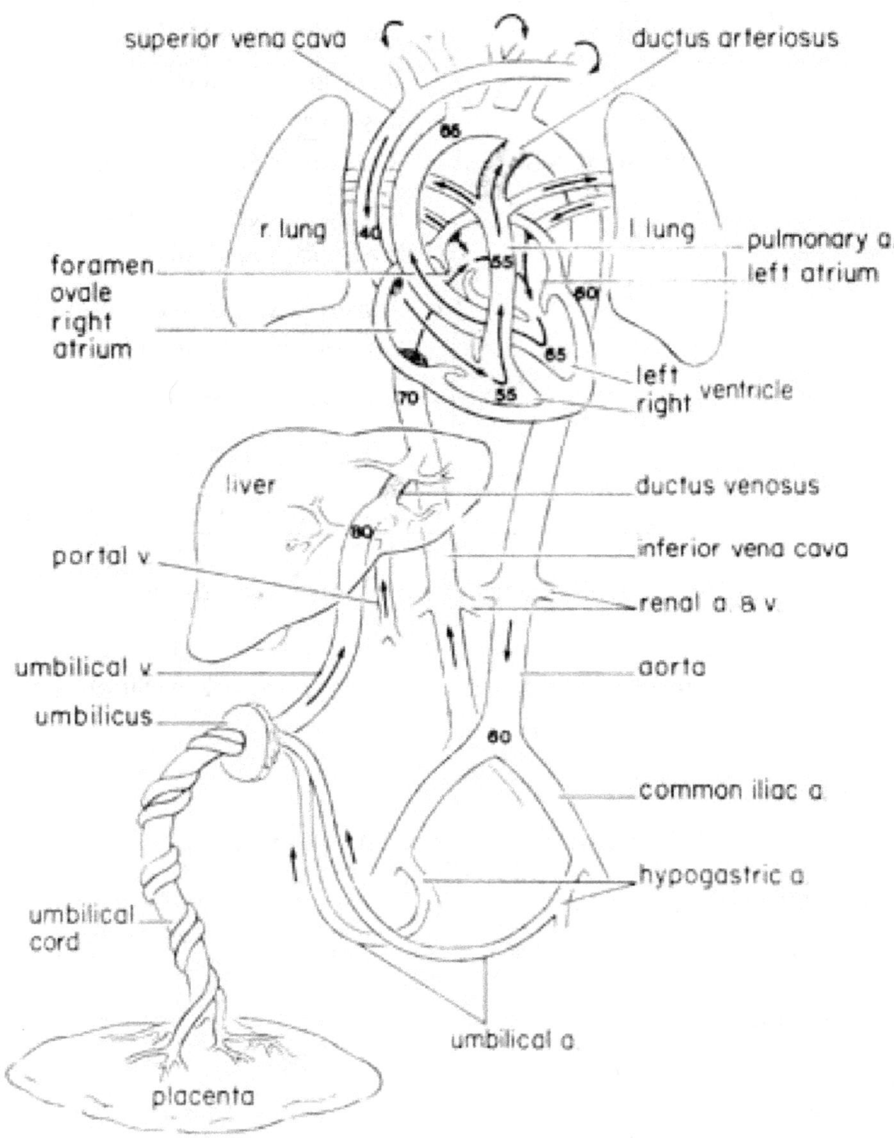

Changes at birth

- No blood flow in the umblical vein → Closure of the ductus venosus
- Lung expansion→ increased O2 tension→ closure of ductus arteriosus
- Increase in systemic vascular resistance and decrease in pulmonary vascular resistance

- Closure of the ductus arteriosus
  - Functional closure 10-15 hrs after birth
  - Anatomic closure after 2-3 weeks
  - Oxygen is the strongest stimulus for closure of the ductus arteriosus
  - Premature neonate- ductus not responsive to O2
  - responsive to NSAID (Indomethacin) for closure and PGE2 for dilation
  - Mature neonate with PDA – poor response to Indomethacin/PGE2

Foetal structure	Adult derivative/remnant
Ductus venosus	Ligamentum venosus
Ductus arteriosus	Ligamentum arteriosus
Umblical vein	Ligamentum teres
Foramen ovale	Fossa ovalis
Left anterior cardinal vein	Left SVC
Intracardiac part of left anterior cardinal vein	Vein/ligament of Marshall

Cardiac anatomy-Highlights

Triangle of Koch

Bounded by

- Tendon of Todaro
- Tricuspid annulus
- Coronary sinus ostium

The AV node lies at the apex of this triangle and anatomical landmark for catheter ablation

Coronary anatomy

Left Main Coronary Artery (LMCA) divides into LAD and LCX

Left Anterior Descending (LAD)

- Courses in the anterior interventricular groove.
- Supplies: Anterior 2/3 of the interventricular septum, anterior wall and apex of LV
- Branches: Diagonal and septal

Left Circumflex (LCX)

- Courses in the left atrioventricular (AV) groove.
- **Supplies:** Lateral/posterior wall of LV and LA
- **Branches:** Obtuse marginal (OM) branches

- Oclusion of the LMCA or proximal LAD is associated with increased mortality
- Occlusion of the RCA has a high chance of AV block and bradycardia

Right Coronary Artery (RCA)

- Courses in the right AV groove
- Supplies: RA, RV, Inferior wall of LV, Posterior 1/3 of interventricular septum, SA node (in 60%) and AV node (in 85–90%)
- Branches - Conus branch, SA nodal branch (60%), acute marginal artery (to RV), Posterior descending artery (PDA) (in most individuals) and AV nodal branch

Cardiac structures with dual blood supply

- Interventricular septum
- Papillary muscles
- Left posterior fascicle of the left bundle

Ramus intermedius- sometimes an extra branch from LMCA between LAD and LCX

Dominance

Defined by the artery that gives rise to the **PDA**:

- **Right dominant** (85%): PDA from RCA
- **Left dominant** (8–10%): PDA from LCX
- **Co-dominant** (7–10%): PDA from both

Venous drainage

Coronary sinus

- The major venous drainage of the heart, situated along the posterior AV groove and opens into the right atrium
- It is guarded by the **Thebesian valve**
- Tributaries of CS are
    - Great cardiac vein- Runs along LAD and drains anterior LV, septum, apex. This vein continues posteriorly as the coronary sinus
    - Middle cardiac vein- Runs with PDA and drains the posterior septum, inferior LV wall
    - Small cardiac vein- Runs with RCA and drains RA, RV
    - Posterior vein of LV- drains posterior LV
    - Oblique vein of Marshall- drains LA
- **Anterior cardiac veins-** small veins from the RV that directly open to the RA
- **Thebesian veins/Vena cordis minimi-** small veins that directly open to cardiac chambers
- **Clinical importance**
    - Coronary sinus catheterisation is important for **EP study**

- The coronary sinus develops from the left horn of the sinus venosus
- The oblique vein of Marshall is a remnant of the left anterior cardinal vein

- Coronary sinus canulation is important for **retrograde cardioplegia** during cardiac surgery
- **CRT- LV lead** is placed via the coronary sinus to the posterolateral vein
- **Persistent LSVC** causes a dilated coronary sinus

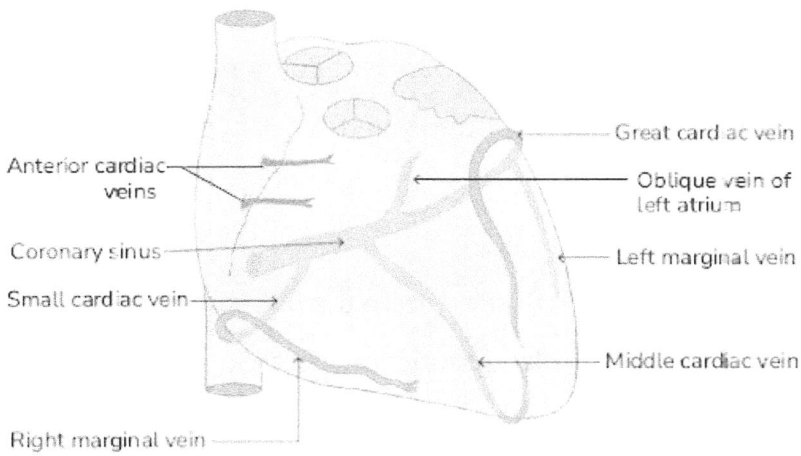

35. Syndromes in Cardiology

1. Alagille Syndrome

- Cardiac: Peripheral pulmonary stenosis, Hypoplastic Pulmonary arteries
- Non-cardiac: intrahepatic Cholestasis, Butterfly vertebrae, hypertension, pointed Chin
- JAG 1 Gene

2. Bland White Garland Syndrome

- Anomalous origin of the left coronary artery from the pulmonary artery
- Usually manifests as severe ventricular dysfunction in a child secondary to severe Ischemia
- Reimplantation of the coronary to the aorta/ Takeuchi repair is the treatment of choice.

3. DiGeorge Syndrome

- Microdeletion of the 22q11 chromosome
- Cardiac: conotruncal defects (TOF (MC), Truncus arteriosus, DORV)
- Non-cardiac: Abnormal facies, Thymic Aplasia, Hypocalcaemia (low PTH), cleft palate

CATCH 22: Cardiac, Abnormal facies, Thymic aplasia, cleft palate, Hypocalcaemia, Ch no 22.

4. CHARGE Syndrome (Eye, Ear, Heart)

- Cardiac: TOF, TGA, DORV
- Non-Cardiac: Coloboma, Growth Retardation, Choanal Atresia, Genital Abnormalities, ear abnormalities.

5. DOWN Syndrome

- Cardiac: AV Canal Defect (MC)/ Endocardial Cushion Defect/ AVSD, VSD, PDA, TOF

Early and more severe PAH in the left-to-right shunt.

6. Holt-Oram Syndrome

- Cardiac: OS ASD, VSD, Conduction disease.
- Non-Cardiac: Radial abnormality (forearm, hand)

7. Noonan Syndrome

- Cardiac: Valvular Pulmonary stenosis (Dysplastic Valve), Peripheral Pulmonary Artery stenosis, HCM
- Non-Cardiac: Male Turner Syndrome, Congenital Lymphoedema.

8. Congenital Rubella Syndrome (CRS)

- Cardiac: Pulmonary Artery stenosis, PDA, TOF.
- Non-Cardiac: Cataract, Retinopathy, Deafness, Bone lesion.

9. Shone Complex

- A series of left heart Obstructive lesions **(NOTCH 1 mutation)**
- Mitral Stenosis (Parachute mitral valve, supramitral membrane), LV Outflow obstruction (Valvular AS, Subvalvular LVOTO), CoA.

10. Scimitar Syndrome

- A type of partial anomalous pulmonary venous connection (PAPVC)
- Anomalous right pulmonary vein drains into the IVC, producing a typical X-ray Sign (Scimitar / Turkish Sword Sign)
- Associated with right lung hypoplasia and pulmonary hypertension.

11. William Syndrome

- 7q11 deletion (loss of function of elastin)
- Cardiac: supravalvular AS, Peripheral PS, Renal artery stenosis, dilated coronaries.
- Non cardiac : Hypercalcemia, Elfin Facies, Microdontia, Enamel Hypoplasia, Inguinal hernia, Mental retardation
- **COANDA Effect:** BP in Rt UL > Lt UL seen in **supravalvular AS.** Occurs due to preferential streaming.

12. Turner syndrome

- Cardiac: Post ductal CoA, PAPVC

13. Cardiocutaneous syndrome

NAXOS Syndrome	Carvajal Syndrome
Plakoglobin Mutation	Desmoplakin Mutation
Hyperkeratosis of Palms and sole with wooly hair	Epidermolytic Keratoderma (like pemphigus)
ARVC	ARVC

14. Carney Complex

- Cardiac Myxoma
- Skin Lesion: Lentiginosis, Skin myxoma
- Endocrine Abnormalities: Primary Pigmented Nodular Adrenocortical Disease

15. Stokes-Adams syndrome

- Sudden unconsciousness in AV block before the escape rhythm resumes

16. Lutembacher syndrome

- Congenital ASD, when associated with acquired mitral stenosis
- Severe left-to-right shunt due to mitral stenosis

36. Cardiac Tumors

- Myxoma is usually associated with constitutional symptoms such as weight loss, myalgia, arthralgia, anaemia, polycythemia, leukocytosis, clubbing, raised ESR, and CRP
- Mimics IE/CTD disorders

Metastatic cardiac tumours (pericardial deposit) are more common than primary cardiac tumours.

Amongst primary cardiac tumours, benign tumours (75%) are much more common than malignant (25%)

Myxoma

- The most common primary cardiac tumour
- Female >> male
- Can be sporadic (90%) or familial (10%), with differences in clinical profile and presentation.
- Surgery is the treatment of choice, irrespective of size

Sporadic	Familial
Usually solitary from interatrial septum in left atrium and Pedunculated with fibrovascular stalk	Multiple tumors and unusual location, can be ventricular location
Middle Age	Young age at presentation, with family history
Less recurrence after surgery (1%-2%)	High recurrence after surgery (10%-20%)

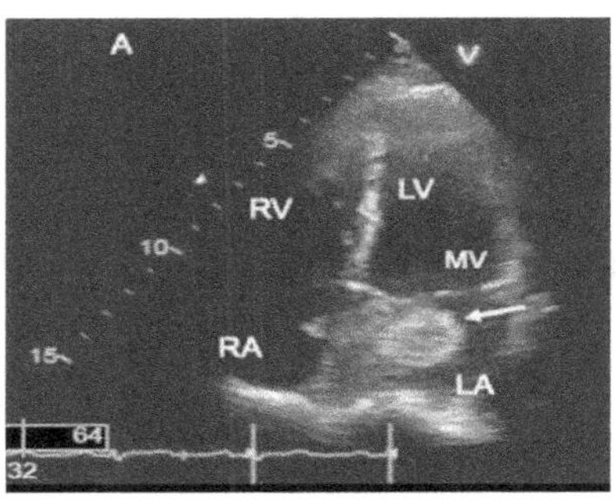

- Familial type may be associated with a **PRKAR1A** (Protein Kinase A) mutation

CARNEY complex

- Myxoma
- Lentigines in skin
- Endocrine overactivity (adrenal, testis, pituitary)

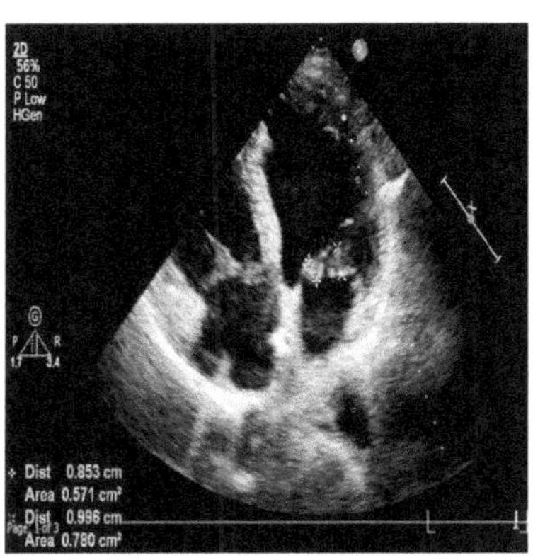

NAME Syndrome

- Nevi
- Atrial Myxoma
- Myxoid Neurofibroma
- Ephelides

LAMB Syndrome

- Lentigines
- Atrial myxoma
- Blue Nevus

Papillary fibroelastoma

- Commonly seen over the valve leaflets
- Can cause valvular dysfunction (stenosis, regurgitation) or embolisation

- Cardiac rhabdomyoma may regress spontaneously in children

Cardiac Rhabdomyoma

- Common in infants and children
- Can cause LVOT/ RVOT obstruction, causing CHF
- Multiple rhabdomyomas are seen in **Tuberous Sclerosis**
- May **resolve spontaneously** on follow-up

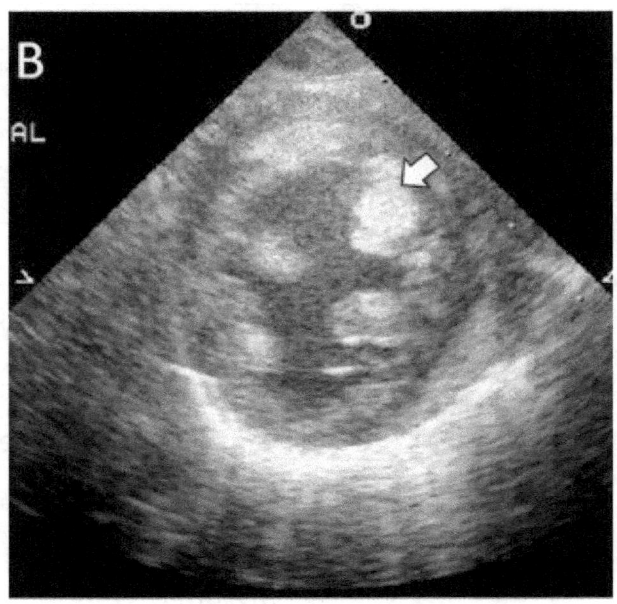

- Cardiac rhabdomyosarcoma MC primary malignant tumor of heart with very poor prognosis

Hemangioma

- Mostly intramyocardial
- Common near the AV node, causing conduction defect

Sarcoma

- The most common malignant primary cardiac tumour
- Rapidly growing and very poor prognosis
- Poor response to chemotherapy and radiation, except for lymphosarcoma

Metastatic cardiac tumour

- Pericardium is commonly involved than the myocardium and endocardium
- A tumour with a high propensity for cardiac metastasis is **melanoma**
- The most common sources of cardiac metastases are breast and lung carci

37. Infective Endocarditis

- Streptococcus bovis (Gallolyticus) related IE seen in the elderly with colonic carcinoma

Microbiology of infective endocarditis

Based on clinical course-

- **Acute-** Staphylococcus aureus, Streptococcus pneumoniae, gram-negative bacilli
- **Subacute-** Viridans streptococci, Enterococcus, HACEK group, fungal, CONS.

Streptococcus

- Indolent infection
- Normal mouth flora as a source
- Usually penicillin-sensitive
- Streptococcus bovis (Gallolyticus) related IE seen in the elderly with colonic carcinoma.

- Listeria endocarditis is commonly associated with pregnancy, delivery, and abortion.

Staphylococcus

- Mostly hospital-acquired.
- Rapidly progressive course.
- CONS are usually subacute and associated with prosthetic valve.

Enterococcus

- Genito-urinary source and common in the elderly.
- Multidrug resistance is common.

- Most common Organism NVE- Streptococcus viridans
- Most common Organism PVE-Staph aureus

Listeria

- Associated with genitourinary infection and following pregnancy, delivery, and abortion.

- Staph aureus- overall, the most common cause of IE

  Most common in IV drug abusers

  The most common cause of early prosthetic Valve
- Staphylococcus epidermidis-Most common cause of late prosthetic valve endocarditis.
- Staphylococcus viridans-Most common community cause of acquired infective endocarditis.

- **MVP** - Most common predisposition for IE in the Western world
- **RHD** - Most common in India.

Culture-negative infective endocarditis

- Mostly secondary to prior antibiotic usage.
- A few organisms, such as Bartonella, Brucella, Coxiella, Legionella, and Tropheryma, do not grow in routine culture media.
- Serology/special culture media are useful for such organisms.

Predispositions

- Mitral Valve> Aortic Valve > Tricuspid Valve >Pulmonary Valve

  Regurgitant lesion > stenotic Lesion (predisposition)
- myxomatous MVP >MR>RHD>Secondary

Skin lesions

Immunological manifestation of IE

- RA factor
- Osler node
- Roth spot

- Petechiae- the most common peripheral sign
- Janeway lesion-

  painless hemorrhagic maculae over palms/soles

  secondary to septic emboli

  Commonly seen in Staphylococcus aureus.
- Splinter haemorrhage

  painless linear haemorrhage in the nail bed.
- Osler node -painful nodules in the pad of fingers

  An immunological phenomenon.
- Roth spot -circular retinal haemorrhage with a pale centre.

  An immunological phenomenon

  Also seen in SLE, NBTE, and Leukaemia.

Diagnosis

Embolisation of vegetation is common in

- Mitral>Aortic
- NVE>PVE
- Staphylococci > Other bacteria

- Diagnosis by DUKE criteria-80% sensitive and 90% specific.
- Procalcitonin has a less reliable role in the diagnosis.
- TEE has a better diagnostic value than TTE.
- Cardiac CT is suitable for the assessment of paravalvular complications, such as an abscess.
- FDG-PET- better role in diagnosis of PVE &CIED infection.
- Aortic IE-conduction abnormality(AV blockage) is common.

Management

- IV antibiotics main stay of therapy
  - Should send appropriate blood culture before starting treatment according to sensitivity

- Empirical antibiotic

  NVE- combination of ampicillin, gentamicin, and flucloxacillin or oxacillin/ceftriaxone

  PVE- vancomycin and gentamicin

POET STUDY-Oral antibiotics in IE

- In patients with endocarditis on the left side of the heart who were in stable condition, changing to oral antibiotic treatment was non-inferior to continued intravenous antibiotic treatment.
- **Indications of surgery in IE-**
  - Hemodynamically unstable valvular lesions/heart failure

    e.g. severe MR
  - Large vegetation/recurrent embolisation
  - para valvular extension/abscess
  - Prosthetic valve endocarditis

Indications of infective endocarditis prophylaxis (AHA)

- Prosthetic heart valve/valve repair with prosthetic material.
- Previous IE
- Congenital heart disease
  - unrepaired CCHD
  - Palliative CCHD (Shunt/conduit)
  - Complete repair with prosthesis (intervention/surgery)
  - Partially repaired for 6 months, conduit
- Post-cardiac transplantation with valvulopathy.

Left-to-right shunt is **NOT** an indication for IE prophylaxis

38. Cardiac Transplantation

- Considered in patients with end-stage structural heart disease with poor functional capacity and no other medical contraindications.
- Cardiopulmonary exercise testing and 6 MWT done to assess functional capacity before transplantation.
- Peak O2 consumption (VO2) of less than 50% of predicted (<10 ml/Kg/min) and a 6 MWT distance of less than 300 m is considered very poor functional capacity and an indication for transplant.

> Peak O2 consumption (VO2) less than 50% of predicted (<10 ml/Kg/min) and 6 MWT distance less than 300 m considered an indication for cardiac transplantation

Surgical Approach

- Two types of allograft anastomosis: biatrial and bicaval
- Bicaval technique is now commonly used with 5 anastomoses, i.e., SVC, IVC, PA, Aorta, LA.

Immunosuppression

- A combination of glucocorticoids, Calcineurin Inhibitors (Cyclosporin, Tacrolimus) and antiproliferative (MMF/ Azathioprine) is used for maintenance Immunosuppression.
- Induction therapy with Rasiliximab (Anti CD 25) or Anti-thymocyte Globulin (ATG) may be used immediately following transplantation.
- Sirolimus and Everolimus slow the progression of transplant coronary vasculopathy.

> Sirolimus and Everolimus slow progression of transplant coronary vasculopathy

Rejection

- Endomyocardial biopsy is considered the gold standard for diagnosis
- Imaging (Echo/MRI) has poor diagnostic value
- Gene expression Assay (Allomap): newer modality to diagnose cellular rejection with a blood test, only to avoid repeated biopsies

Cellular	Humoral/ Ab Mediated
Usually asymptomatic and detected on routine surveillance biopsy	Associated with graft dysfunction and hemodynamic compromise
Bx: lymphocyte infiltration Myocyte damage	Bx: Less lymphocyte infiltration Complement Deposition
Rx:escalation of Immunosuppression ATG	Rx: Plasmapheresis

Outcome / Survival

- Significant improvement in QOL and functional capacity
- Recent successful US registries suggest a post-transplant 1-year. survival >90% and 3 yrs. survival >85%.
- Median survival is approximately 12 years

Cardiac allograft vasculopathy

- Development of obstructive coronary artery disease (CAV) is the most important long-term complication after transplant.
- Seen in 20% patients after 1 year. and 40%-50% at 5 years.
- Yearly CAG with/ without IVUS/OCT done for screening.
- Statins and Aspirin are used for all patients post-transplant, irrespective of lipid level.
- Sirolimus/Everolimus, as part of an immunosuppression regimen, has been shown to slow the progression of CAV.

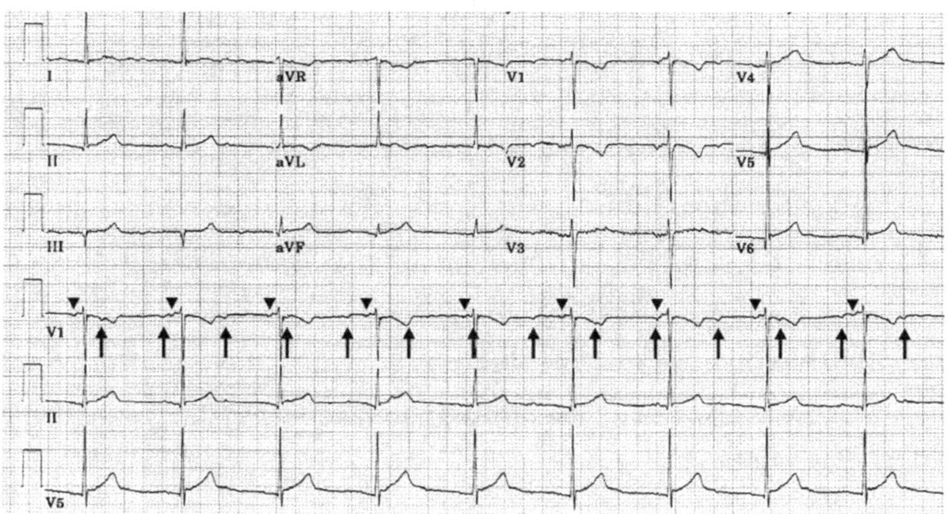

ECG after cardiac transplant showing two types of P waves from the dual SA node of the donor and recipient heart.

39. Pregnancy and Heart Disease

- PCWP, PA pressure, and JVP remain normal in pregnancy

Physiological changes in pregnancy

- HR-Increase by 10 beats/min over prepregnancy level
- BP(MAP) shows a small drop in BP (5-10mmhg) during early pregnancy, and returns to baseline in the third trimester.
- PVR and SVR decrease.
- Cardiac output increases 30-50%. (Both stroke volume and heart rate increase)
- Increases in blood volume (plasma volume>RBC volume)
- PCWP, PA pressure, and JVP remain normal.
- Heart failure is common at the end of the 2nd trimester and the immediate post op period (sudden addition of placental autotransfusion and removal of IVC compression)

Normal CV findings in pregnancy

Clinical

- Collapsing pulse, prominent jugular pulse (normal jugular venous pressure), cardiomegaly, (lateral apical impulses), Palpable RV/ PA impulse, faint ESM in the pulmonary area, S3

ECG

- PAC, PVC, left axis deviation, Q waves in inf leads.

Echo

- dilated all cardiac chambers, LVH, TR (mild to moderate)

- Cardiac stenotic lesion (MS, AS) is less well tolerated than regurgitant lesion (MR, AR) (with decreasing SVR in pregnancy, regurgitation may decrease)

Heart disease in pregnancy

Risk stratification of pregnancy with cardiac illness is done using the

- WHO risk classification
- CARPREG II score

Conditions considered **extremely high risk** for pregnancy are (40-100% maternal mortality)

- Severe PAH/ES,
- Severe MS/AS,
- LVEF< 30%

- Past h/o PPCM,
- Aortic lesion (ED syndrome, aortic aneurysm, COA)-very high risk of dissection.

General management principles in pregnancy with heart disease

- Drugs contraindicated-

  ACEI/ARB-teratogenic

  Atenolol-fetal growth retardation,

  statin,

  VKA/warfarin

  Bosentan
- NSAIDs are not safe in late pregnancy, early ductus closure
- Hydralazine is used for vasodilation in place of ACE inhibitors for heart failure during pregnancy.
- Electrical cardioversion is safe during pregnancy
- Cardiac surgery is usually avoided unless absolutely indicated (20% fetal loss)
- Balloon dilation of valvular stenosis can be done with obstetric backup

> - Vaginal delivery is usually preferred over CS except few unusual scenarios

Mode of delivery-

- Vaginal delivery is generally preferred over CS (to minimise blood loss)
- Indications of C Section
  - on warfarin-high risk of fetal ICH
  - Dilated thoracic aorta -dissection
  - Refractory heart failure
  - Hemodynamic instability

Specific conditions

Hypertension

> - Ideal time for BMV during pregnancy: 24-30 weeks of gestation

- Hypertension in pregnancy – BP>140/90 mmHg, Severe HTN-BP>160/110 mmHg
- Drug therapy for all pregnant females with confirmed BP > 140/90
- Safe Drugs: Beta blocker (Most evidence for Labetalol, Metoprolol, bisoprolol also safe), DHP CCB (Most evidence for Nifedipine, Amlodipine, Felodipine, nicardipine also used) and Methyl dopa
- Severe HTN (BP>160/110) should be hospitalised

- IV Labetalol DOC, Other drugs- IV Nicardipine, IV Hydralazine (2nd line)
- Safety data of thiazide diuretics is not clear.

Mitral stenosis

- Usually worsens during pregnancy with an increase in HF and cardiac output.
- There is a high chance of pulmonary oedema during delivery/immediate postpartum
- BMV/MV replacement should be done before conception if MS- severe, even asymptomatic
- BMV can be done during pregnancy if severe MS.
- Ideal time for BMV: 24-30 weeks

Pulmonary arterial hypertension

- Idiopathic severe PAH/Eisenmenger syndrome is associated with a very high mortality risk,
- Considered a contraindication for pregnancy, and a good contraceptive should be used.

Peripartum cardiomyopathy

- PPCM is defined as heart failure developing in the last trimester/5 months postpartum and LVEF< 45%
- Oxidative stress, prolactin cleavage product (16k PRL), and impaired VGEF signalling have been attributed to pathogenesis.
- Age>30, multiparous, twin pregnancy, preeclampsia, tocolytic therapy, and GDM are considered risk factors

  Management-

  - Bromocriptine (inhibits prolactin) can be used; however, the risk of thromboembolism is high, and anticoagulation should be combined.
  - Routine anticoagulation for all patients is not recommended.
  - Prompt delivery in advanced heart failure.
- Complete recovery in 20-60% patients.
- High chance of recurrence, should avoid multiple pregnancy.

Warfarin embryopathy

- If exposed during 6-12 weeks of gestation.
- Manifest as nasal hypoplasia, short limbs and digits, stippled epiphysis
- Up to 5mg warfarin risk is negligible

Anticoagulation during pregnancy (mechanical heart valve)

- **Warfarin** crosses the placenta and is associated with embryopathy when exposed in the first trimester and fetopathy when used later.
  - The risk of embryopathy is very less if the warfarin dose is <5mg
- **UFH** does not cross the placenta and has no effect on the fetus; however, it needs constant IV infusion and aPTT monitoring

- **LMWH** crosses the placenta, requires daily subcutaneous injection, has less effective anticoagulation and needs anti-Xa level monitoring.
- NOAC- no safety information available, currently contraindicated in pregnancy.

Suggested anticoagulation approach (ESC2018/AHA2014)

- 1st Trimester-VKA (if warfarin <5mg), LMWH or UFH if warfarin >5mg
- 2nd Trimester-VKA-warfarin until 36 weeks
- Before delivery-stop VKA and start SC LMWH or UFH infus

40. Clinical Cardiology

Jugular venous pressure (JVP)

- Reflects **right atrial pressure** via pulsation of the **internal jugular vein**
- Normal JVP: ≤ **3–4 cm above the sternal angle** (~8–9 cm H_2O from RA)
- Best examined with the patient at a **45° angle**, using the **right IJV**

Waveform Components

- a wave – Atrial contraction
- c wave – Tricuspid valve bulging during ventricular systole
- x descent – Atrial relaxation
- v wave – Passive venous filling of RA
- y descent – RA emptying into RV

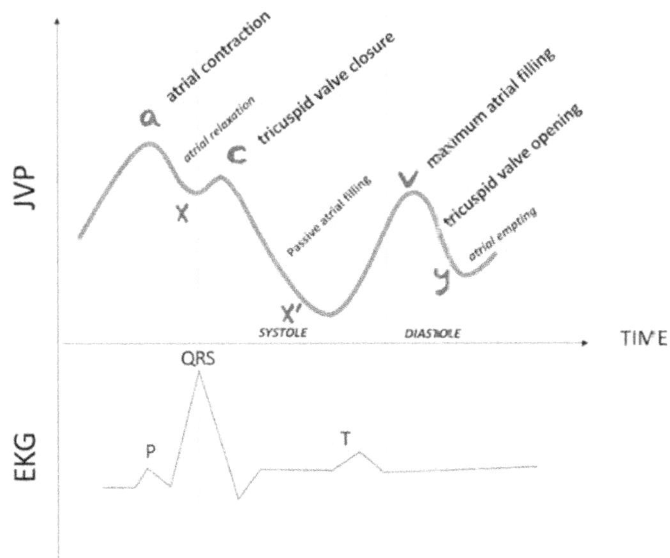

Clinical Abnormalities

Kussmaul's sign: ↑ JVP on inspiration (constrictive pericarditis, RV infarct)

Finding	Condition
Prominent a wave	Pulmonary HTN, TS, RVH
Absent a wave	Atrial fibrillation
Cannon a wave	AV dissociation (e.g., complete heart block, VT)
Prominent v wave	TR
Rapid y descent	Constrictive pericarditis
Slow y descent	Cardiac tamponade
Elevated JVP	RHF, fluid overload, constrictive pericarditis, tamponade

Arterial Pulse

Normal Arterial Pulse Waveform (dicrotic pulse)

- **Upstroke**: Rapid systolic ejection
- **Peak**: Systolic blood pressure
- **Dicrotic notch**: Aortic valve closure
- **Dicrotic wave**: Early diastolic rebound
- **Downstroke**: Diastolic runoff

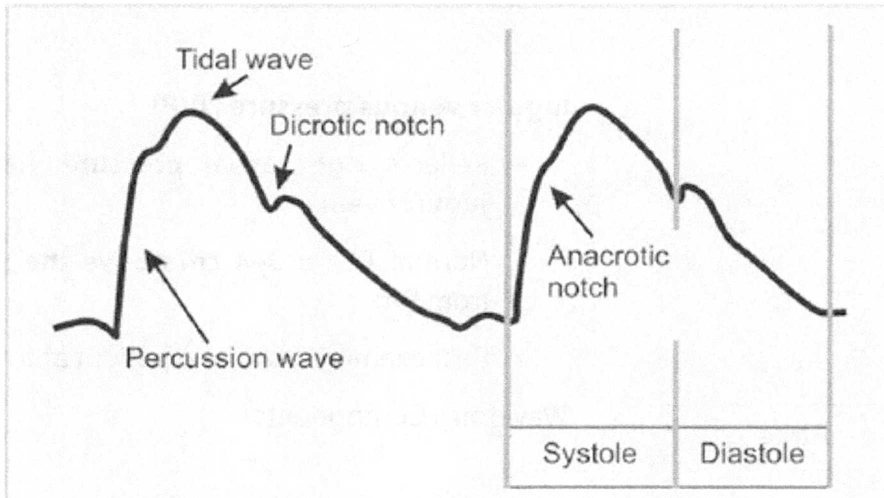

Pulsus paradoxus is an exaggeration of normal physiology (a decrease in SBP during inspiration due to a decrease in filling of the LV during inspiration)

seen in

- Cardiac tamponade
- CCP sometimes
- Severe Asthma/COPD

Pulsus paradoxus is **absent** in tamponade when there is associated severe AR/ASD

Reverse pulsus paradoxus is seen in (an increase in SBP during inspiration)

- HOCM
- Positive pressure ventilation

Abnormal Pulse Types

Anacrotic (slow-rising)	Delayed upstroke	Aortic stenosis
Bisferiens	Two systolic peaks	HCM, AR + AS
Dicrotic	Two peaks (systole + diastole)	Low output states, sepsis
Pulsus parvus et tardus	Small and delayed	Severe AS
Collapsing (water hammer)	Rapid upstroke & fall	AR, PDA, high-output states
Pulsus alternans	Alternating strong/weak beats	LV failure
Pulsus paradoxus	↓ SBP >10 mmHg on inspiration	Cardiac tamponade, CCP, severe asthma
Pulsus bigeminus	Normal + premature beat pattern	PVCs, digitalis toxicity

Cardiac Auscultation

First heart sound (S1)

- Closure of **mitral and tricuspid valves**
- Best heard at the **apex**
- **Loud S1:** MS, short PR. **Soft S1:** MR, long PR, reduced LV function

Second heart sound (S2)

- Hangout interval of pulmonary circulation is longer than systemic circulation, causing physiological splitting of S2

- Closure of semilunar valves (aortic and pulmonary valves)
- Best heard at the base (left upper sternal border)
- Components: **A2** (aortic), **P2** (pulmonary)
- Physiologic splitting of S2 secondary to a longer hangout interval of the pulmonary valve and delayed closure
- Physiological splitting is audible during inspiration and a single S2 during expiration
- Pathological split
  - **Wide split:** RBBB, PS
  - **Fixed split:** ASD
  - **Paradoxical/reverse split:** LBBB, AS

Hangout interval

- Time interval between the end of ejection and semilunar valve closure.
- It is longer for the pulmonary valve than the aortic valve due to lower pulmonary resistance.
- leads to physiological splitting of S2 (A2 precedes P2)
- Shortened in pulmonary hypertension, leading to a narrow or single S2.

Third heart sound (S3) Early diastole (rapid filling phase)

- Normal in: young, pregnancy
- Pathological: LV failure, DCM, MR

Fourth heart sound (S4)

- Late diastole due to atrial contraction against a stiff ventricle
- Seen in: LVH, HCM, ischemia.
- Absent in: AF

Added sounds

Ejection Click	High-pitched systolic	(Bicuspid AV, PS)
Tumor Plop	Low-frequency early diastole	(Atrial myxoma)
Pericardial Friction Rub	Triphasic scratchy sound	Acute pericarditis

Systolic Murmurs

- **Aortic stenosis (AS)**: Ejection systolic, right 2nd ICS, radiates to carotids
- **Mitral regurgitation (MR)**: Holosystolic, apex to axilla
- **Tricuspid regurgitation (TR)**: Holosystolic, increases with inspiration
- **Ventricular septal defect (VSD)**: Harsh holosystolic at LLSB
- **Mitral valve prolapse (MVP)**: Midsystolic click ± late systolic murmur
- **Hypertrophic cardiomyopathy (HCM)**: Harsh systolic, increases with Valsalva/standing

Diastolic Murmurs

- **Mitral stenosis (MS)**: Mid-diastolic with opening snap, heard best at the apex
- **Aortic regurgitation (AR)**: Early diastolic decrescendo at LSB
- **Pulmonary regurgitation (PR)**: Early diastolic (Graham Steell murmur in pulmonary HTN)
- **Tricuspid stenosis (TS)**: Mid-diastolic at LLSB, increases with inspiration

Continuous murmur

- PDA
- RSOV
- AV fistula
- Collaterals in Coarctation
- Venous hum
- Mammary suffle
- MS with ASD
- TAPVC
- Peripheral PS

Dynamic auscultation

- Involves changing preload, afterload, or position to distinguish murmurs.
- Helps differentiate murmurs that sound similar at rest.

Key manoeuvres and effects:

- **Inspiration**: ↑ right-sided murmurs (TR, PS)
- **Expiration**: ↑ left-sided murmurs (MR, AS)
- **Valsalva**(strain phase) ↓preload ↓ most murmurs; ↑ **HCM, MVP**
- **Standing**: ↓ preload; ↑ **HCM, MVP**, ↓ AS, MR
- **Squatting**: ↑ preload/afterload; ↑ **MR, AS**, ↓ HCM, MVP
- **Handgrip**: ↑ afterload; ↑ **MR, AR**, ↓ AS, HCM

41. Mechanical Circulatory Support

Devices designed to assist or replace the function of the left or right ventricle in patients with cardiogenic shock or advanced heart failure.

Indications / Strategies

1. **Bridge to recovery**
   - In situations of acute reversible cardiac conditions such as Acute MI, Myocarditis, and Post-cardiac-surgery.
   - Device preferred: IABP, Impella, ECMO (both cardiac and pulmonary), tandem Heart, Centrimag
   - Devices are removed once ventricular function recovers
2. **Bridge to transplant**
   - In chronic irreversible cardiac conditions, those who are eligible for transplantation, e.g., end-stage CAD/cardiomyopathy, or congenital heart disease.
   - Preferred devices: Heart Mate, HeartWare, Total Artificial Heart
3. **Destination therapy**
   - In chronic irreversible cardiac conditions, those who are not eligible for transplantation
   - Preferred devices: Heartmate, Heartware, TAH placed surgically

IABP (Intraaortic balloon pump)

- Most commonly used MCS device.
- Consists of a balloon catheter placed in DTA commonly via the femoral artery and attached to a console outside, which controls inflation and deflation.
- Helium gas is used for balloon inflation because of its low viscosity, allowing rapid inflation/deflation and absored rapidly if the balloon bursts.
- Balloon inflates during diastole **(starts at the middle of the T wave as a dicrotic notch in the pressure waveform)** and deflates at the end diastole **(peak of the R wave)**
- Inflation of the balloon during diastole increases filling pressure and improves coronary blood flow. Deflation of the balloon during systole decreases SBP and decreases afterload, which helps in improving cardiac output.

IABP mainly functions to unload the left ventricle and help in effective contraction

SHOCK II Trial

- Role of IABP in cardiogenic shock with MI
- No Difference in 30-Day Mortality with or without use of IABP
- Routine use after MI is not recommended

- Hemodynamic effects: -

SBP	decrease	CO	increase
DBP	increase	PCWP	decrease
MAP	increase	Afterload	decrease

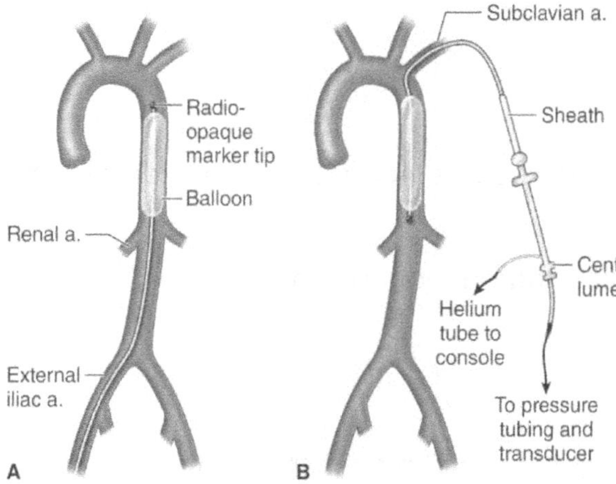

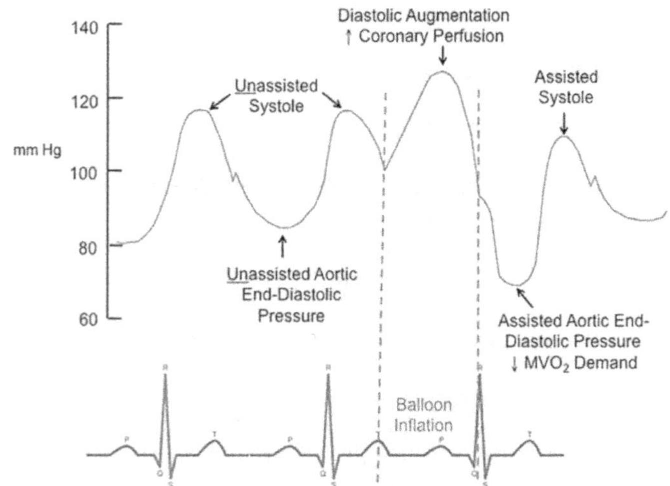

IMPELLA

Impella directly pumps blood from LV to aorta

- Micro axial pump placed across aortic valve, which pumps blood continuously from LV cavity into Aorta.
- Unloads LV cavity increases forward flow and improves coronary perfusion.
- Improvement in cardiac output higher than IABP
- Various versions available based on improvement in cardiac output.
    - Impella 2.5, CP, 5.0, 5.5
    - RV Impella (specially designed for Right ventricle)

Although used in situations of cardiogenic shock for temporary benefit, mortality benefit has not been established

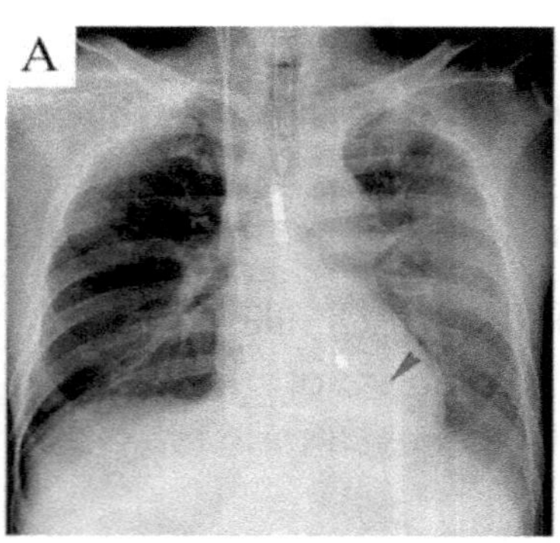

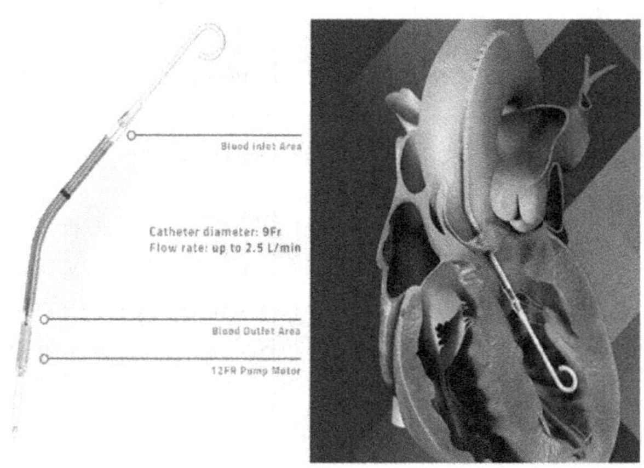

TANDEM HEART

- Left atrium to aorta.
- Assist device stays outside the body, pumps blood from, LA via a transeptally placed cannula (input) into the femoral artery.
- The oxygenator is also attached to the pump, allowing both LV unloading and oxygenation.
- Improvement in MAP and Cardiac output is higher than with IABP
- No study has shown a mortality benefit.

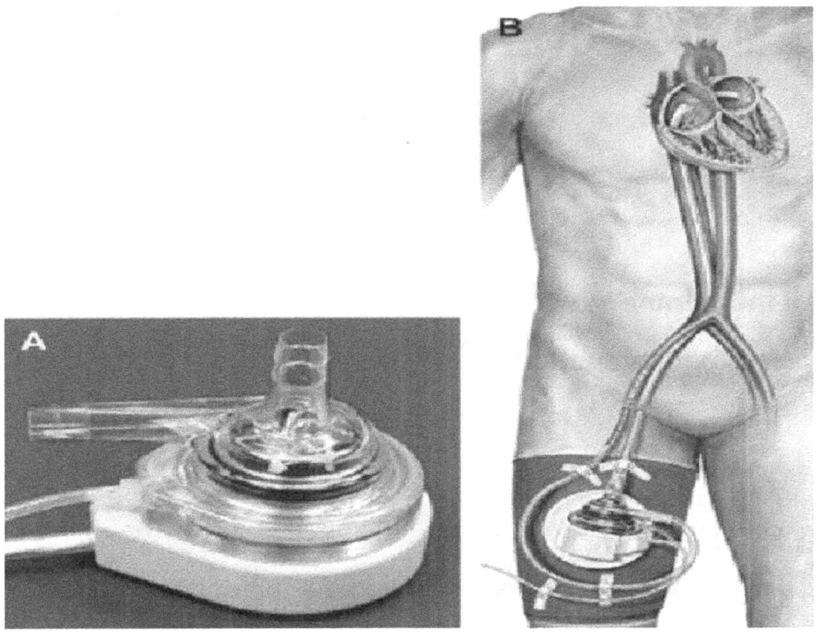

HEARTMATE

- A continuous flow pump is implanted surgically into the pericardial cavity.
- Receives blood from the LV and the output is to the aorta.
- Mostly used for long-term support. (BTT, DT)
- Heartmate III is more favourable than Heartmate II (Momentum Trial)

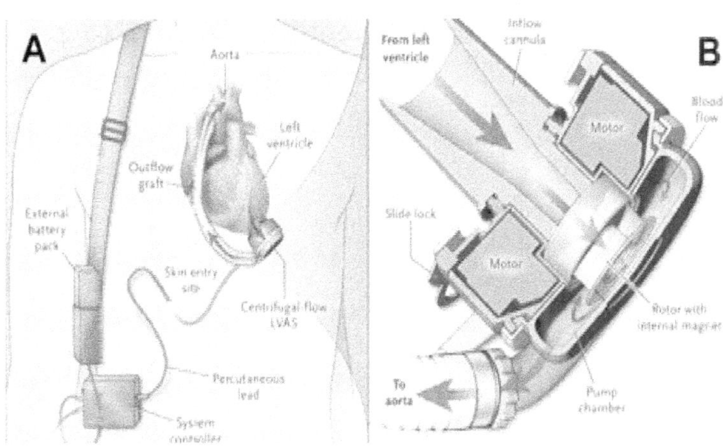

TOTAL ARTIFICIAL HEART (TAH)

- Consists of right and left prosthetic ventricles (50-70 ml capacity) designed to eject blood with the help of pneumatic air sac compression.
- Outflow is connected to the aorta and pulmonary artery

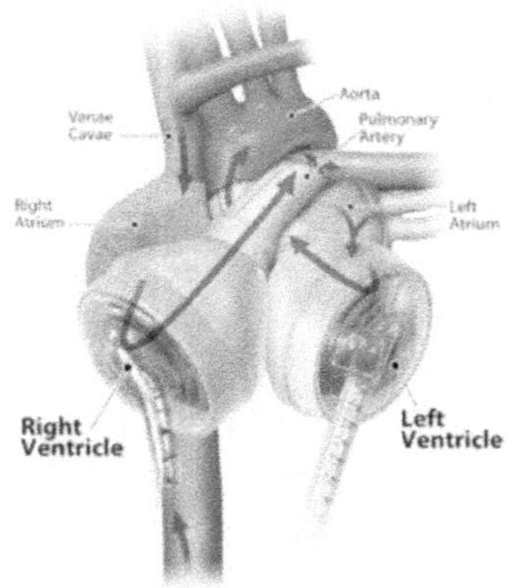

Total artificial heart

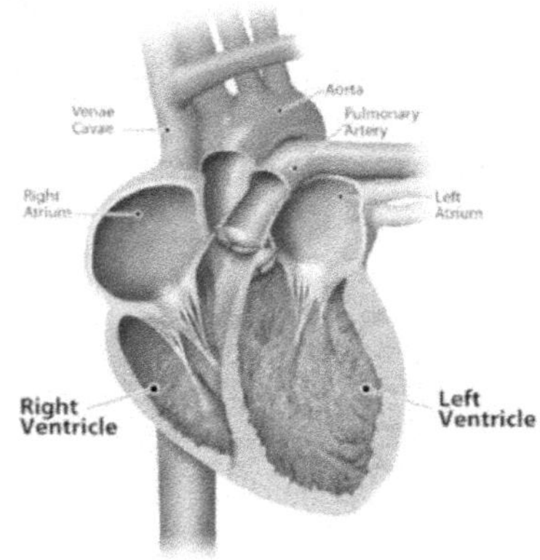

Human heart

ECMO (Extra-corporeal membrane oxygenator)

Provides complete cardiopulmonary support.

2 types

VV ECMO

- Input from the vein (femoral) and output to the vein.
- When only respiratory support is required (oxygenation only)

VA ECMO

- Input from vein and output to artery
- Both circulatory and respiratory support.
- More commonly used.

- A continuous flow pump with a membranous oxygenator stays outside between the input and output.
- Disadvantages: increased afterload for the ventricle, leading to poor ventricular recovery / coronary perfusion.

42. Cardiac Pacemaker

Indications of a permanent pacemaker

- **SA nodal disease**
  - Symptomatic sinus bradycardia/sinus pause
  - Chronotropic incompetence
  - Symptomatic bradycardia secondary to essential drugs (e.g. beta blocker in CHF)
- **AV nodal disease**
  - Complete AV block, Second degree type 2, infranodal 2:1 block, high degree AV block, irrespective of symptoms
  - Symptomatic second-degree type 1 block/ bifascicular block/ trifascicular block
  - Alternating bundle branch block (alternating RBBB and LBBB)

> Pacing is contraindicated when AV block is reversible or transient secondary to an identifiable cause
>
> - Hyperkalemia
> - MI

Pacemaker- Device and lead

- A pacemaker device **(Pulse generator)** contains a long-lasting battery (7-10 years) and electronic circuits.
- Flexible insulated wires **(Lead)** connected from the device to the desired cardiac chambers
- Types of pacemakers depending upon the number of leads
  - **Single chamber-** Single lead in RA or RV
  - **Dual chamber-** Lead in RA and RV
  - **Biventricular/triple lead-** Lead in RA, RV and coronary sinus (LV)

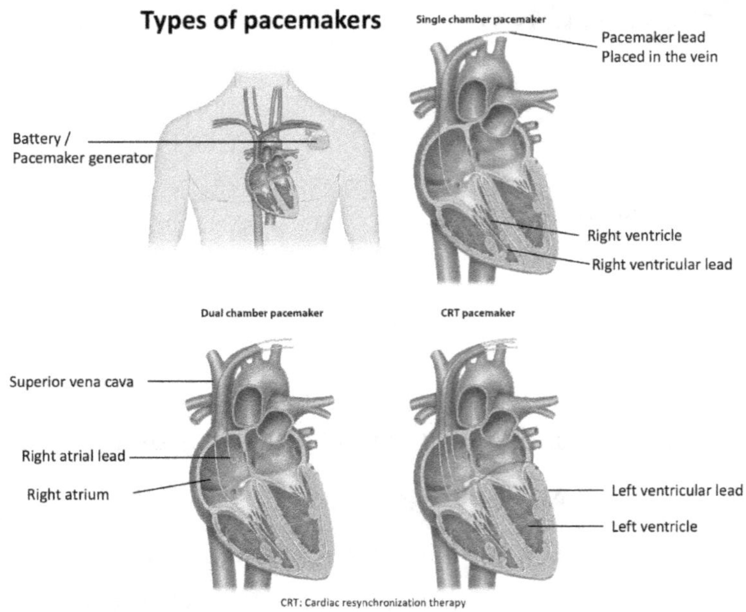

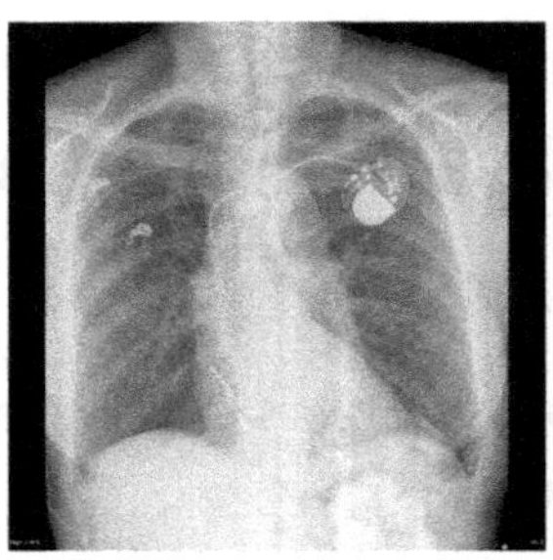

Pneumothorax after pacemaker implantation

Pacemaker Procedure

- Leads are placed via axillary or subclavian puncture using venogram and fluoroscopic landmarks.
- The device is implanted in a subcutaneous pocket created over the pectoral area.

Possible complications

- Pneumothorax/hemothorax (injury to lungs during venous puncture)
- Cardiac tamponade (RV perforation by lead)
- Long-term complications
    - Device infection
    - Lead dislodgement
    - Device/lead malfunction

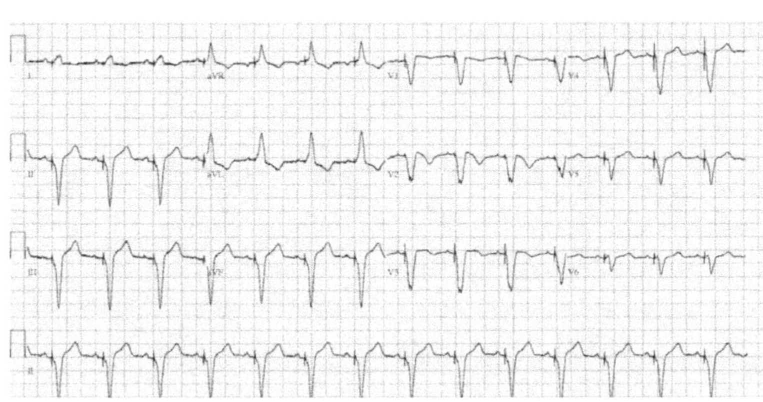

- ECG after a permanent pacemaker showing LBBB pattern, as pacing is usually done via the RV side of the septum. Rule out lead perforating the septum if there is RBBB.

Pacemaker function and modes

- **Important functions of a pacemaker are**
  - **Sensing:** Detects the heart's intrinsic electrical activity.
  - **Pacing:** Sends impulses when the heart rate is too slow or absent.
- **Modes of a pacemaker**

  NBG Pacemaker Code **(5-letter naming system)-** This standardised code describes the function of a pacemaker using up to 5 positions, though the first 3 are most commonly used.

Position	Function	Options
1st	Chamber Paced	O = None, A = Atrium, V = Ventricle, D = Dual (A+V)
2nd	Chamber Sensed	O, A, V, D
3rd	Response to Sensing	O = None, T = Triggered, I = Inhibited, D = Dual (T + I)
4th	Rate Modulation	O = None, R = Rate-responsive
5th	Multisite Pacing	O = None, A, V, D

Rate modulation- allows the pacemaker to increase the pacing rate during exercise or stress by detecting body motion or respiration.

Common Pacemaker Modes

VVI	Ventricle paced, ventricle sensed, pacing inhibited if native beat sensed
AAI	Atrium paced and sensed, pacing inhibited by native atrial activity
DDD	Both chambers paced and sensed; response is dual (trigger or inhibit as needed)
VOO	Ventricle paced only, no sensing (asynchronous) – used during surgery

- DDD mode standard of care
- VVI- in permanent AF
- AAI- Sick sinus syndrome with normal AV conduction

Choice of pacing mode

- **Dual-chamber pacing with DDD mode** is the **standard of care** in almost all patients
- Patients with permanent atrial fibrillation and AV block, where atrial sensing is not required, single-chamber pacing with VVI mode is preferred
- AAI pacing (atrial only) is preferred in some patients with sick sinus syndrome with normal AV nodal conduction

Pacemaker syndrome

- Atrioventricular dysynchrony in patients with single-chamber ventricular pacing (VVI) causing heart failure
- Atria contracts against closed valves and loss of atrial kick
- Dual-chamber pacing with DDD mode is preferred to prevent pacemaker syndrome

Pacing-induced cardiomyopathy

- Pacing via the RV septum, the ventricular depolarisation spreads via the myocardium and causes ventricular dysynchrony (LBBB)
- This leads to ventricular dysfunction in the long run
- This led to the concept of conduction system pacing (more physiological)

Conduction system pacing (CSP)

Directly pacing at the conduction system to achieve a more synchronous/physiological ventricular activation

Advantages

- Preserves **narrow QRS** and **ventricular synchrony**
- Prevents or reverses **pacing-induced cardiomyopathy**

Types of CSP:

His Bundle Pacing (HBP)	Direct pacing of the His bundle
Left Bundle Branch Area Pacing (LBBAP)	Pacing near/in the left bundle branch

Current Indications:

- Patients with **AV block** needing permanent pacing
- Patients with **heart failure and LBBB** (as an alternative to CRT)
- Patients with previous **RV pacing–induced cardiomyopath**

43. Cardiac Physiology

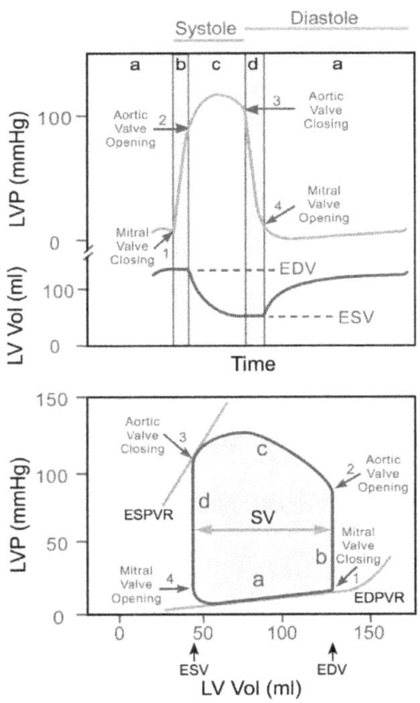

- Width of loop – suggest stroke volume
- Area of loop- suggest stroke work
- **ESPVR** –Best load-independent measure of cardiac contractility

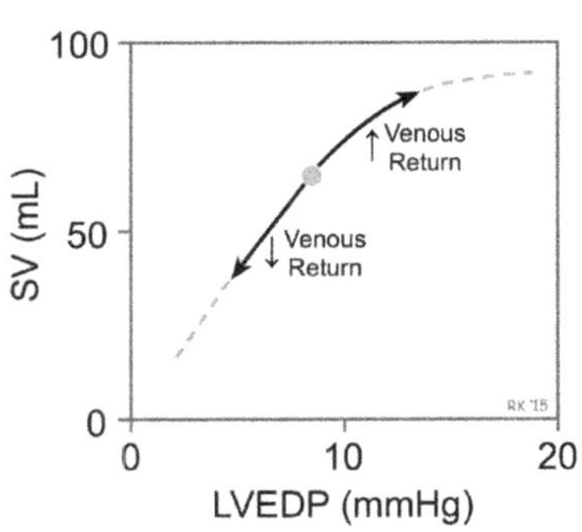

I. Cardiac pressure-volume loop (p-v loop)

- Left ventricular pressure plotted against left ventricular volume during complete cardiac cycle to produce the PV loop.
- Provide many physiological properties of the ventricle.

A single cardiac cycle is divided into four stages.

- **Ventricular filling** (a)

  mitral valve open, aortic valve closed; ventricular pressure rises slowly with an increase in volume.

- **Isovolumetric contraction** (b)

  Both valves are closed, and pressure rises while volume remains constant till the opening of the aortic valve.

- **Ejection** (c)

  The aortic valve opens and mitral valve closes; ventricular pressure increases with a decrease in volume.

- **Isovolumetric relaxation** (d)

  Both valves are closed, and pressure decreases without a change in volume.

ESPVR (End Systolic Pressure Volume Relationship)

The slope of the curve at end diastole represents the inotropic (systolic) state of the ventricle.

Decreases in the slope of ESPVR suggest a decrease in contractility.

EDPVR (End Diastolic Pressure Volume Relationship)

The slope of the curve at end diastole represents ventricular compliance. (lusiotropy)

An increase in slope suggests a less compliant ventricle (e.g. HCM

Frank Starling's law

- The stroke volume of the heart increases in response to an increase in the volume of blood in the ventricles, before contraction (LVEDV)

<table>
<tr><th>Systolic dysfunction (DCMP)</th><th>Diastolic dysfunction (HCM, RCM)</th></tr>
<tr><td>Decrease in slope of ESPVR</td><td>Increase in slope of EDPVR</td></tr>
<tr><td>Shift of PV loop to right and width reduced</td><td>Position remains same width reduced</td></tr>
<tr><td>Increase in end diastolic and end systolic volume and low stroke volume</td><td>Decrease in end diastolic volume and stroke volume</td></tr>
<tr><td>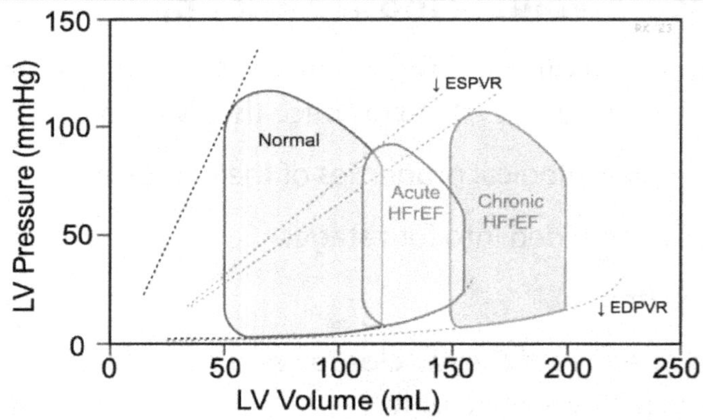
</td><td>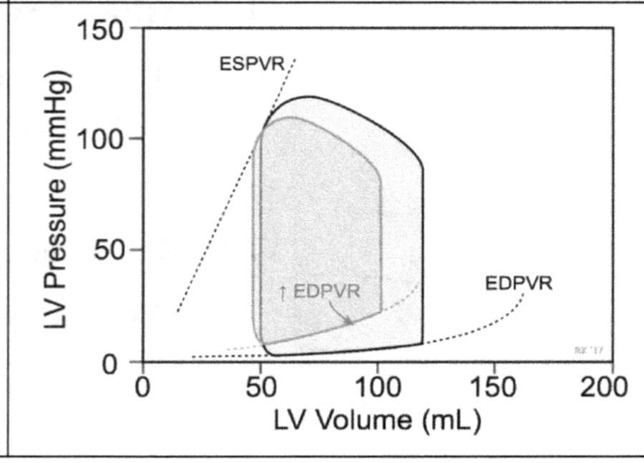
</td></tr>
</table>

PV loop pictures adapted from cardiovascular physiology concepts by Richard E Klabunde

II. Action potential

- The action potential of cardiac myocytes is different from that of pacemaker cells (SA node, AV node)

Cardiac myocyte action potential

- **Phase 4 (Resting Potential):** The cell is at rest, with a membrane potential of approximately -90 mV. This is maintained primarily by an **outward flow of potassium (K+) ions** through potassium channels.
- **Phase 0 (Rapid Depolarisation):** Opening of fast voltage-gated **sodium (Na+) channels**, rapid influx of sodium ions. This rapid inflow causes the membrane potential to become positive, creating the "spike" of the action potential.
- **Phase 1 (Initial Repolarisation):** The fast sodium channels inactivate, and a transient outward **potassium (K+)** current opens. This brief outward movement of positive ions causes a small drop in the membrane potential.
- **Phase 2 (Plateau Phase):** It is caused by the balance between two opposing currents: a slow, inward flow of **calcium (Ca2+) ions** through L-type calcium channels and a continued outward flow of **potassium (K+**) ions. This plateau prolongs the action potential, which in turn prolongs the refractory period, preventing the heart muscle from being restimulated too quickly and allowing for a coordinated, effective contraction.
- **Phase 3 (Repolarisation):** The L-type calcium channels close, voltage-gated **potassium (K+) channels** open, causing a strong, outward flow of potassium ions.

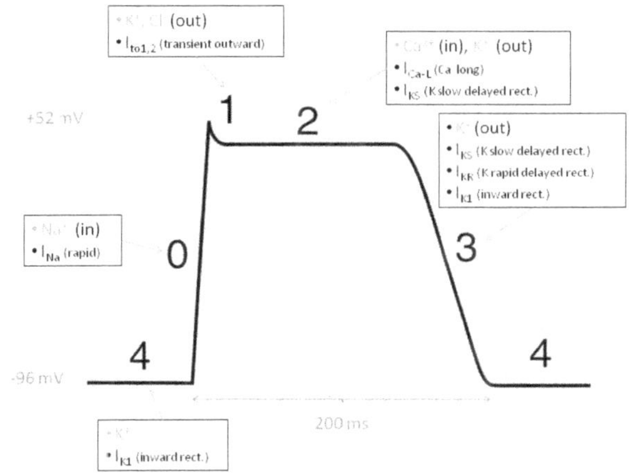

Pacemaker Action Potential

The action potential in pacemaker cells (SA node) is different. They have a characteristic **automaticity**, meaning they can spontaneously generate their own action potentials without an external stimulus.

- **Phase 4 (Spontaneous Depolarisation):** Pacemaker cells do not have a stable resting potential. Instead, they exhibit a slow depolarisation, or "pacemaker potential." This is caused by a slow inward current of sodium ions, often called the "funny current" (If). As the membrane potential slowly becomes more positive, it approaches the threshold for the next phase.
- **Phase 0 (Depolarisation):** When the threshold is reached, voltage-gated L-type **calcium (Ca2+) channels** open, and the influx of calcium ions causes the rapid upstroke of the action potential. This upstroke is not as steep as in contractile cells because calcium channels open more slowly than sodium channels.
- **Phase 3 (Repolarisation):** Voltage-gated **potassium (K+) channels** open, leading to a net outward flow of potassium ions that brings the membrane potential back to its most negative point before the next spontaneous depolarisation begins.

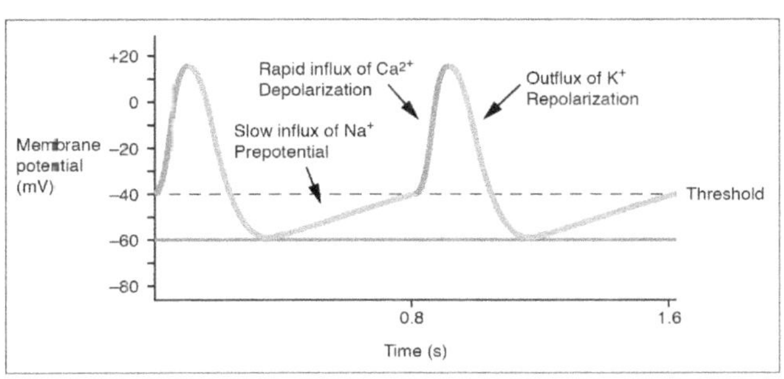

Phase 4 is solely responsible for cardiac automaticity. There are no phase 1 and 2 in automatic cells.

The slope of phase 0 determines the conduction velocity of the myocyte.

Treppe phenomena/Staircase effect/Bowditch effect

- Increased force of contraction with an increase in heart rate (force frequency relationship)
- This is secondary to the rise in intracellular calcium load in a healthy heart
- This effect is absent in a failing heart

Bezold Zarisch Reflex

- The cardioinhibitory vagal reflex, as bradycardia, vasodilation, and hypotension, results from stimulation of cardiac mechanoreceptors in the left ventricle. Usually triggered by myocardial ischemia (mostly inferior wall MI), intra-arterial nitroglycerin, and neuraxial anaesthesia.

Anrep effect

- Increased afterload → ↑ contractility (homeometric autoregulation)

Laplace law

- Wall stress = (Pressure × Radius) / (2 × Wall thickness).
- Explains LV hypertrophy with chronic pressure overload

Windkessel effect

- Elastic recoil of aorta maintains diastolic flow.

Bainbridge reflex

- Venous return → stretch RA → ↑ HR (via vagal inhibition).

Keep in mind **Wiggers' diagram** of the cardiac cycle to have a comprehensive idea of the pressure change in different chambers during the cardiac cycle

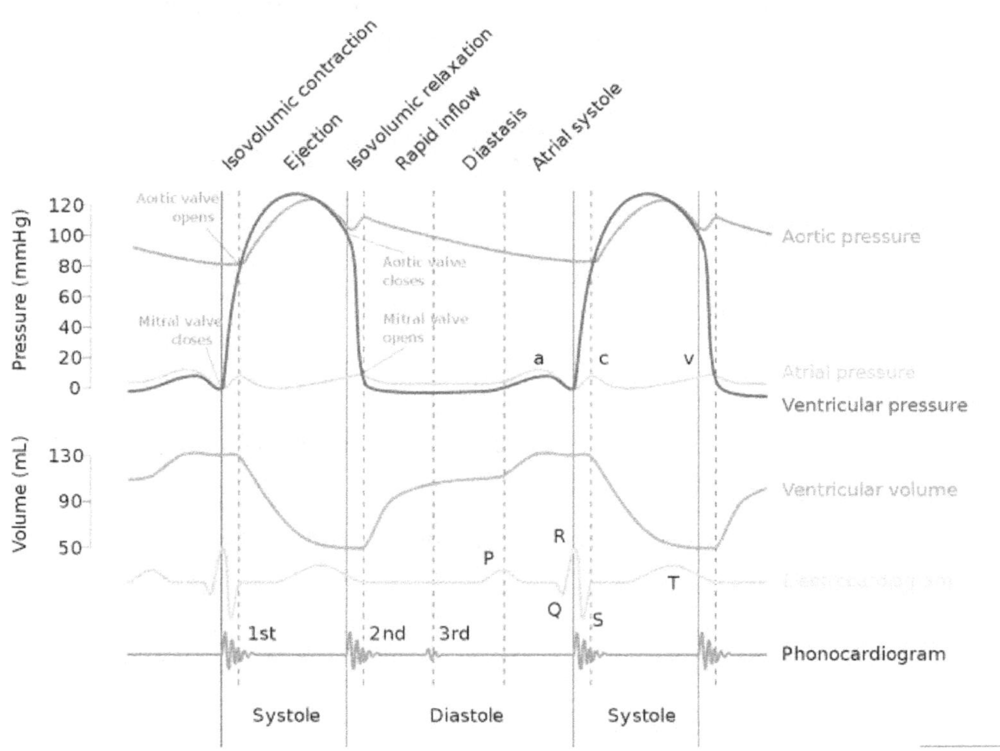

44. Miscellaneous Topics

1. Endothelial function test

Endothelial dysfunction, an early sign of atherosclerosis and a strong predictor of future cardiovascular events. This is primarily characterised by reduced bioavailability of nitric oxide (NO), a vital vasodilator.

- Most tests quantify the ability of blood vessels to dilate in response to stimuli that normally cause the endothelium to release NO. A blunted or paradoxical response (vasoconstriction) indicates dysfunction.

Non-Invasive Methods

- **Flow-Mediated Dilation (FMD):** Uses high-resolution ultrasound to measure the diameter change in a major conduit artery, typically the brachial artery, following a temporary occlusion of blood flow (reactive hyperemia).
- **Peripheral Arterial Tonometry (PAT):** Measures changes in the pulse wave amplitude in the finger during reactive hyperemia, reflecting microvascular function.

Invasive Method (Coronary Circulation):

- **Intracoronary Acetylcholine Testing:** Used in a catheterisation lab to assess coronary artery diameter changes in response to an infused drug (acetylcholine), considered the gold standard for directly assessing coronary endothelial function. Normal response is vasodilation with acetylcholine, and there is vasoconstriction with endothelial dysfunction

Pulse wave velocity (PWV)

- PWV is the speed at which the pressure wave, generated by the heart's contraction, travels along the arteries. **A higher** PWV indicates **stiffer** arteries, meaning they have lost elasticity.
- **Pulse Wave Velocity (PWV)** is a measure of **arterial stiffness** and an independent predictor of cardiovascular risk.
- **Measurement:**
    - Carotid-Femoral PWV (cfPWV). This is calculated by dividing the distance between the carotid artery and the femoral artery by the time delay it takes for the pulse wave to travel that distance.
    - brachial-ankle PWV (baPWV)

2. Anticoagulation in AF post-PCI/ACS patients

- Anticoagulation (NOAC/VKA) has better stroke prevention potential than antiplatelets in patients with AF.
- DAPT has shown benefit in the prevention of recurrent MI/stent thrombosis/ mortality in ACS/ post-PCI patients
- However, when patients have both conditions, combining DAPT with anticoagulation (triple therapy) is associated with a very high bleeding risk.

- In such patients
  - Triple therapy (aspirin+clopidogrel+OAC) for 1-4 weeks
  - Dual therapy (OAC +clopidogrel)- for 6month-1 year
  - NOAC/ OAC only- after 1 yea

3. Mechanism of arrhythmia

Enhanced automaticity	Re-entry	Triggered activity	
		EAD	DAD
• EAT, MAT • AIVR • Parasystole	• Scar VT • Atrial flutter • AVRT/AVNRT • Fascicular VT • Brugada • (phase II re-entry)	• LQT/Torsades	• CPVT • Digoxin toxicity • Outflow VT • RVOT/LVOT VT

- DC Cardioversion usually terminates re-entry arrhythmia. Enhanced automaticity usually does not respond to DC cardioversion
- Adenosine, a potent and short-acting AV nodal blocker, terminates arrhythmias involving the AV node, such as AVNRT/AVRT

4. Drug interactions in cardiology

- **Warfarin + Amiodarone**
  - Amiodarone inhibits CYP2C9, leading to decreased warfarin metabolism and increased INR/ bleeding risk. Reduce the warfarin dose by 30-50%.
- **Clopidogrel + Omeprazole/esomeprazole**
  - Omeprazole inhibits CYP2C19 and reduces clopidogrel activation. This combination should be avoided.
- **Amiodarone + Digoxin**
  - P-gp inhibition by amiodarone leads to increased digoxin levels. Reduce the digoxin dose and monitor digoxin level.
- **Statin (simvastatin/lovastatin) + Amiodarone**
  - Amiodarone inhibits statin metabolism (CYP3A4) and increases the chance of myopathy
- **DOACs (apixaban/rivaroxaban) + ritonavir/ketoconazole**
  - Strong P-gp/CYP3A4 inhibitors decrease metabolism and increase the risk of bleeding

- **Statin (simvastatin/lovastatin) and CYP3A4 inhibitors**
  - Increase statin level and myopathy
- **Loop diuretics + digoxin**
  - Hypokalemia/hypomagnesemia caused by loop diuretics increases the chance of digoxin toxicity
- **Beta blocker, CCB and digoxin**
  - Risk of severe bradycardia
- **Nitrate with PDE4 inhibitor (Sildenafil)**
  - Risk of severe hypotension

5. Metabolic syndrome

Defined as **three or more** of the following five risk factors (based on National Cholesterol Education Program, NCEP-ATP III):

Risk Factor	Defining Measurement
Abdominal Obesity	≥ **40 inches** (102 cm) for men or ≥ **35 inches** (88 cm) for women
Elevated Triglycerides	≥ **150 mg/dL** (1.7 mmol/L) or being on medication for high triglycerides.
Low HDL	< **40 mg/dL** for men or < **50 mg/dL** for women, or being on medication for low HDL.
High Blood Pressure	≥ **130/85 mm Hg** or being on medication for high blood pressure.
Elevated Fasting Glucose	≥ **100 mg/dL** (5.6 mmol/L) or being on medication for high blood glucose.

6. Anticoagulants

i. Indirect Thrombin Inhibitors

A. Unfractionated Heparin (UFH)

- Source: Animal origin (porcine/bovine mucosa).
- **Mechanism:** Binds to **antithrombin III** → accelerates its action → inhibits **thrombin (IIa)** and **factor Xa.**
- **Administration:** IV or SC (not oral).
- **Monitoring:** aPTT (target 1.5–2.5× control). Unpredictable dose response and need monitoring with apTT
- **Adverse effects:**
  - Bleeding
  - Heparin-induced thrombocytopenia (HIT type II)
  - Osteoporosis (long-term)
- **Antidote:** Protamine sulfate.

B. Low Molecular Weight Heparins (LMWHs)

- Examples: **Enoxaparin, Dalteparin, Tinzaparin**.
- **Mechanism:** Preferentially inhibits **factor Xa** > thrombin.
- **Advantages:** Predictable dose-response, less HIT, no need for routine monitoring.
- **Antidote:** Partial reversal by protamine.

C. Fondaparinux

- Synthetic pentasaccharide; selectively inhibits **factor Xa** via antithrombin.
- **No antidote**; minimal risk of HIT.

ii. Vitamin K Antagonists

Warfarin, Acenocoumarol

- **Mechanism:** Inhibits **vitamin K epoxide reductase,** blocking synthesis of **vitamin K-dependent factors II, VII, IX, X** and proteins C, S.
- **Onset:** Delayed (36–72 hrs) due to existing clotting factors.
- **Monitoring:** INR (therapeutic range 2–3; 2.5–3.5 for mechanical valves).
- **Adverse effects:**
  - Bleeding
  - Skin necrosis (due to protein C depletion)
  - Teratogenicity (contraindicated in pregnancy)
- **Antidote:** Vitamin K, Fresh frozen plasma (FFP), or Prothrombin complex concentrate (PCC).

iii. Direct Oral Anticoagulants (DOACs / NOACs)

A. Direct Thrombin Inhibitor:

- **Dabigatran** (oral prodrug)
- **Mechanism:** Directly inhibits **thrombin (IIa)** → prevents fibrin formation and platelet activation.
- **Antidote:** Idarucizumab.

B. Direct Factor Xa Inhibitors:

- **Rivaroxaban, Apixaban, Edoxaban, Betrixaban**
- **Mechanism:** Directly inhibits **factor Xa** (free and clot-bound).
- **Advantages:**
  - Rapid onset/offset
  - Fixed dose, no monitoring
  - Fewer drug/food interactions
- **Antidote:** Andexanet alfa.

iv. Parenteral Direct Thrombin Inhibitors

- **Bivalirudin, Argatroban, Lepirudin**
- Used mainly in **HIT** and **PCI** settings.
- **Monitoring:** aPTT.
- **No specific antidote** (short half-life).

7. Universal definition of MI (Fourth Universal Definition of Myocardial Infarction 2018)

The clinical criteria for an **acute MI** require the detection of a **rise and/or fall** of cardiac troponin (cTn) values, with at least one value above the **99th percentile Upper Reference Limit (URL)**, AND at least one of the following:

1. Symptoms of acute myocardial ischemia (e.g., chest pain, shortness of breath).
2. New ischemic ECG changes (e.g., new ST-T wave changes or new left bundle branch block).
3. Development of pathological Q waves on the ECG.
4. Imaging evidence of new loss of viable myocardium or new regional wall motion abnormality in a pattern consistent with an ischemic aetiology.
5. Identification of a coronary thrombus by angiography (including intracoronary imaging) or by autopsy.

Clinical classification

MI Type	Underlying **Mechanism**
Type 1	**Spontaneous MI** related to a primary coronary event, such as plaque rupture/erosion
Type 2	**Secondary to Ischemic Imbalance** due to oxygen supply/demand mismatch, unrelated to acute plaque instability. Examples include coronary spasm, embolism, severe anaemia, sustained tachyarrhythmia, or hypotension.
Type 3	**Sudden unexpected cardiac death.**
Type 4	**MI Related to Coronary Intervention**
Type 4a	MI related to **Percutaneous Coronary Intervention (PCI).**
Type 4b	MI related to **Stent Thrombosis.**
Type 4c	MI related to **Restenosis** after PCI.
Type 5	MI related to **Coronary Artery Bypass Grafting (CABG)** surgery.

8. Coarctation of the aorta

- **Congenital narrowing of the aortic lumen**, usually located just distal to the origin of the **left subclavian artery** near the **ductus arteriosus** (juxtaductal region).
- **Accounts for 5-8% congenital heart disease**
- **Common association**
    - **Bicuspid aortic valve is associated with 50-60% of CoA**

- **Turner syndrome**
- **Intracranial aneurysms and risk of**

- Varied clinical presentation
  - Shock in a neonate
  - Uncontrolled upper limb hypertension (an important cause of secondary hypertension in adults)
  - Heart failure in adults, if untreated
  - Risk of aortic aneurysm and dissection
- Management
  - Surgical repair in neonate/childhood
  - Balloon dilation/stent in adult
- Persistent hypertension even after repair/surgery in some patients

9. Supravalvular aortic stenosis

- Narrowing of the aorta just above the aortic valve
- **Common causes**
  - **Williams syndrome-** microdeletion of chromosome 7/mutation of the elastin gene, Elfin facies, mild intellectual disability
  - **Familial hypercholesterolemia-** deposition of lipids along the ascending aortic wall
- **Coanda sign-** Differential Blood Pressure in arm-significantly higher systolic blood pressure in the right arm compared to the left arm due to preferential streaming of blood after stenosis towards the right subclavian.
- Surgical repair is the treatment of choice

10. CABG (Coronary artery bypass graft) Summary

CABG is a **surgical revascularisation procedure** designed to restore blood flow to ischemic myocardium by bypassing obstructed coronary arteries using **arterial or venous grafts**

- Indications
  - Complex triple vessel disease/left main stenosis
  - Diabetes with multivessel disease
  - Ischemic cardiomyopathy (severe CAD with reduced LV ejection fraction)

Types of grafts

Arterial Grafts:

- **Left Internal Mammary Artery (LIMA):** gold standard; most commonly anastomosed to LAD. Patency >90% at 10 years.

- **Right Internal Mammary Artery (RIMA):** used for additional targets; bilateral use increases sternal wound risk.
- **Radial Artery:** good long-term patency if the target vessel has >70% stenosis; requires perioperative calcium channel blockers to prevent spasm.
- **Gastroepiploic Artery:** used occasionally for inferior wall targets.

Venous Grafts:

- **Great Saphenous Vein (GSV):** easy to harvest but prone to intimal hyperplasia and atherosclerosis; 10-year patency ~50%.
- **Small saphenous or arm veins** are rarely used.

Surgical Techniques

- **On-pump CABG:** traditional method using cardiopulmonary bypass; the heart is arrested with cardioplegia. Provides a stable field and complete revascularisation.
- **Off-pump CABG (OPCAB):** performed on a beating heart without bypass; reduces systemic inflammation and renal/neuro complications, but is technically more challenging.
- **Minimally invasive or robotic CABG:** used for isolated LAD lesions or hybrid revascularisation with PCI.

11. Cardioplegia

Induced, reversible **cardiac arrest** during surgery to provide a still, bloodless field and **protect the myocardium** from ischemia.

- **Mechanism:** High-potassium solution causes **diastolic arrest** by membrane depolarisation; **hypothermia** lowers metabolic demand.
- **Goals:** Reduce oxygen consumption, preserve ATP, limit ischemic and reperfusion injury.

Types:

- **By composition:** *Crystalloid* (e.g., St. Thomas) or blood cardioplegia (better oxygen and buffering).
- **By temperature:** *Cold (4–10°C)* most common; warm for reperfusion or intermittent use.
- **By route:** *Antegrade* (aortic root), retrograde (coronary sinus), or *combined.*
- **By dosing:** Intermittent, continuous, or single-dose (e.g., Custodiol HTK).

Key components: High K^+, Mg^{2+}, buffers, glucose, minimal Ca^{2+}, ± lidocaine/mannitol

12. Primary prevention of CVD

Risk Assessment

- Use the **ASCVD Risk score**(10-year risk of MI, stroke, or cardiovascular death).
- Reassess every **4–6 years** in adults aged **40–75 years**.

- **Risk categories (ACC/AHA 2019–2024):**
  - **Low:** <5%
  - **Borderline:** 5–7.4%
  - **Intermediate:** 7.5–19.9%
  - **High:** ≥20%

Management

Lifestyle Measures (First-line for all)

- **Healthy diet:** Mediterranean or DASH diet.
- **Physical activity:** ≥150 min/week of moderate or 75 min/week of vigorous exercise.
- **Weight:** Maintain BMI < 25 kg/m^2.
- **Avoid tobacco and limit alcohol.**
- **BP control:** Target <130/80 mmHg.
- **Glycemic control:** HbA1c <7% (if diabetic).

Pharmacotherapy

A. Statins

- **High-intensity statin:**
  - For adults 40–75 years with **LDL-C ≥190 mg/dL**, **diabetes**, or **10-year ASCVD ≥ 20%.**
- **Moderate-intensity statin:**
  - For **intermediate-risk (7.5–19.9%)** after shared decision-making.
- **Consider the CAC score** if low/moderate risk score:
  - CAC = 0 → may defer statin (unless diabetes, smoking, family history).
  - CAC ≥ 100 → statin indicated.

B. Aspirin (2022 USPSTF & ACC/AHA updates)

- **Routine aspirin NOT recommended** for primary prevention due to bleeding risk.
- **Consider low-dose aspirin (75–100 mg/day)** only if:
  - Age **40–70 years,**
  - **High ASCVD risk** but **low bleeding risk.**
- **Avoid** in adults >70 years or with any **increased bleeding risk** (GI bleed, CKD, anticoagulant

45. ECG in ACS

The culprit vessel for MI is predicted based on the ST-elevation pattern. ST-depression is not a good predictor of the culprit vessel.

- Identification of the culprit vessel helps in planning PCI in an emergency setting
- ST elevation criteria

New ST elevation at the J-point in **≥2 contiguous leads**:

- **≥ 1 mm (0.1 mV)** in all leads other than V2–V3
- **≥ 2 mm in men ≥40 yrs**, ≥ **2.5 mm in men <40 yrs**, ≥ **1.5 mm in women** (V2–V3)

Infarct Site	ST Elevation	Reciprocal Depression	Likely Artery
Inferior	II, III, aVF	I,aVL	RCA (80%), LCx (20%)
Lateral	I, aVL, V5–V6	III, aVF	LCx, diagonal branch of LAD
Anteroseptal	V1–V3		LAD (proximal)
Anterolateral	V3–V6, I, aVL	III, aVF	LAD or LCx
Posterior	ST depression + tall R in V1–V3	ST elevation in V7–V9	RCA or LCx
Right ventricular (RV)	V3R–V6R (especially V4R)		Proximal RCA

Special ECG Patterns in Acute MI

Wellen's syndrome

- Deeply inverted or biphasic T waves in V2–V3 during the pain-free period. Suggestive of critical proximal LAD stenosis and requires prompt revascularisation.
- Wellens Type I- Biphasic T waves, Type II – Deep symmetric inverted T waves

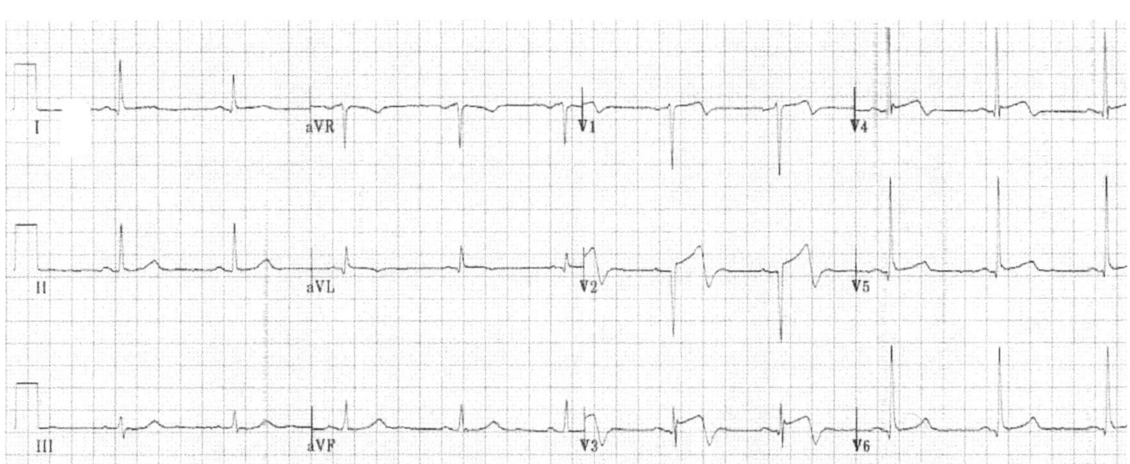

De winter pattern

- Up-sloping ST depression with tall symmetrical T in precordial leads. Suggestive of critical proximal LAD stenosis and requires prompt revascularisation.

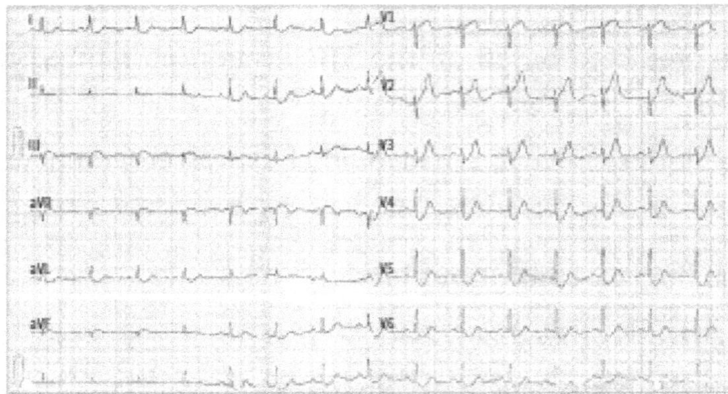

Posterior wall MI

- ST depression with tall R in V1–V3.
- Occlusive STEMI, which mimics NSTEMI with ST depression only
- Confirmed with ST elevation in posterior leads (V7–V9)

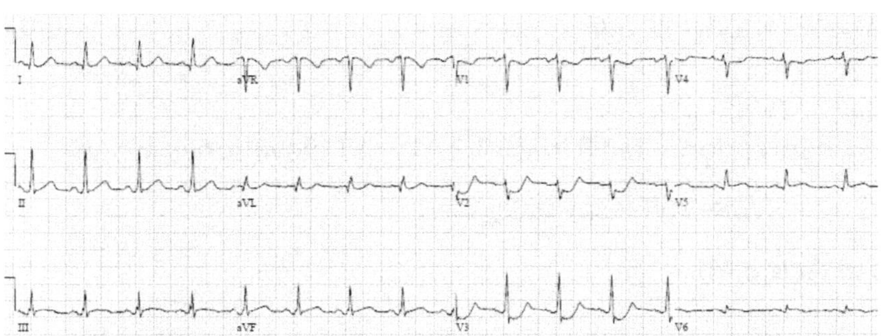

RV MI

- ST elevation in V4R, often with inferior MI
- Usually secondary to occlusion in the proximal RCA
- Management implications- when RV infarction is suspected in inferior MI, avoid nitrates and give IV fluid to maintain adequate preload.

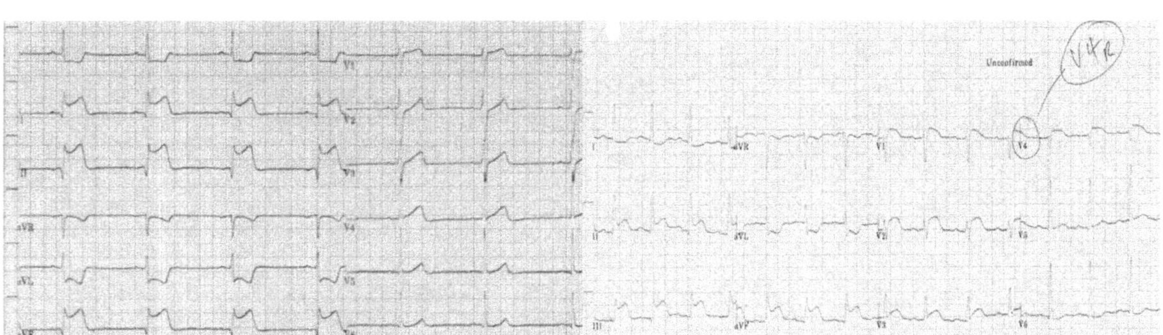

Left main disease/Triple vessel disease

- Diffuse ST depression + ST elevation in aVR/V1
- Suggestive of severe global myocardial ischemia secondary to Left main/severe triple vessel disease

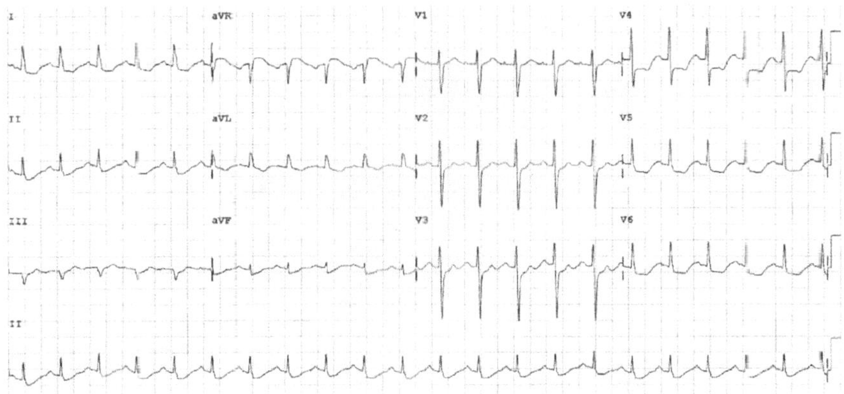

LBBB in MI (Sgarbossa Criteria)

- LBBB is normally associated with discordant ST-T changes and making it difficult to diagnose MI in the presence of LBBB
- **Sgarbossa Criteria-** to diagnose MI in the presence of MI

	Score
ST elevation ≥ 1 mm concordant (same direction as QRS) in any lead	5
ST depression ≥ 1 mm in V1–V3	3
ST elevation ≥ 5 mm discordant (opposite direction to QRS)	2

Score ≥ **3 points** → **diagnostic for MI** (specificity ~90%, sensitivity ~36%)

- Smith modified the 3rd criterion to → Discordant ST elevation with ST/S ratio ≥ 0.25 suggests MI

  Increase sensitivity
- RBBB does not cause much alteration in ST-T, and the diagnosis of MI is not problematic

ECG changes during childhood

- Normal HR in a neonate is 120-230 bpm and gradually decreases with age to reach the adult rate in 15 years
- Right axis deviation at birth. The axis becomes normal by 1y age [normal axis at birth is abnormal]
- Dominant R in V1/ right precordial leads at birth. Normalises by 6 months to 8 years
- Q wave seen in inferior leads (II, III, aVF) & V5 V6 at birth s/o clockwise loop. Counter-clockwise loop (q in I, aVL) seen in AVSD, inlet VSD
- The T wave in lead V1 is upright at birth, becomes inverted by 7 days and persists till 7 years of age. An upright T wave in V1 during 7 days to 7 years suggests RVH

MCQ Level II

401. False about Lutembacher syndrome?

   A. ASD ameliorates the clinical signs of MS

   B. MS ameliorates features of ASD

   C. More chance of developing AF

   D. Soft mid-diastolic murmur and OS

402. False statement regarding BAV?

   A. Aortopathy is related to the severity of AS/AR

   B. Right and left cusp fusion is the most common type

   C. Type of fusion and presence of raphe affect outcome

   D. Associated coarctation of the aorta increases the chances of aortic dissection

403. Causes of supraventricular tachycardia with a wide QRS complex, all except?

   A. AF with WPW

   B. AF with bundle branch block

   C. Antidromic AVRT

   D. Orthodromic AVRT

404. Which of the following characteristics doesn't differentiate between AVNRT and AVRT?

   A. Pre-excitation in baseline ECG

   B. Very fast tachycardia

   C. RP<PR interval

   D. P wave over the ST segment

405. Which of the following doesn't differentiate the CCP from the RCMP?

   A. Equalisation of filling pressure

   B. Significant elevation of JVP

   C. Systolic area index

   D. Exaggerated ventricular interdependence

406. False about LQTS?

   A. Triggered activity underlies arrhythmogenesis

   B. Prolonged action potential duration

   C. Transmural dispersion of repolarisation

   D. Sympathetic stimulation reduces arrhythmogenic potential

407. False statement regarding management of Torsades de Pointes (polymorphic VT with LQT)?
   A. Amiodarone is the antiarrhythmic drug of choice
   B. Magnesium is helpful in acute settings
   C. Beta blocker and ICD in congenital LQTs
   D. Temporary pacing and isoproterenol help to suppress bradycardia-induced polymorphic VT

408. False statement regarding Short QT syndrome
   A. Decrease the incidence of AF
   B. Predisposes to VF and sudden cardiac death
   C. Digitalis can cause acquired SQT
   D. KCNH2 mutation-gain of function & Quinidine-treatment of choice

409. False about Brugada syndrome?
   A. Sodium channel blockade unmask ECG sign
   B. Phase-3 re-entry
   C. RVOT ablation is a treatment option
   D. Quinidine suppresses recurrent VT

410. In which inherited arrhythmia is RF ablation a therapeutic option?
   A. Brugada
   B. SQTS
   C. LQTS
   D. CPVT

411. False statement regarding early repolarisation syndrome
   A. Spectrum of J-wave syndrome
   B. ER pattern common in anterior and lateral leads
   C. Quinidine is useful in recurrent VT/VF
   D. ICD indicated for secondary prophylaxis

412. True statement regarding idiopathic VT?
   A. Poor response to ablation therapy
   B. Fascicular VT responds to verapamil
   C. Associated with myocardial scar
   D. ECG has no localising value

413. False statement regarding LQTS?

A. Post-partum period triggers in LQT2

B. Beta blockers are more effective in LQT1

C. Genetics determines outcome

D. AR inheritance common

414. False statement regarding the genetics of LQTS?

A. Mutation-specific triggers for ventricular arrhythmia

B. The efficacy of beta-blocker therapy doesn't depend upon genotype

C. ECG pattern depends upon genotype

D. Ranolazine as genotype-targeted therapy for LQT3

415. AAD of choice in Atrial fibrillation with pre-excitation?

A. Amiodarone

B. Procainamide

C. Digoxin

D. Adenosine

416. Commonest cause of severe pulmonary stenosis?

A. Congenital

B. RHD

C. Carcinoid syndrome

D. Noonan syndrome

417. Melody value is used in?

A. Transcatheter pulmonary valve replacement

B. Surgical AVR

C. Transcatheter AVR

D. Valved VSD patch closure

418. Critical pulmonary stenosis in a neonate, the treatment of choice is?

A. Pulmonary valve balloon dilation

B. Surgical valvotomy

C. Shunt surgery

D. PGE infusion

419. Cause of supravalvular pulmonary stenosis?

   A. Alagille syndrome

   B. William syndrome

   C. Noonan syndrome

   D. All of the above

420. Which of the following ECHO parameters doesn't differentiate pseudo-normal from normal diastolic function?

   A. E/e' ratio

   B. E/A ratio

   C. Pulmonary vein Doppler

   D. Flow propagation velocity

421. Wrong statement regarding physiology of diastolic dysfunction?

   A. Hypertension is a common predisposition

   B. Increased filling pressure

   C. LA size usually remains normal

   D. Reduced annular velocities during diastole

422. False statement regarding omega-3-FA?

   A. The REDUCE-IT trial didn't show any cardiovascular benefit of 4gm of EPA

   B. EPA & DHA are two common omega-3-FA

   C. Marine fish are exclusive source of omega-3-FA

   D. The STRENGTH trial was neutral about the cardiovascular benefit of omega-3-FA

423. False statement about alcohol septal ablation for HCM?

   A. More chances of causing LBBB

   B. Contrast ECHO useful

   C. Done in symptomatic LVOT obstruction

   D. Absolute alcohol is injected in the septal branch of LAD

424. False statement about SGLT2 inhibitor?

   A. Sotagliflozin inhibits both SGLT2 &SGLT1

   B. Cardioprotective effect in patients without DM

   C. Hypotension as a side effect

   D. Not recommended in patients without DM

425. PET-CT useful in cardiology in all except?

A. Myocardial viability

B. Prosthetic valve IE

C. Cardiac sarcoidosis

D. Cardiac amyloidosis

426. False statement regarding primary prevention of CVD?

A. The ASCVD risk score is useful

B. CAC for risk stratification of high-risk

C. Statins most useful drug

D. Aspirin may be used

427. Very high risk for pregnancy, all except?

A. Eisenmenger syndrome

B. Aortic aneurysm

C. Severe MR

D. Severe PAH

428. False statement about BNP &pro-BNP?

A. NT pro-BNP levels are usually not elevated in HFpEF

B. Reduced level in obesity

C. NT pro-BNP is more useful in patients on ARNI

D. Protective in heart failure

429. Exercise ECG not advised in?

A. Atypical chest pain

B. Baseline normal ECG

C. Severe asymptomatic AS

D. Acute coronary syndrome

430. False statement regarding exercise ECG?

A. Good prognostic value and poor diagnostic value

B. Exercise-induced hypotension indicates underlying severe CAD

C. Baseline ST-T changes are a relative contraindication

D. Better modality to diagnose obstructive CAD than stress echocardiography

431. False statement regarding mechanical complications of acute MI?

A. Increased mortality

B. Free wall rupture is most fatal

C. Loud murmur in ventr cular septal rupture

D. Pansystolic murmur in papillary muscle rupture

432. False statement about flecainide?

A. First choice in structural heart disease in VT

B. A sodium channel blocker

C. Contraindicated in patients with coronary artery disease

D. Less propensity for QT prolongation

433. The wrong matching of the action potential of the cardiac myocyte?

A. Stage 0- Fast inward Na channel

B. Stage 1- Transient outward K channel

C. Stage 2- Inward Ca channel

D. Stage 3- Outward. Na channel

434. Incorrectly matched the cerivative of the pharyngeal arch vessel?

A. 3rd arch- common carotid

B. Left 4th arch- arch of the aorta

C. Left 6th arch- subclavian artery

D. 5th arch vessel- disappear

435. Which vein continues as the coronary sinus?

A. Great cardiac vein

B. Middle cardiac vein

C. Great coronary vein

D. Vein of Marshall

436. The second heart field develops into?

A. Left atrium

B. Left ventricle

C. Mitral valve

D. Aortopulmonary trunk

437. False statement regarding the embryology of the cardiovascular system?

A. The oblique vein of Marshall is the remnant of the vitelline vein

B. Pulmonary veins are responsible for the development of the left atrium

C. Sinus venosus develops into the smooth part of the right atrium

D. Migration of neural crest cells is important for the outflow tract development

438. False about supravalvular aortic stenosis?

A. Left upper limb blood pressure is higher

B. LVH seen

C. William syndrome common

D. Maybe associated with peripheral PS

439. Cardioprotective antidiabetic drug, all except?

A. Empagliflozin

B. Pioglitazone

C. Sitagliptin

D. Insulin

440. False statement about Coarctation of Aorta?

A. Less often associated with BAV

B. Surgery is the treatment of choice in infants

C. Associated with an intracranial berry aneurysm

D. Rib notching is less common in infants

441. BAV false statement?

A. Aortopathy is proportionate to the severity of the valvular lesion

B. TAVI can be done

C. Presents younger than degenerative AS

D. Right and left cusp fusion is the most common

442. False statement regarding hang-out interval?

A. Depends on the capacitance of circulation

B. Depends on the resistance of circulation

C. Shorter for pulmonary circulation than systemic

D. Explain the basis of the second heart sound (S2) split

443. High-sensitivity troponin (Hs troponin) false statement?

A. More sensitive assay method

B. More likely to detect troponin levels in normal people

C. Most useful in an emergency setting

D. Less negative predictive value

444. False statement about iFR?

A. Correlates well with FFR

B. Adenosine is needed for maximum hyperemia

C. DEFINE-FLAIR study supported the role of iFR

D. Wave free period used

445. False statement about Eisenmenger syndrome?

A. Anticoagulation commonly prescribed

B. Pulmonary vasodilators useful

C. Closure of the shunt is an absolute contraindication

D. Reversal of the shunt

446. Metabolic alkalosis is common with the use of?

A. Loop diuretics

B. Metformin

C. Statin

D. I/V beta blocker

447. False about the condition shown in the X-ray of an infant?

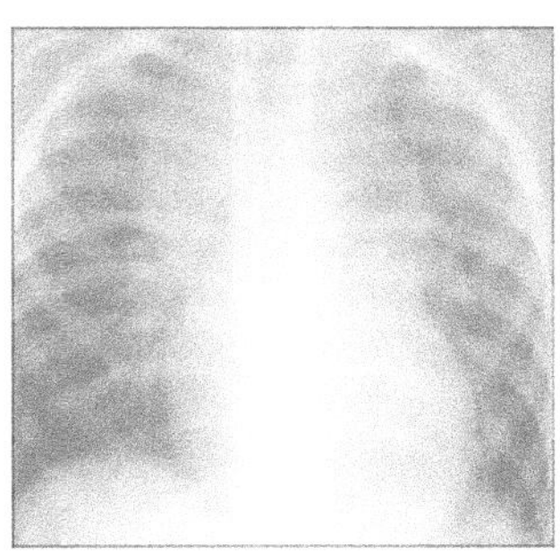

A. Similar oxygen saturation in all four cardiac chambers

B. Heart failure is common

C. The infracardiac type is the most common

D. Infracardiac type is usually obstructive

448. Fontan surgery is contraindicated in?

   A. Low PVRI

   B. Severe LV dysfunction

   C. Sinus rhythm

   D. Competent AV valve

449. Which is considered a management option for HOCM

   A. High-dose beta blocker

   B. Avoid diuretics

   C. Avoid vasodilators

   D. All of these

450. Which of the following is not considered a high-risk factor for SCD in patients with HCM

   A. LVOT gradient of more than 40 mm Hg

   B. Massive LVH

   C. LGE burden > 15 %

   D. Hypotension with exercise

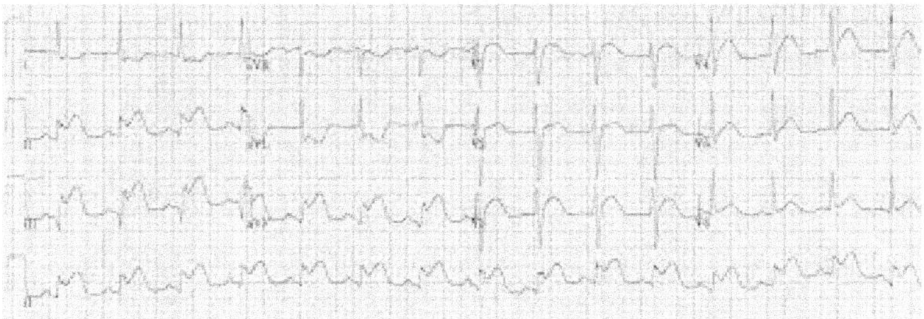

451. A patient with an acute onset of rest angina comes to the emergency room with the following ECG. What is the likely culprit occluded artery?

   A. Proximal RCA

   B. Proximal LAD

   C. Mid LAD

   D. Circumflex artery

452. A patient with an acute onset of rest angina and an episode of syncope comes to the emergency room with a heart rate of 35 beats/minute. What is the likely culprit artery occlusion?

   A. RCA

   B. Proximal LAD

   C. LCX

   D. Diagonal artery

453. A 40-year-old male had one episode of unstable tachycardia requiring defibrillation. ECG during and after defibrillation is shown below. What is the next best management strategy

   A. Check electrolyte

   B. Early RF ablation

   C. Chronic beta-blocker therapy

   D. Amiodarone

454. A 34-year-old female presented with multiple episodes of syncope with the following ECG. The most likely diagnosis is

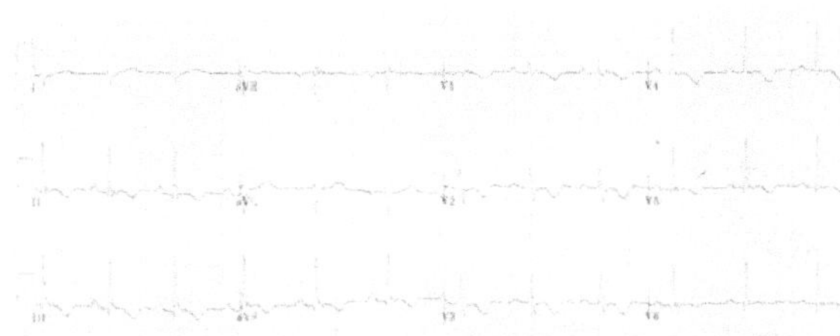

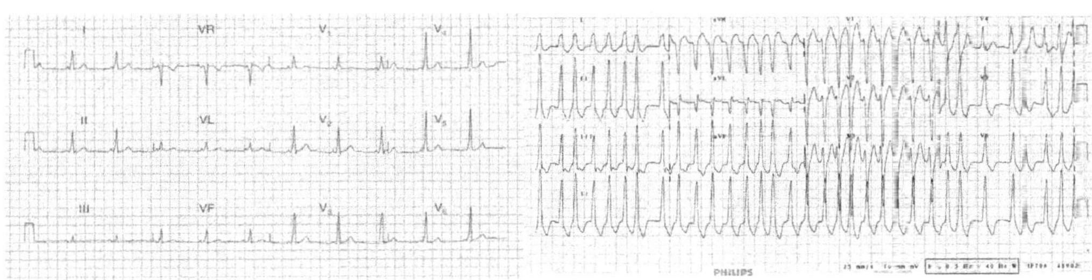

   A. RVOT VT

   B. ARVC

   C. HCM

   D. Ebstein anomaly

455. A 26-year-old male presented with multiple episodes of syncope with the following ECG. The drug of choice for this condition is

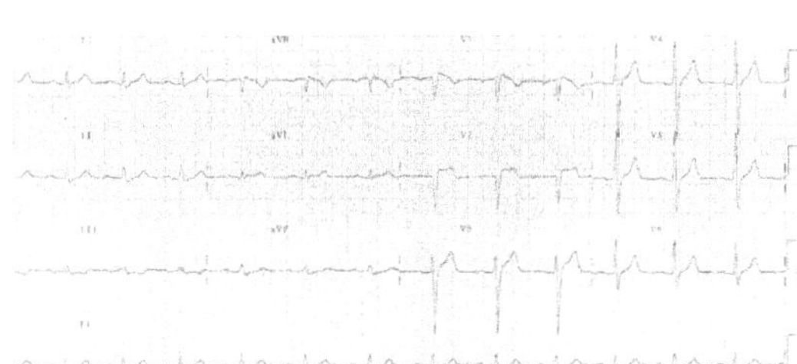

   A. Quinidine

   B. Procainamide

   C. Amiodarone

   D. Metoprolol

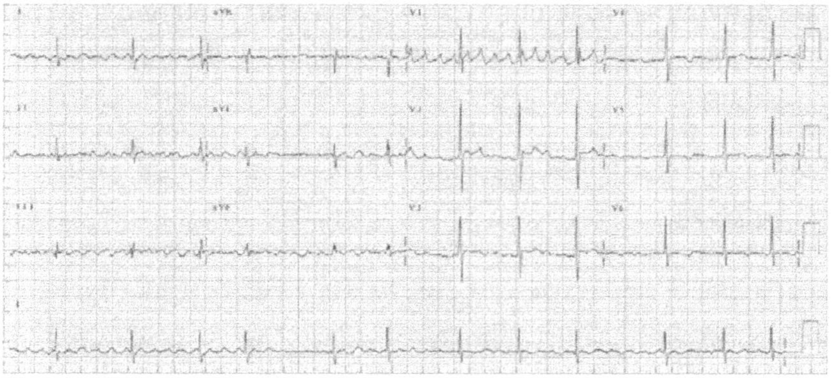

456. All are true about LQT3, except

A. Gain-of-function Na channel

B. Exercise precipitates syncope

C. Beta blockers are less useful

D. Long ST segment with narrow-based T wave

457. This is a 33-year-old female with a history of multiple episodes of self-limiting palpitations. The ECG during the OPD visit is shown below. The most likely diagnosis is

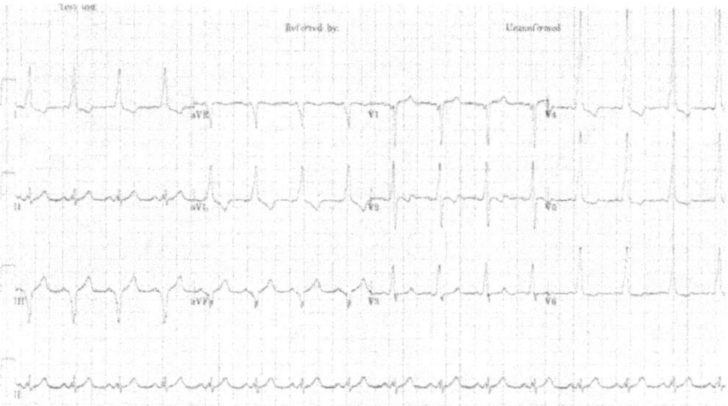

A. AVRT

B. AVNRT

C. EAT

D. AF-FVR

458. A 34-year-old female with progressive dyspnea for the last 10 years now came with worsening symptoms and the following ECG. The most likely diagnosis is-

A. Atrial fibrillation

B. Atrial flutter

C. MAT

D. EAT

459. A 29-year-old male came to the emergency with palpitation for the last 4 hours in a hemodynamically stable condition. What is the preferred drug in this condition?

A. Amiodarone

B. Procainamide

C. Digoxin

D. Flecainide

460. Which of the following veins accompanies left anterior descending artery

A. Middle cardiac vein

B. Great cardiac vein

C. Vein of Marshall

D. Anterior cardiac vein

461. A patient with severe mitral stenosis had an episode of dizziness with vomiting. ECG recorded at the casualty shown below. What is the most likely diagnosis?

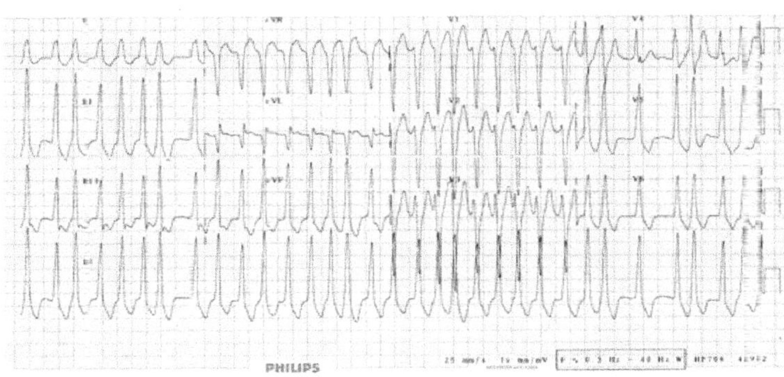

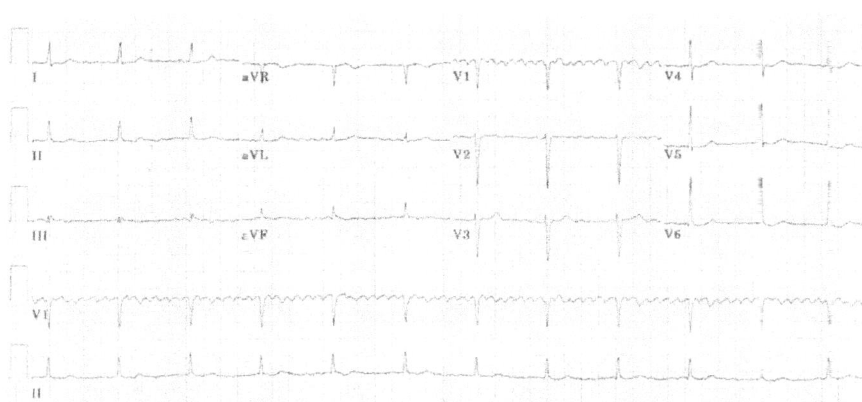

A. Cerebral embolism

B. Complete heart block

C. New onset atrial fibrillation

D. Digoxin toxicity

462. Wrong statement regarding the following ECG pattern

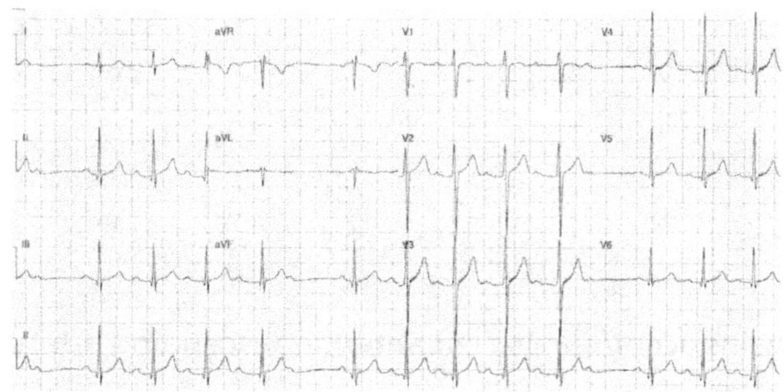

A. It can be physiological in athletes

B. Needs a permanent pacemaker if associated with syncope

C. The site of block is usually in the His-Purkinje system

D. Progressive prolongation of the PR interval

463. Which of the following is not a hemodynamic consequence of the device shown below

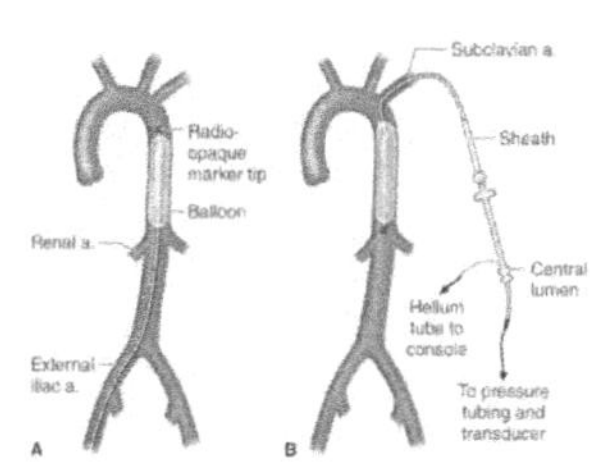

A. Increase SBP

B. Increase DBP

C. Increase MAP

D. Increase CO

464. ECG finding indicates

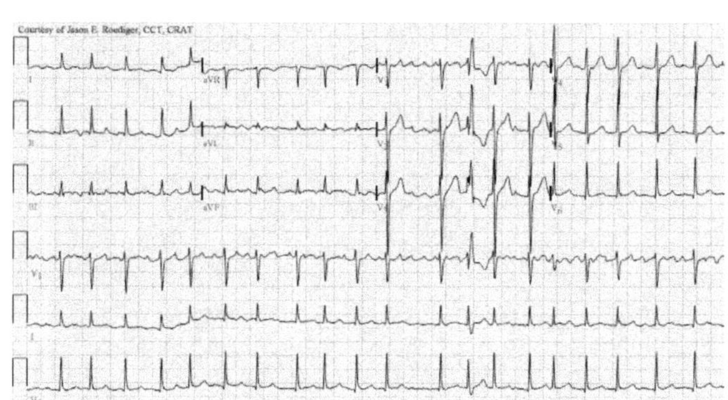

A. Bowditch phenomena

B. Ashman phenomena

C. Wenkebach phenomena

D. De-Winter phenomena

465. A 47-year-old male with recent febrile illness presents with progressive dyspnoea and orthopnea for the last few days. The ECG obtained in the casualty is shown below. What should be the appropriate next step for this patient?

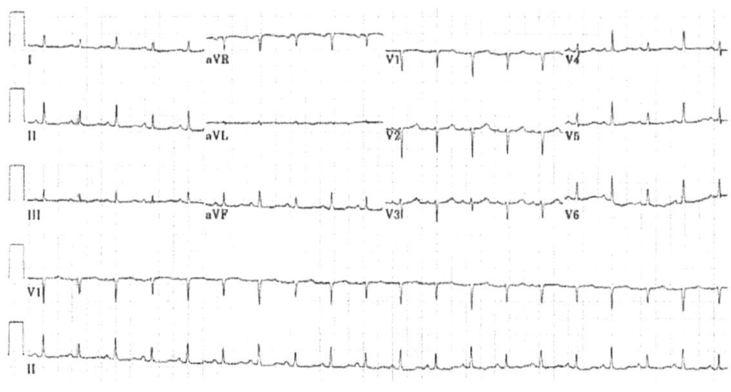

A. CT chest

B. Cardiac MRI

C. Endocardial biopsy

D. pericardiocentesis

466. A 32-year-old primigravida in the first trimester of pregnancy visited for consultation regarding anticoagulation. She had undergone cardiac surgery with a mitral mechanical prosthesis 2 years back and was taking warfarin 4mg daily. Her current INR is 2.7. What should be the next step

A. Continue the same dose of warfarin

B. Switch to heparin

C. Switch to Dabigatran

D. Switch to bivalirudin

467. A 50-year-old male with recurrent vomiting and the following ECG in the casualty. What should be the next step in management?

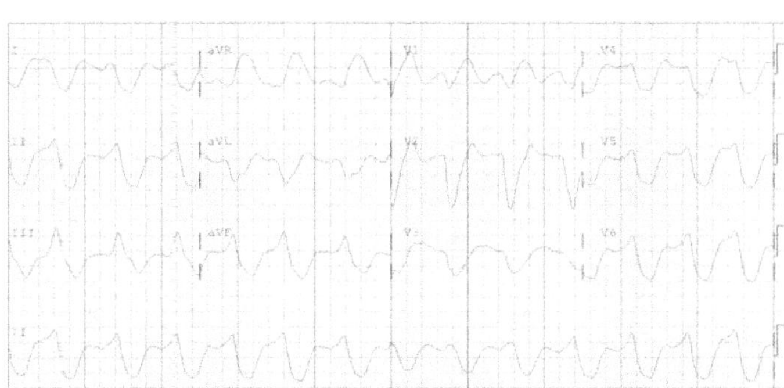

A. IV Calcium gluconate

B. Insulin and dextrose solution

C. IV Glucagon

D. IV Atropine

468. The following ECG recorded in a patient with STEMI after thrombolysis suggests

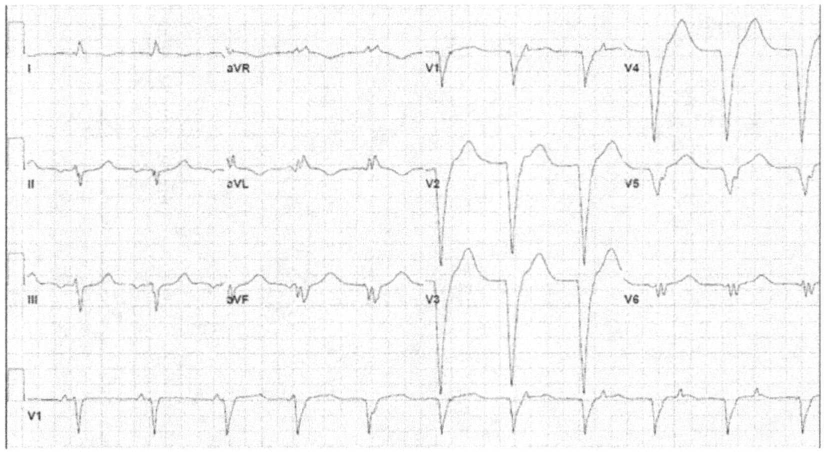

A. Ventricular tachycardia

B. Complete heart block

C. Accelerated idioventricular rhythm

D. VT

469. A 30-year-old female visited the emergency department with retrosternal chest pain worsening on deep inspiration. The initial ECG is shown below. What should be the next plan

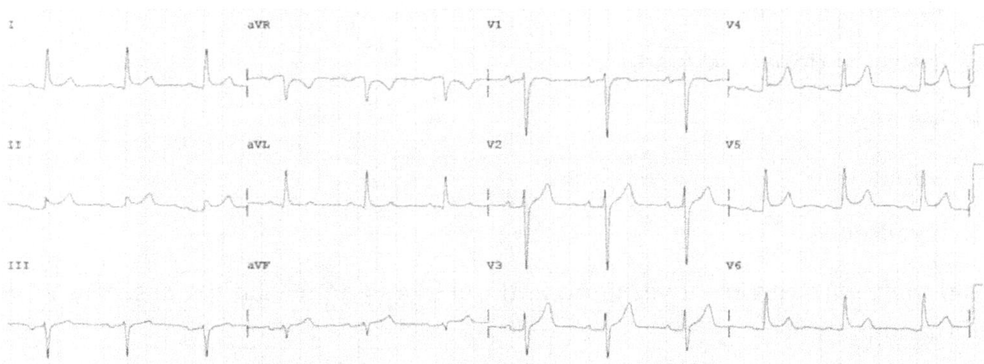

A. Primary angioplasty

B. NSAID

C. Ceftriaxone

D. pericardiocentesis

470. A 55-year-old female had multiple episodes of dizziness and one episode of fainting at rest. Holter monitoring showed the following findings. She will require

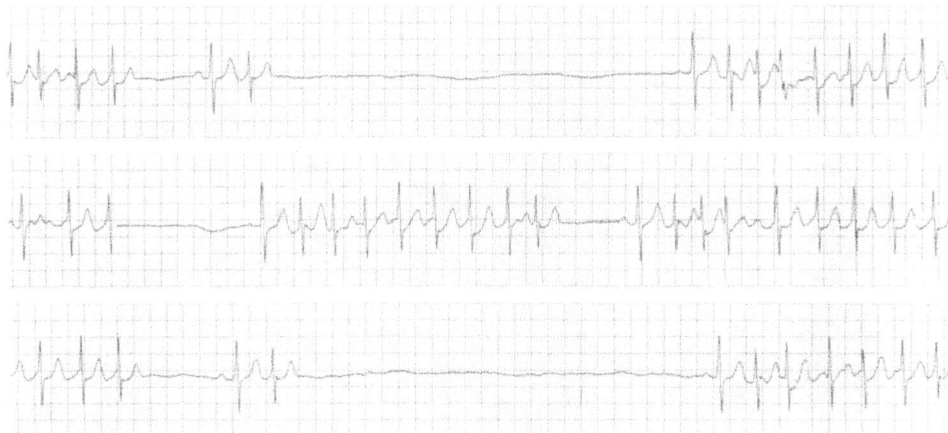

A. Medical observation

B. Permanent pacemaker

C. AICD

D. Orciprenaline

471. Mismatch in perfusion and metabolism scan in cardiac PET suggests

A. Hibernating myocardium

B. Scarred myocardium

C. Normal myocardium

D. All of these

472. Which is a SPECT tracer for myocardial perfusion imaging

A. Thallium

B. N-ammonia

C. 18FDG

D. 82 Rubidium

473. Myocardial PET is useful in

A. Viability assessment after MI

B. ATTR amyloidosis

C. Sarcoidosis

D. All of these

474. Which is not an advantage of 99Tc over Thallium for myocardial perfusion imaging

   A. Less radiation exposure

   B. Can assess viability

   C. No redistribution

   D. Imaging can be done hours after injection

475. The PLATO trial evaluated the efficacy of which drug

   A. Clopidogrel

   B. Ticagrelor

   C. Cangrelor

   D. Prasugrel

476. A false statement regarding the management of NSTEMI is

   A. Early invasive strategy preferred in high-risk patients

   B. GRACE score guides timing of revascularisation

   C. P2Y12 inhibitors are usually avoided before CAG

   D. 1-3 months DAPT preferred if PCI not done

477. The GRACE score is used for

   A. NSTEMI risk stratification

   B. Bleeding risk of DAPT

   C. Risk of stent thrombosis

   D. Anatomical complexity of CAD

478. Which of the following is considered as J wave syndrome

   A. Brugada

   B. Early repolarization

   C. Idiopathic VF

   D. All of these

479. The DK crush method is used for which type of coronary lesion

   A. Bifurcation

   B. Chronic total occlusion

   C. Acute total occlusion

   D. Tortuous artery

480. Permanent atrial fibrillation refers to

  A. AF more than 7 days

  B. AF persisting for more than 1 year

  C. AF where no rhythm control strategy planned

  D. AF in the presence of structural heart disease

481. Atrial fibrillation in one of the following conditions considered most dangerous

  A. Mitral stenosis

  B. Accessory pathway

  C. HOCM

  D. CHB

482. Which of the following DOACs is considered safer in the presence of renal dysfunction

  A. Apixaban

  B. Edoxaban

  C. Rivaroxaban

  D. Dabigatran

483. Which of the following DOACs has more GI bleeding as an adverse event

  A. Rivaroxaban

  B. Dabigatran

  C. Apixaban

  D. Edoxaban

484. False statement regarding DOAC

  A. Efficacy and safety studied in non-valvular AF

  B. No need for INR monitoring

  C. More risk of intracranial bleeding

  D. Reversal agent available

485. In which condition is long-term anticoagulation advised, irrespective of the CHADS-VAS score

  A. HOCM

  B. Hypertension

  C. Severe MR

  D. Mild MS

486. False statement regarding cardiac transplantation
   A. Post-transplantation 1-year survival is more than 90%
   B. Bi-atrial anastomosis is commonly done
   C. Sirolimus has been shown to reduce transplant vasculopathy
   D. The Allomap test is used to detect cellular rejection

487. Which of the following immunosuppressants has been shown to reduce transplant vasculopathy
   A. Sirolimus
   B. Tacrolimus
   C. Azathioprine
   D. ATG

488. Which of the following methods is used for assessing the effect of heparin during coronary intervention
   A. ACT
   B. APTT
   C. PT
   D. D-dimer level

489. The ACT level desired during coronary intervention is
   A. 250-300
   B. 100-150
   C. >400
   D. ACT monitoring not required

490. False statement regarding primary prevention of cardiovascular events
   A. ASCVD score assesses 10-year risk of MI/death
   B. Statin therapy guided by the ASCVD score
   C. CAC needs to better risk-stratify borderline risk individuals
   D. ASCVD score assesses the lifetime risk

491. Treatment of choice for CTEPH
   A. Pulmonary endarterectomy
   B. Riociguat
   C. Balloon pulmonary angioplasty
   D. Sildenafil

492. False statement regarding various types of lipids

   A. HDL has an inverse relation with CV disease

   B. LDL has a causal role in atherogenesis

   C. Direct LDL measurement is inaccurate in hypertriglyceridemia

   D. Fasting lipid profile has more prognostic significance than non-fasting evels

493. Which is not an indication for high-intensity statin

   A. LDL Cholesterol > 190 mg/dl

   B. Diagnosed ASCVD

   C. ASCVD score 7.5 %

   D. Homozygous familial hypercholesterolemia

494. Which is not a PCSK9 inhibitor

   A. Alirocumab

   B. Evolocumab

   C. Mipomersan

   D. Incliseran

495. Coronary Artery Calcium (CAC score) is useful in the risk stratification of

   A. High risk

   B. Borderline risk

   C. Low risk

   D. All of the above

496. Which is an option for the management of end-stage idiopathic PAH

   A. Lung transplantation

   B. Balloon atrial septostomy

   C. Pott shunt

   D. All of these

497. False statement regarding management of IPAH

   A. Routine anticoagulation is not useful

   B. A combination pulmonary vasodilators is inferior to monotherapy

   C. Calcium channel blockers help in vasoreactive PAH

   D. Balloon atrial septostomy is a palliative procedure

498. Which is an oral prostaglandin analogue approved for PAH

A. Selexipag

B. Riociguat

C. Tripostinil

D. Epoprostenol

499. False statement regarding prosthetic heart valves

A. Lifelong anticoagulation for mechanical valves

B. NOAC preferred over VKA

C. Durability is less with bioprosthetic valves

D. The Ross procedure involves an aortic autograft

500. Which of the following type of mechanical valve is most commonly used nowadays

A. Homograft

B. Ball in a cage

C. Monoleaflet mechanical

D. Bileaflet mechanical

501. Which is not an indication for IE prophylaxis

A. Unrepaired TOF

B. 3 months following ASD device closure

C. Previous episode of endocarditis

D. Restrictive VSD

502. Which of the following trial assessed the role of TAVI

A. PARTNER

B. ISCHEMIA

C. SPRINT

D. All of these

503. Which of the following cardiac tumor is commonly seen over the valve leaflets

A. Fibroelastoma

B. Mesothelioma

C. Myxoma

D. Metastatic deposits

504. False statement regarding cardiac myxoma

A. Fever and constitutional symptoms are common

B. Multiple tumours seen in the sporadic type

C. Surgery is the treatment of choice

D. High recurrence rate in familial tumours

505. False statement regarding stress testing in stable CAD

A. Exercise ECG has better diagnostic value than stress MPI

B. Exercise ECG should not be done when there are baseline ST-T changes

C. Functional capacity can be assessed in exercise ECG testing

D. Up-sloping ST depression can be normal

506. Functional capacity assessed during exercise ECG is measured in terms of

A. Woods unit

B. Metabolic equivalents

C. Peak vo2

D. Distance travelled

507. A poor response to CRT (cardiac resynchronisation therapy) is expected n all except

A. RBBB

B. CHB

C. Atrial fibrillation

D. Ventricular pacing <97%

508. Which of the following drug has shown CV benefit in patients with HFpEF?

A. SGLT2 inhibitor

B. ARNI

C. Beta blocker

D. Spironolactone

509. PA (pulmonary artery) banding is not useful in

A. DCM

B. D-TGA

C. CCTGA

D. Ebstein

510. A wrongly matched mechanism of action is

   A. Incliseran- PCSK9 inhibition

   B. Bempedoic acid- CETP Inhibition

   C. Rosuvastatin- HMGCoA inhibition

   D. Evolocumab- PCSK9 inhibition

511. Arterial pulse tracing is shown in the figure is seen in

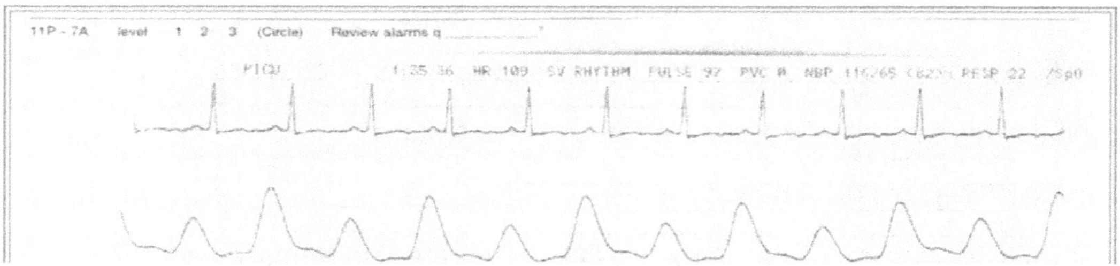

   A. LV failure

   B. Severe AR

   C. Cardiac tamponade

   D. hemopericardium

512. Which anticancer drug does not cause cardiomyopathy

   A. Cisplatin

   B. Cyclophosphamide

   C. Trastuzumab

   D. Herceptin

513. The wrong match is

   A. Mexiletine

   B. Verapamil

   C. Quinidine

   D. Propranolol

514. Sildenafil useful in

   A. CTEPH

   B. PVOD

   C. COPD

   D. PAH due to schistosomiasis

515. Which does not cause paradoxical embolism

   A. Platypnoea orthodeoxia

   B. PFO

   C. Pulmonary AV malformation

   D. Coronary sinus fistula

516. Early systolic murmur is seen in all except

   A. Acute MR

   B. Low-pressure TR

   C. Muscular VSD

   D. Aortic stenosis

517. Drug used as a "pill in pocket" in atrial fibrillation

   A. Amiodarone

   B. Propafenone

   C. Vernakalant

   D. Quinidine

518. Coronary myocardial oxygen consumption is

   A. 60-80 %

   B. 80-100%

   C. 20-30%

   D. 40-50%

519. Pregnancy well well-tolerated with

   A. Severe MS with MVA <1 cm^2

   B. PS with a gradient of 60 mm Hg

   C. ASD with severe PAH

   D. AS with a gradient of 60 mm Hg

520. Which of the following suggests inoperability in cardiac shunts

   A. Significant shunt murmur

   B. ECG -Katz Wachtel phenomena

   C. CXR- cardiomegaly

   D. Qp : Qs = 1.2

521. Large VSD is usually inoperable by

   A. Less than 6 months

   B. 2yrs

   C. 10yrs

   D. 20yrs

522. Juvenile mitral stenosis is associated with all except

   A. More subvalvular involvement

   B. More thromboembolism

   C. Rapid progression

   D. Severe PAH

523. All are predictors of chronic RHD following an episode of ARF except

   A. Severe arthritis

   B. Recurrent ARF

   C. CHF in the first episode

   D. Severe carditis

524. Balloon atrial septostomy is useful in all except

   A. TGA

   B. TAPVC

   C. End-stage idiopathic PAH

   D. Truncus arteriosus

525. Left heart disease presenting with early right heart failure

   A. Lutembacher syndrome

   B. AS +MS

   C. Severe MS

   D. Acute MR

526. The LODOCO trial was done to evaluate the role of

   A. Colchicine

   B. Canakimumab

   C. Methotrexate

   D. Trastuzumab

527. Diastolic flow reversal in DTA is seen in all except

A. Vein of Galen malformation

B. Abbernathy malformation

C. RSOV to RV

D. PDA

528. The REVEAL score is used for risk stratification of

A. PAH

B. PS

C. PTE

D. HOCM

529. All are associated with increased risk of thromboembolism except

A. Chicken wing LAA

B. LAA blood flow < 20 cm/s

C. Spontaneous echo contrast in LA

D. LAA thrombus

530. Which of the following trials involved a sham procedure for the evaluation of coronary revascularisation

A. ORBITA

B. COURAGE

C. ISCHEMIA

D. STITCH

531. Which of the following does not require exercise testing for provoking arrhythmia?

A. CPVT

B. Brugada

C. LQT

D. SQT

532. Which of the following is most frequently seen in children with long RP tachycardia

A. AVNRT

B. PJRT

C. JET

D. AVRT

533. A patient of DCMP with CHF was admitted with worsening dyspnea. Investigation reveals Na 128, K 3.4, and urea 69. All are correct except

A. Chronic hyponatremia has a poor prognosis

B. 3% saline can be infused slowly

C. Diuretics can be given

D. Can be volume repleted or depleted

534. Treatment options for diltiazem toxicity, all except

A. Inj calcium gluconate

B. Inj glucagon

C. Inj insulin

D. Inj aminophylline

535. Drug of choice for beta-blocker intoxication

A. Inj glucagon

B. Inj sodabicarbonate

C. Specific monoclonal ab

D. Idarucizumab

536. Relative risk of which of the following is highest with hypertension

A. Heart failure

B. Stroke

C. MI

D. Death

537. SGLT2 inhibitors – all are true except

A. Reduce mortality in HFrEF

B. Reduce CV mortality in HFpEF

C. Reduce stroke incidence

D. Should be avoided when GFR < 15

538. 70 yr old type 2 DM, all are considered as useful preventive measures except

A. Aspirin

B. Atorvastatin

C. Ramipril

D. SGLT2 inhibitor

539. Ideal gestational age to perform foetal echocardiography for congenital cardiac anomaly

    A. 18-22 week

    B. 20-24 week

    C. After 30 weeks

    D. First trimester

540. Risk stratification tool for asymptomatic WPW pattern in routine ECGs done by

    A. Holter

    B. Exercise testing

    C. EP study

    D. All of the above

541. HFrEF with renal dysfunction, the drug of choice is

    A. ACEI

    B. ARNI

    C. CCB

    D. Hydralazine and isosorbide dinitrate

542. In which of the conditions is pulsus paradoxus not seen in a patient with cardiac tamponade

    A. ASD

    B. Severe AR

    C. Both a and b

    D. None

543. In which of the following valvular heart diseases, surgery indicated even without symptoms

    A. Severe AR, EF >60%

    B. Severe AR, LVESD <50 mm

    C. Severe MR, LVESD <40mm

    D. Severe MR, EF <60%

544. Which of the following parameters not included in the Duke treadmill score

    A. Exercise duration

    B. ST deviation

    C. BP change

    D. Angina severity

545. Cyanotic spell in TOF precipitated by all except

A. Anaemia

B. Tachycardia

C. Phenylephrine

D. Fever

546. Character of vulnerable plaque, all except

A. Microcirculation

B. Macrophage infiltration

C. Large lipid core

D. High vascular smooth muscle

547. Drug contraindicated in pregnancy

A. Nifedipine

B. Labetalol

C. Hydralazine

D. Sodium nitroprusside

548. All are covered by the pericardium except

A. Left atrium

B. SVC

C. Right atrium

D. Right atrial appendage

549. False about the condition shown in the schematic diagram?

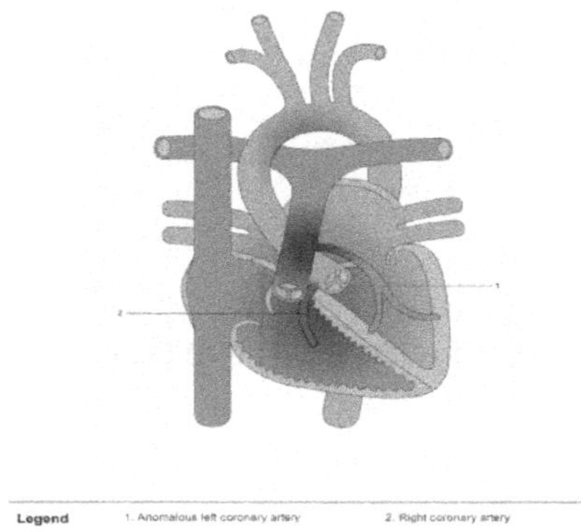

A. Heart failure a common presentation

B. Takeuchi repair done

C. ECG changes uncommon

D. Mimic dilated cardiomyopathy

550. Management option for late-presenting d-TGA

A. Atrial switch

B. Staged arterial switch

C. PDA stent

D. All of these

551. Pulmonary mitral continuity is seen in

A. TOF

B. D-TGA

C. Ebstein

D. Tricuspid atresia

552. Right heart catheterisation revealed Mean PA pressure of 45 mm Hg, Oxygen saturation of RA-67, PA-83, and Aorta-99. Qp: Qs =

A. 2

B. 3.2

C. 4

D. 1.2

553. Hoffman variant TOF, which is true

A. VSD is restrictive

B. PS is less severe

C. Pulmonary atresia

D. No aortic override

554. True about TOF with absent pulmonary valve-

A. Recurrent respiratory tract infection is common

B. PS usually severe

C. Mild PR seen

D. Pulmonary arteries are usually of normal size

555. False about primary hyperaldosteronism-

A. Adrenal adenoma common than hyperplasia

B. Spironolactone is the drug of choice

C. Aldosterone-renin ratio is a screening method

D. Hyperkalemia is common

556. False about heart failure pathogenesis

A. Increased SERCA activity

B. Decreased Beta-2 activity

C. Increased RyR activity

D. Reduced Na-K ATPase activity

557. A false statement about acute rheumatic fever is

A. More common in females

B. Long latent period for chorea

C. Secondary prevention with Penicillin reduces disease progression

D. Carditis is most common

558. False statement regarding anticoagulation in pregnancy

A. Heparin does not cross the placenta

B. Warfarin less than 5mg is safe in the first trimester

C. NOACs are safe in pregnancy

D. Wardarin crosses the placenta and causes embryopathy

559. ECG suggestive of-

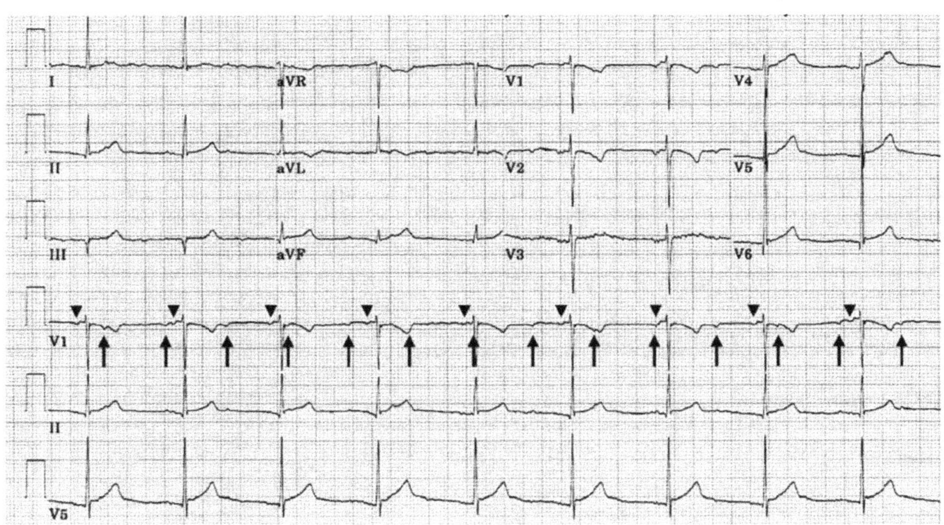

A. Post-cardiac transplantation

B. EAT

C. Wandering pacemaker

D. SA nodal exit block

560. A 34-year-old asymptomatic female found to have pulmonary stenosis (peak gradient 40mm Hg and mean 24mm Hg) during screening echocardiography before job recruitment. What is best management?

A. Clinical monitoring

B. Balloon dilation of PV

C. Surgery

D. Transcatheter PV replacement

561. False about coarctation of the aorta

A. Relief of coarctation usually normalises BP

B. Surgery is indicated in infants and neonates

C. Associated with IC aneurysms

D. Bicuspid aortic valve is a common association

562. Homograft not useful in

A. Arterial switch in TGA

B. Rastelli

C. Ross procedure

D. TOF with pulmonary atresia

563. Which is not true regarding coronary vasodilators

A. Regadenoson- newer selective A2a agonist

B. Adenosine- nonselective

C. Adenosine- short half-life

D. Regadenoson- more side effects

564. Correct order of consequence after myocardial ischemia

A. Diastolic dysfunction> systolic dysfunction> ECG change> chest pain

B. Systolic dysfunction> diastolic dysfunction> ECG change> chest pain

C. Chest pain> diastolic dysfunction> systolic dysfunction> ECG change

D. Chest pain> systolic dysfunction >diastolic dysfunction> ECG change

565. ISCHEMIA trial- false statement is

A. An ischemia-guided approach decreases mortality

B. ACS patients excluded

C. LM stenosis excluded

D. Randomised controlled trial

566. Load independent measure of cardiac contractility

A. Ejection fraction

B. Fractional shortening

C. Tei index

D. Isovolumetric relaxation time

567. A 3-month-old child was found to have rhabdomyoma on screening echo. What should be the next line of management?

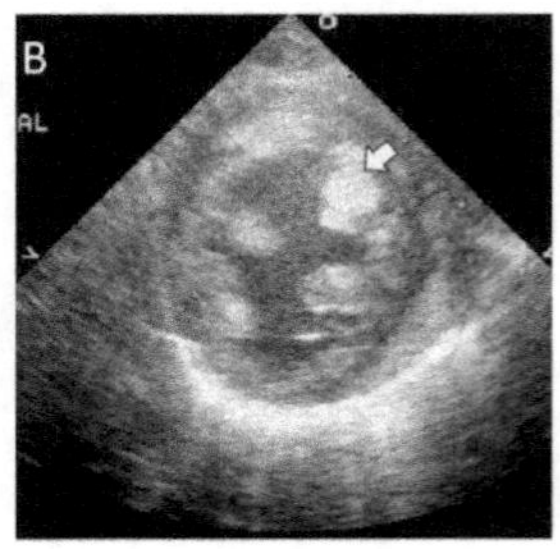

A. Emergency surgical excision

B. Elective surgical excision

C. Wait and watch with echocardiography monitoring

D. Chemotherapy

568. Patient with metastatic Ca breast presents with gross pericardial effusion and hypotension. Which is seen in the echo in this patient-

A. Systolic RV collapse

B. Decreased tricuspid respiratory variation

C. Increased mitral respiratory variation

D. Collapsed IVC

569. Correct about pulsus paradoxus

A. Exaggerated respiratory variation of systolic blood pressure

B. SBP fall of more than 18 mm Hg are significant

C. Seen even in the presence of severe AR

D. Needs invasive BP measurement

570. Mixed venous saturation 64%, aortic saturation 100%, and PA saturation 88%. What is the value of Qp: Qs

A. 3:1

B. 1:3

C. 2:1

D. 4:1

571. Very small VSD with jet velocity 2m/s. all are possible except

    A. Pulmonary hypertension

    B. Pulmonary stenosis

    C. Gerbode defect

    D. Double-chambered right ventricle

572. False statement in differentiating HCM Vs an athlete's heart

    A. LV cavity size is usually dilated with normal contractility and hypertrophy in athletes

    B. Diastolic dysfunction in HCM

    C. Abnormal ventricular strain parameters in athletes

    D. Increased ejection fraction in sarcomeric HCM

573. False statement regarding the physiological effect of isotonic and isometric exercise

    A. Isotonic exercise is associated with eccentric LVH

    B. Isometric exercise is associated with concentric LVH

    C. Isotonic exercise is associated with a decrease in peripheral resistance

    D. Isometric exercise is associated with a decrease in diastolic BP

574. Post PVC arterial pressure tracing is shown below. Diagnosis is

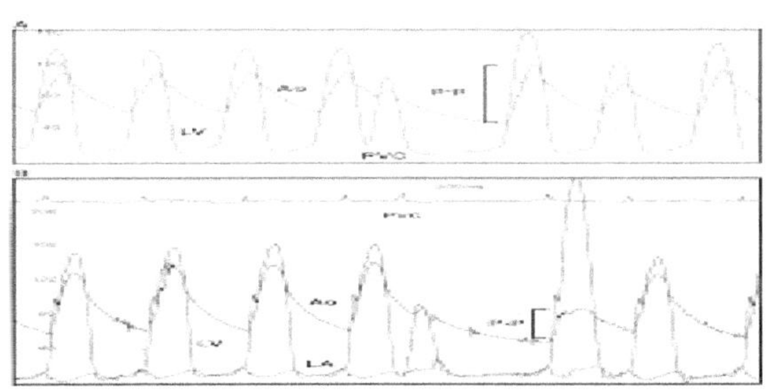

    A. Aortic stenosis

    B. HOCM

    C. HCM without obstruction

    D. Supravalvular AS

575. The wrong statement regarding the pericardium is

    A. Protects against unusual distension of cardiac chambers

    B. Congenital absence is usually fatal

    C. Supplied by the phrenic nerve

    D. Usually, 2-layered- serosal

576. Wrong statement regarding pericardiocentesis

A. Subxiphoid access is commonly done

B. Remove the pigtail once the drain output is 100ml /24hr

C. Echo guidance before drainage is a must

D. Drainage of hemopericardium is avoided if no hemodynamic compromise

577. Balloon atrial septostomy (BAS)- most commonly done in

A. D-TGA

B. Ebstein

C. Tricuspid atresia

D. TOF

578. Which is not a feature of RVH

A. Rsr with r >0.5mv

B. qR pattern in V1

C. p pulmonale

D. RAD

579. Wrong statement regarding CPVT

A. Early morning syncope at rest

B. RyR receptor mutation

C. Beta blocker useful

D. Bidirectional VT seen

580. The drug not useful in CPVT

A. Amiodarone

B. Carvedilol

C. Flecainide

D. Verapamil

581. Listeria endocarditis is common in

A. IV drug abuser

B. Dental procedure

C. Ureteric stent implantation

D. Prosthetic heart valve

582. A false statement regarding the SPRINT trial is

A. Reduction in CV mortality with aggressive BP control

B. Applicable to the non-diabetic population

C. Aggressive BP control is associated with more AKI

D. Aggressive SBP control to less than 120 mmHg in diabetics reduces CV mortality

583. True about FFR is

A. Depends on HR and BP

B. Less than 0.9 suggests significant stenosis

C. Depend upon the amount of viable myocardium supplied

D. NTG is used as a coronary vasodilator

584. Lung uptake during stress thallium indicates

A. Raised LVEDP

B. Pulmonary parenchymal disease

C. Pulmonary hypertension

D. Alveolar hemorrhage

585. False statement regarding adequate chest compression as per the ACLS guideline

A. 80-100 per minute

B. 5-6 cm depth compression

C. Compression ventilation ratio 30:2 without an advanced airway

D. One breath every 6 seconds with an advanced airway

586. Thrill in the left 2nd intercostal space in a patient with ASD is seen in all except

A. Associated with severe MR

B. Lutembacher

C. Associated PS

D. Eisenmenger syndrome

587. PCI in a patient with stable CAD is done mainly for

A. Reduce sudden death

B. Reduce MI

C. Angina relief

D. Prevent LV dysfunction

588. False statement regarding aortic stenosis echocardiography

A. Peak instantaneous gradient measured by echocardiography

B. Peak-to-peak gradient measured by cardiac catheterisation

C. Peak instantaneous gradient is usually less than the peak-to-peak gradient

D. Severe AS can be there with a low gradient

589. Contraindication to rotational atherectomy

A. SVG graft

B. Ostial lesion

C. Superficial calcium

D. Bifurcation stenosis

590. All are true about HITT except

A. Early HIT good prognosis

B. Platelet transfusion crucial

C. PF4 assay is used for diagnosis

D. Thrombogenic tendency despite low platelet count

591. Acute heart failure in a 50-year-old male and X-ray chest showing pulmonary oedema without cardiomegaly. The most probable cause is

A. Multivalvular heart disease

B. Hypertensive heart disease

C. Pneumonia

D. Pulmonary embolism

592. ECG in a patient with a structurally normal heart and h/o syncope is shown below. The next plan is

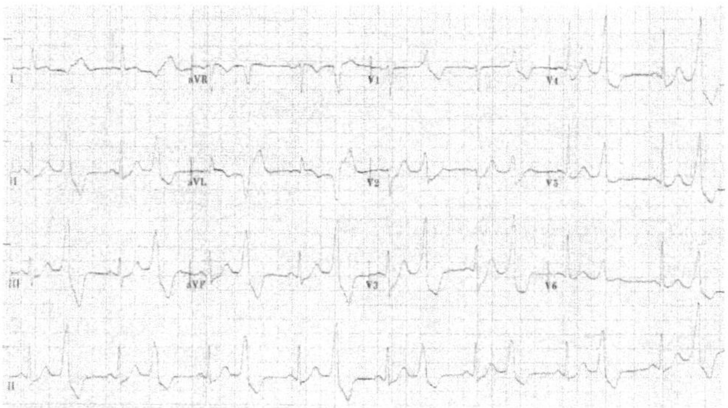

A. EPS

B. HUTT

C. TMT

D. CAG

593. Cardiac surgery is not possible on a beating heart in

A. Aortic arch repair

B. Closed mitral valvotomy

C. Pericardiectomy

D. CABG

594. Pregnancy with heart disease, all are true except

A. Caesarean section is usually preferred

B. Pulmonary oedema is common after delivery

C. Blood loss is more with CS than with vaginal delivery

D. Increased risk of aortic dissection

595. A false statement regarding primary PCI is

A. Superior to thrombolysis if the window period is less than 12 hours

B. Culprit artery only revascularisation if hemodynamically unstable

C. Complete revascularisation can be done if hemodynamically stable

D. Routine thrombus aspiration decreases mortality

596. TOTAL trial in coronary intervention is

A. Rheolytic thrombectomy done

B. Mortality benefit

C. Manual thrombectomy useful

D. Increases stroke risk

597. INVICTUS trial

A. Warfarin is superior to rivaroxaban in rheumatic AF

B. Warfarin is non-inferior to dabigatran in patients with a mechanical heart valve

C. Warfarin is non-inferior to clopidogrel in mild DVT

D. Warfarin is superior to rivaroxaban in non-valvular AF

598. The most sensitive modality to detect cardiac allogenic vasculopathy

A. IVUS

B. Angiography

C. CT angiography

D. Dobutamine stress echocardiography

599. Which is a high-risk feature in a patient with asymptomatic WPW pattern in the ECG
   A. SPERRI during AF < 250ms
   B. Sudden loss of preexcitation during TMT
   C. Intermittent preexcitation
   D. Refractory period of bypass tract > 250 ms
600. Which is not a treatment option for ATTR amyloidosis
   A. Tafamidis
   B. Patisiran
   C. Mipomersan
   D. Inotersan
601. False statement regarding sitosterolemia
   A. LDL levels elevated
   B. Statins as first-line treatment
   C. Dietary restriction useful
   D. Episodes of hemolysis seen
602. False statement regarding management of homozygous familial hypercholesterolemia
   A. Statin as first-line therapy
   B. PCSK9 inhibitors are useful in the LDL receptor null variant
   C. LDL apheresis useful
   D. Liver transplant in the late stage
603. Which of the following factor is not considered while choosing between a mechanical and a bioprosthetic valve
   A. Contraindication to anticoagulation
   B. Life expectancy
   C. History of endocarditis
   D. planning of pregnancy
604. False statement regarding the cardiac neoplasm
   A. More recurrence with familial myxoma
   B. Rhabdomyoma may regress completely
   C. Melanoma most common cause of secondary
   D. Papillary fibroelastoma usually involves the papillary muscle of the mitral valve

605. Young boy with a history of syncope and following ECG. What is the next best investigation

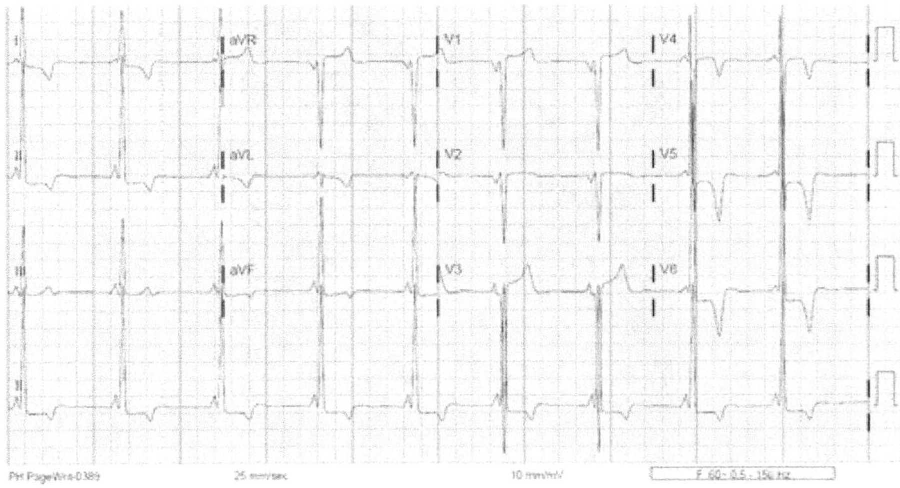

A. 24hr holter monitoring

B. CT angiography

C. EP study

D. Cardiac MRI

606. False statement regarding mechanical circulatory support

A. IABP increases systolic BP

B. Impella increases stroke volume

C. VV-ECMO provides only respiratory support

D. Tandem heart pumps from the left atrium to the aorta

607. A 4-day-old neonate with severe respiratory distress with the following CXR. Most likely diagnosis

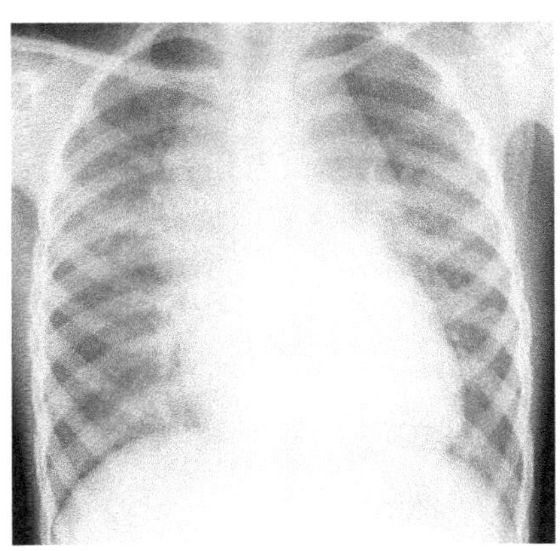

A. Large PDA

B. TGA -VSD

C. VSD -pulmonary atresia

D. Obstructed TAPVC

608. What is the device shown in the chest X-ray

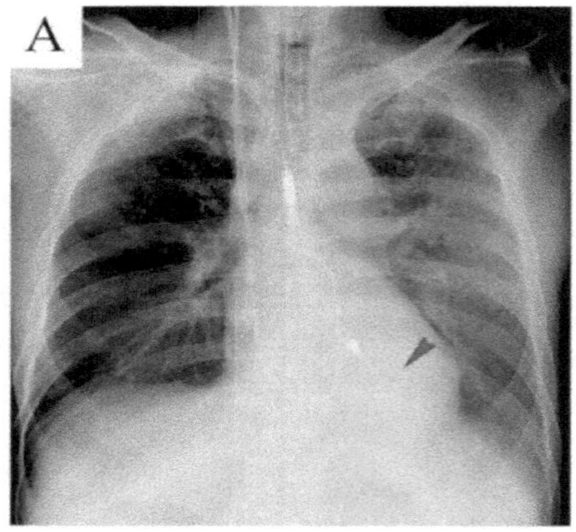

A. LV-Impella

B. Intra-aortic balloon pump

C. pacemaker

D. LVAD

609. Echo picture shown below. Which is not seen in this condition?

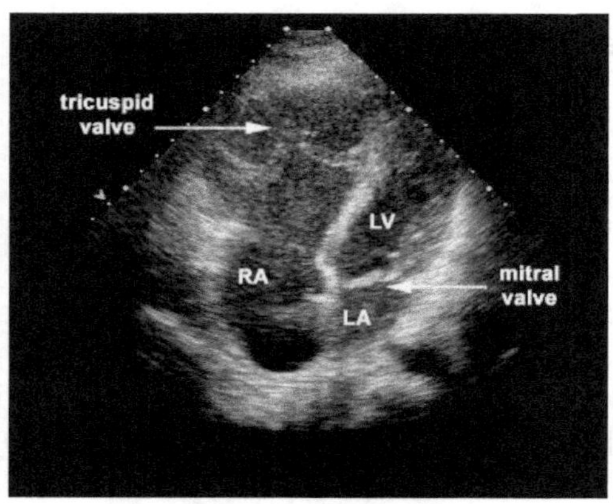

A. Most patients have ASD

B. Multiple heart sounds heard

C. Central Cyanosis

D. Loud P2

610. Correct anticoagulation strategy after prosthetic heart valve implantation

A. After mechanical valve- life-long Warfarin

B. After bioprosthetic valve- anticoagulation for 6 months

C. After TAVI- single antiplatelet

D. After mitral valve repair- lifelong anticoagulation

611. Wrongly matched combination

    A. Anrep effect- increase in contractility with an increase in afterload

    B. Treppe effect- force-frequency relationship

    C. Laplace law- wall tension is directly proportional to chamber dimension

    D. Bernoulli equation- wall stress inversely proportional to wall thickness

612. After complete occlusion of the epicardial artery, all of the following are correct except

    A. Myocyte dysfunction within minutes

    B. Complete necrosis in 6 hours

    C. ATP depletion within seconds

    D. Irreversible injury starts in 20-40 minutes

613. STICH Trial

    A. CABG is non-inferior to medical therapy in ischemic heart failure at 5 years

    B. PCI is superior to medical therapy in low EF

    C. PCI has a survival benefit in high ischemia

    D. CABG is inferior to PCI in diabetes with multivessel CAD

614. An increased A-a gradient suggests

    A. Hypoventilation

    B. V/Q mismatch

    C. High altitude

    D. hypoxemia

615. Which of the following correctly characterises high-output heart failure

    A. Increased cardiac output

    B. Peripheral vasodilation

    C. Increased metabolic demand

    D. All of the above

616. In a patient with mitral stenosis, the LA pressure is not elevated in

    A. Tachycardia

    B. Anaemia

    C. Pregnancy

    D. ASD

617. Continuous murmur is seen in all except

A. Mitral stenosis with ASD

B. TOF with absent pulmonary valve

C. TAPVC

D. Peripheral PS

618. Eisenmengerization involves all except

A. Increase in PA pressure

B. Decrease PVRI

C. Bidirectional shunt

D. Cyanosis

619. Lung uptake in SPECT MPI suggests

A. LV dysfunction

B. No ischemia

C. Mild ischemia

D. Critical LM stenosis

620. All are contraindications of rotational atherectomy except

A. High thrombus burden

B. Significant tortuosity

C. Ostial stenosis

D. Saphenous venous graft

621. Which of the following condition is least associated with CHD

A. Situs inversus with dextrocardia

B. Situs ambiguous with mesocardia

C. Situs inversus with levocardia

D. Situs solitus with dextrocardia

622. CHF is seen in day 1 of life in all except

A. Vein of Galen malformation

B. Hypoplastic left heart syndrome

C. Severe aortic stenosis

D. Large VSD

623. False statement regarding natriuretic peptides

A. BNP level increases with age

B. BNP level increases with BMI

C. Distinguish cardiac Vs non-cardiac dyspnea

D. BNP level is elevated with the use of ARNI

624. False about the use of ARNI

A. Always require a demonstration of prior tolerability of ACEI

B. Increases the level of BNP

C. Risk of AKI

D. Withhold ACEI/ARB for at least 48 hrs before starting ARNI

625. Which of the following drug has not shown any mortality benefit in patients with heart failure

A. Digoxin

B. Isosorbide dinitrate and hydralazine

C. ACEI

D. Metoprolol succinate

626. False statement regarding cardiopulmonary exercise testing

A. Peak VO2 is a marker of cardiac output

B. Peak VO2 may increase up to 18-fold with maximal exercise

C. Peak VO2 and VCO2/VO2 (anaerobic threshold) are useful markers of exercise capacity

D. Peak VO2 <12 ml/kg/min indicates a good prognosis

627. False statement regarding amiodarone

A. Mean elimination half-life is 53 days

B. Dose adjustment not required for renal dysfunction

C. PFT monitoring for chronic use

D. Mortality benefit in patients with ventricular tachycardia after MI

628. False statement regarding supraventricular arrhythmia

A. Short RP- Typical AVNRT and AVRT

B. Typical AVNRT-antegrade conduction to the ventricle via slow pathway

C. Typical atrial flutter usually left atrial origin

D. Pulmonary veins are a common source of atrial fibrillation

629. Patient with a history of syncope while running. ECG at rest was normal. ECG recorded at 5 min exercise during TMT as below. Most likely diagnosis

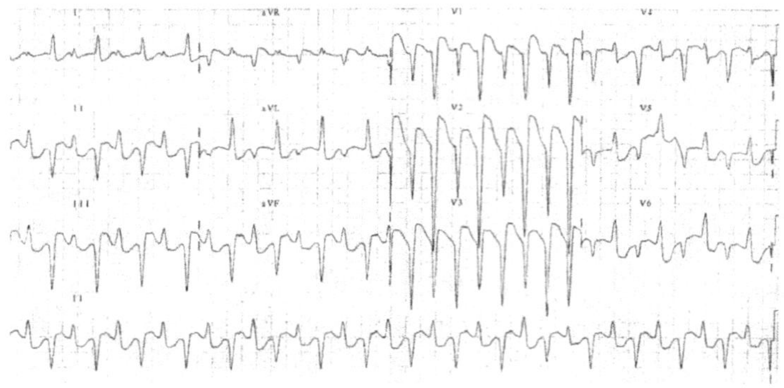

A. Long QT

B. CPVT

C. Brugada

D. RVOT VT

630. Patient with STEMI-AWMI thrombolysis in the community health centre. What should be the next plan?

A. PCI should be performed within 90 minutes

B. Refer to PCI PCI-capable hospital early

C. No further PCI needed

D. Medical stabilization

631. William syndrome, all are true except

A. Mental retardation

B. Hyperthyroidism

C. Hypercalcemia

D. Supravalvular AS

632. Gold standard for RV function estimation

A. Cardiac MRI

B. Speckle tracking echocardiography

C. TEE

D. CT angiography

633. True about ARVC is

A. RBBB morphology VT

B. More common in females

C. Pathological changes are also seen in LV

D. RF ablation is highly successful for treating VT

634. The risk of recurrence of congenital heart disease is highest if the father is affected with

A. Marfan

B. Congenital AS

C. ASD

D. VSD

635. All of the following drugs have shown mortality benefit after MI, except

A. Metoprolol succinate

B. Eplerenone

C. Amiodarone

D. Enalapril

636. True about Takotsubo cardiomyopathy

A. Physical or emotional stress precipitates

B. Common in the elderly

C. ECG evidence of ischemia

D. Normal coronaries

637. A 60-year-old male recently had an extensive anterior wall MI with a large area of akinetic anterior wall on echocardiography. All of the following tests are useful in identifying v able myocardium except

A. Stress echocardiography

B. Exercise ECG

C. Cardiac MRI

D. PET -CT

638. Unequal upper limb pulse can be seen in all except

A. Supravalvular AS

B. NSAA

C. Aortic dissection

D. Marfan

639. All of the following causes hypocalcemia except

A. Acute respiratory alkalosis

B. DiGeorge syndrome

C. Thiazide diuretics

D. Hyperphosphatemia

640. Which is not an indication for surgery in Ebstein anomaly

   A. NYHA II class

   B. Cardiomegaly

   C. Refractory SVT

   D. Paradoxical embolism

641. True about Scimitar syndrome, all except

   A. Systemic arteries from the aorta supply rt lower lung

   B. May be associated with severe PAH

   C. Partial anomalous pulmonary venous drainage to the SVC

   D. The right lung is usually hypoplastic

642. Features of acute severe AR are all except

   A. Normal LV size

   B. Normal pulse pressure

   C. Premature closure of the mitral valve

   D. Long diastolic murmur

643. P2 is not loud in

   A. MS

   B. ASD

   C. Ebstein

   D. Idiopathic PAH

644. Which is not a class I indication for CRT

   A. LBBB with NYHA III

   B. QRS duration > 150ms

   C. LVEF < 35%

   D. RBBB

645. False about coarctation of the aorta

   A. Persistent hypertension is rare after successful treatment

   B. Frequently associated with BAV

   C. May present with LV dysfunction

   D. Mid mid-systolic murmur over the anterior chest may be heard

646. Anticoagulant of choice for HITT

   A. Nadoparin

   B. Fondaparinux

   C. Enoxaparin

   D. Dalteparin

647. True about cardiac involvement in HIV/AIDS

   A. Accelerated atherosclerosis

   B. DCMP is the most common cardiac manifestation

   C. PAH worsen prognosis

   D. All of the above

648. Congenital LQTS is most commonly due to a mutation of which ion channel

   A. Na

   B. K

   C. Ca

   D. Ryr receptor

649. Bundle branch re-entrant tachycardia is characterised by

   A. More common in patients with cardiomyopathy/myocardial scar

   B. Catheter ablation is not useful

   C. RBBB pattern is more common

   D. Common in a structurally normal heart

650. Use of Lithium in the mother is associated with which of the following congenital anomaly in the baby

   A. Ebstein

   B. TGA

   C. ASD

   D. AVSD

651. The most common benign cardiac tumour in children

   A. Papillary fibroelastoma

   B. Atrial myxoma

   C. Rhabdomyoma

   D. Lipoma

652. In heterotaxy, peripheral blood smear are most likely to show

A. Howel Jolly bodies

B. Sickle cell

C. Lymphoblast

D. Spherocyte

653. New onset LBBB during peak exercise suggest

A. Phase 3 block

B. Old MI

C. Coronary spasm

D. Circus movement tachycardia

654. Zilebesiran-False statement is

A. Newer antidiabetic

B. RNA interference of angiotensinogen

C. Six-monthly subcutaneous injections

D. Long-term BP control

655. Which anti-hypertensive agent has been shown to worsen heart failure

A. Doxazocin

B. Lisinopril

C. Chlorthalidone

D. Amlodipine

656. The desmoplakin mutation responsible for

A. Arrhythmogenic cardiomyopathy

B. Dilated cardiomyopathy

C. Cardiac sarcoidosis

D. Ventricular non-compaction

657. Lorundrostat is

A. Aldosterone synthase inhibitor

B. Aldosterone receptor antagonist

C. Newer ACE inhibitor

D. Newer ARB

658. Lorundrostat is evaluated for the management of

A. Resistant hypertension

B. ATTR amyloidosis

C. Adrenal adenoma

D. Heart failure

659. Wilkins' echo score is useful in

A. Mitral valvotomy suitability

B. Aortic valvotomy suitability

C. Mitral valve replacement

D. TAVI

660. The straight left heart border in mitral stenosis is due to

A. LA appendage enlargement

B. Dilated pulmonary trunk

C. Underfilled LV

D. All of these

661. Which is not a contraindication for percutaneous mitral valvotomy in severe MS

A. Large LA clot

B. Severe PAH

C. Moderate MR

D. Severe commissural calcification

662. Which is related to the severity of mitral stenosis

A. S2-OS gap

B. Intensity of MDM

C. Loud S1

D. Loud P2

663. Calculate the mitral valve area with the pressure half-time of 220 ms

A. 1.1 cm2

B. 1.0 cm2

C. 1.2 cm2

D. 2 cm2

664. False statement regarding the hemodynamic consequences of severe mitral stenosis

A. Raised PCWP

B. Raised LVEDP

C. Elevated PA pressure

D. Elevated LA pressure

665. Which of the following auscultatory finding in mitral stenosis suggests a calcified valve

A. Reduced Opening snap intensity

B. Increased s2-os gap

C. Loud S1

D. Loud MDM

666. The primary goal of medical management in severe mitral stenosis is

A. Improve diastole time by controlling heart rate

B. Increase systolic time

C. Reduce LVEDP

D. Improve LA contraction

667. Which of the following trials showed a mortality benefit with MitraClip in heart failure with severe secondary mitral regurgitation

A. MITRA-FR

B. COAPT

C. ISCHEMIA

D. MADIT RIT

668. A 67-year-old male with a history of past inferior wall MI and 2 episodes of heart failure hospitalisation over the last 1 year. He is compliant with optimal medical therapy. Now he is functional class NYHA III and LVEF 27 % with severe secondary MR. What is the next appropriate management?

A. Trans catheter edge-to-edge repair of mitral valve (m-TEER)

B. Mitral valve replacement

C. Continue medical therapy

D. CRT

669. An antiarrhythmic drug contraindicated in coronary artery disease, according to the CAST study

A. Flecainide

B. Amiodarone

C. Sotalol

D. Lidocaine

670. False statement regarding PCWP
    - A. Estimate of LA pressure
    - B. Estimate of RA pressure
    - C. Measured by right heart catheterisation
    - D. A balloon-tipped catheter is useful

671. FINEARTS-HF evaluated the role of
    - A. Evolocumab in HFpEF
    - B. Spironolactone in HFpEF
    - C. Finerenone in HFpEF
    - D. Finerenone in HFrEF

672. False about May-Thurner syndrome
    - A. Recurrent deep venous thrombosis involving the right leg
    - B. The left iliac vein is compressed by the right iliac artery
    - C. Venous stenting may be useful
    - D. Long-term anticoagulation

673. Which of the following is a measure of arterial stiffness
    - A. Pulse wave velocity
    - B. Augmentation index
    - C. Pulse pressure
    - D. All of the above

674. Which of the following methods examines endothelial function
    - A. Brachial artery flow-mediated dilation
    - B. EndoPat
    - C. Invasive coronary angiogram with acetylcholine
    - D. All of the above

675. Role of digitoxin in heart failure with reduced ejection fraction
    - A. Reduces the composite of mortality and heart failure hospitalisation
    - B. Only improve the quality of life
    - C. Does not reduce mortality
    - D. None of these

676. False statement regarding Mavacamten

A. Improve the symptoms in obstructive HCM

B. Similar symptom relief in non-obstructive HCM

C. Cardiac myosin inhibitor

D. Reduces ventricular contractility

677. False statement regarding the use of beta-blocker in MI

A. Routine intravenous metoprolol is recommended during acute MI

B. Not useful in patients after MI with EF >40%

C. Decrease in the incidence of arrhythmic mortality

D. Contraindicated in cardiogenic shock

678. A 22-year-old male complained of progressive dyspnoea for the last 5 years. On probing, his mother revealed a history of recurrent hospitalisation with chest infection during infancy. Examination revealed central cyanosis and oxygen saturation of 86% in the upper limb. Which of the following statement is false about this condition?

A. A shunt murmur is usually absent

B. Cardiomegaly is common

C. Closure of the shunt is not indicated

D. Poor prognosis

679. Which is not a management option in a 21-year-old patient with VSD-Eisenmenger syndrome

A. Shunt closure on priority

B. Iron supplementation

C. Lung transplantation

D. sildenafil

680. Which of the following anti-inflammatory drug has shown benefit in the secondary prevention of CAD

A. Tocilizumab

B. Canakinumab

C. Low dose colchicine

D. All of the above

681. Which of the following is false regarding the management of patients stabilised after acute heart failure

A. ARNI is safe

B. SGLT2 inhibitors should be prescribed

C. Digitoxin has a favourable benefit

D. Rapid (within 2 weeks) uptitration of all drugs detrimental

682. A 58-year-old male with anterior STEMI receives tenecteplase 45 minutes after symptom onset. Thirty minutes later, chest pain subsides, and ECG shows a **wide-complex rhythm at 70 bpm**, QRS morphology similar to LBBB, with occasional sinus capture beats.

A. Failed reperfusion

B. Accelerated idioventricular rhythm (AIVR) — a marker of successful reperfusion

C. Ventricular tachycardia — start amiodarone

D. Junctional rhythm due to inferior MI

683. Which of the following phases is responsible for cardiac automaticity

A. Phase 4

B. Phase 1

C. Phase 3

D. Phase 2

684. Which of the following features differentiates AIVR from ventricular tachycardia

A. Rate <100/min

B. LBBB morphology

C. AV dissociation

D. Presence of fusion beats

685. **The most common site of congenital coronary artery anomaly origin (anomalous coronary from opposite sinus) involves:**

A. Left circumflex from right coronary sinus

B. RCA from left sinus

C. LAD from right sinus

D. LCx from pulmonary artery

686. Treppe phenomena suggest

A. Increase in contractility with an increase in heart rate

B. Increase in contractility with an increase in venous return

C. Increase in contractility with an increase in afterload

D. Increase in contractility with an increase in preload

687. The most specific arrhythmia suggestive of digoxin toxicity

A. Atrial tachycardia with block

B. Regularized AF

C. Multifocal VPC

D. Polymorphic VT

688. The smooth part of the right atrium is developed from

    A. Sinus venosus

    B. Pulmonary veins

    C. Primitive atrium

    D. Septum primum

689. Resting membrane potential of cardiac myocyte

    A. -90 mV

    B. -70 mV

    C. +90 mV

    D. +70 mV

690. **Which coronary artery most commonly supplies the AV node in a right-dominant circulation?**

    A. LAD

    B. LCx

    C. RCA

    D. Posterior descending artery (PDA)

691. a

692. False statement regarding the procedure shown in the picture

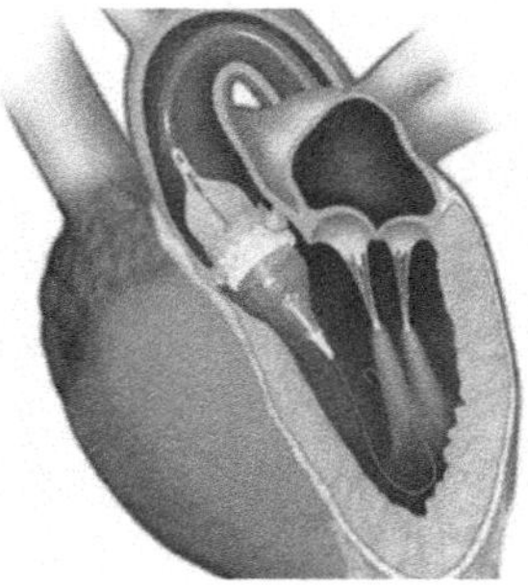

    A. Bioprosthetic valve used

    B. Needs lifelong anticoagulation

    C. Complete heart block is an adverse event

    D. CT assessment of the aortic valve morphology is crucial before the procedure

693. Which is not a predisposition for congenital complete heart block

    A. TOF

    B. Maternal autoantibodies

    C. CCTGA

    D. AVSD

694. False statement regarding the bicuspid aortic valve

A. Aortic stenosis is more common than regurgitation

B. Aortopathy is independent of valvular dysfunction

C. Associated with coarctation of the aorta

D. Right and non-coronary cusp fusion is the commonest type

695. Which trial evaluated the role of TAVI in low surgical risk patients

A. PARTNER 3

B. PARTNER

C. PARTNER2

D. EVEREST

696. Pulse-tracing below indicates

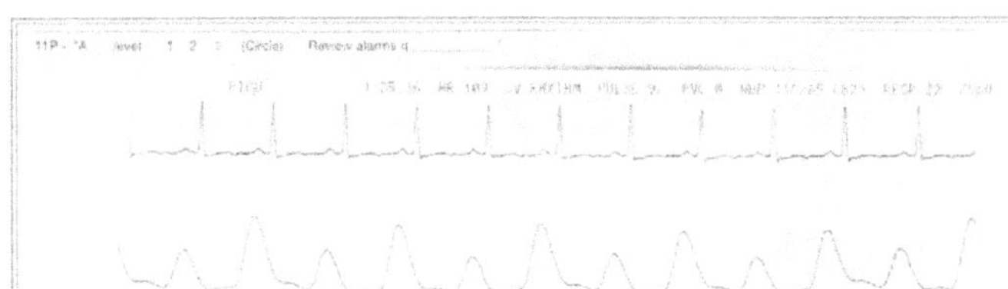

A. Electrical alternans

B. Atrial fibrillation

C. Cardiac tamponade

D. Severe heart failure

697. Pulsus paradoxus is absent despite tamponade in which of the following conditions

A. Severe AR

B. VSD

C. Pericarditis

D. Tubercular effusion

698. A 58-year-old man with hypertension and dyslipidemia presents with exertional chest tightness for the last 6 months. The pain occurs predictably on climbing two flights of stairs and subsides with rest. He denies chest pain or dyspnea at rest. Physical examination is unremarkable. ECG at rest is normal. He is currently on amlodipine 5 mg daily and atorvastatin 20 mg daily. What should be the next step in management?

A. Stress test to assess provokable ischemia

B. Start anti-anginals

C. Decrease statin dose

D. CT coronary calcium assessment

699. A 55-year-old male undergoes primary PCI for proximal LAD occlusion. Angiography reveals an additional 80% RCA and 70% LCx stenosis. Hemodynamically stable post-PCI. What should be the next plan?

A. Leave them untreated

B. Staged PCI of non-culprit lesions before discharge

C. Medical therapy only

D. CABG

700. Wrong statement regarding the following procedure

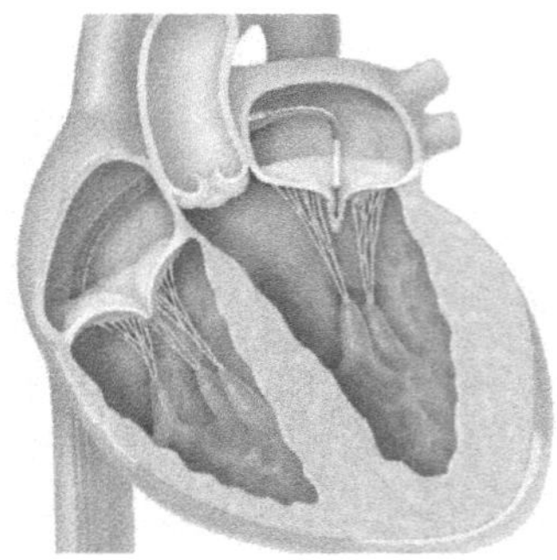

A. Suitable for severe secondary MR

B. Mitral stenosis is a possible complication

C. Alfeiri stitch is a surgical alternative

D. Most suitable for primary MR

701. What is the expected ECG finding of the patient with the following CXR

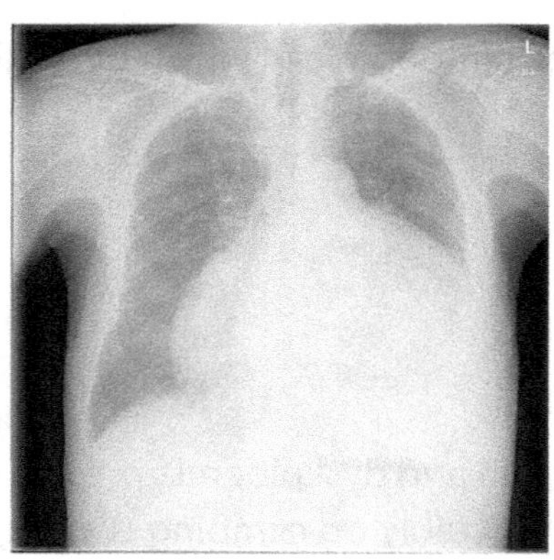

A. Electrical alternans

B. Right axis deviation

C. Biventricular hypertrophy

D. VT

702. Which of the following arrhythmias has the highest success rate for catheter ablation

A. Atrial fibrillation

B. PSVT

C. Atypical flutter

D. MAT

703. The **plateau phase (Phase 2)** of the ventricular action potential is mainly due to:

A. Na^+ influx

B. K^+ efflux

C. Ca^{2+} influx through L-type channels

D. Cl^- movement

704. Which of the following antiarrhythmic drug is contraindicated after MI

A. Esmolol

B. Lidocaine

C. Flecainide

D. Amiodarone

705. A 34-year-old female with progressive dyspnoea visits the OPD. An X-ray of the chest is shown below. What should be the next step in the evaluation?

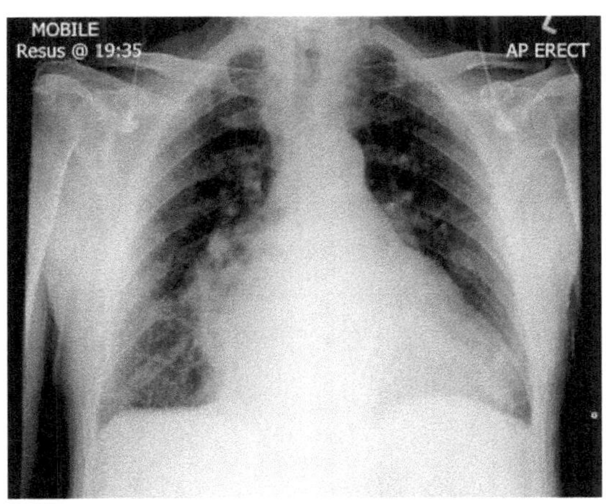

A. Cardiac CT

B. Transthoracic echocardiography

C. Check eosinophil count

D. HRCT Chest

706. Chest compression rate as per ACLS guideline is

A. 100-120/minute

B. 80-100/minute

C. 60-80/minute

D. 90-100/minute

707. **A patient develops hoarseness of voice following percutaneous closure of a patent ductus arteriosus. The most likely cause is injury to:**

A. Right recurrent laryngeal nerve

B. Left vagus nerve

C. Left recurrent laryngeal nerve

D. Thoracic sympathetic chain

708. An 8-month-old infant with a large perimembranous VSD and episodes of hospitalisation with pneumonia. What should be the next line of management?

A. Early surgical closure of VSD

B. Wait till the 1-year completion

C. Medical management and monitoring

D. Cardiac catheterization

709. Katz Wachtel's phenomena indicate

A. Biventricular hypertrophy in VSD

B. Notching of QRS in OS-ASD

C. RBBB after long short cycle

D. R on T phenomena

710. Elderly female in emergency with respiratory distress and hypotension. Bedside POCUS revealed the following image. What should be the next line of management?

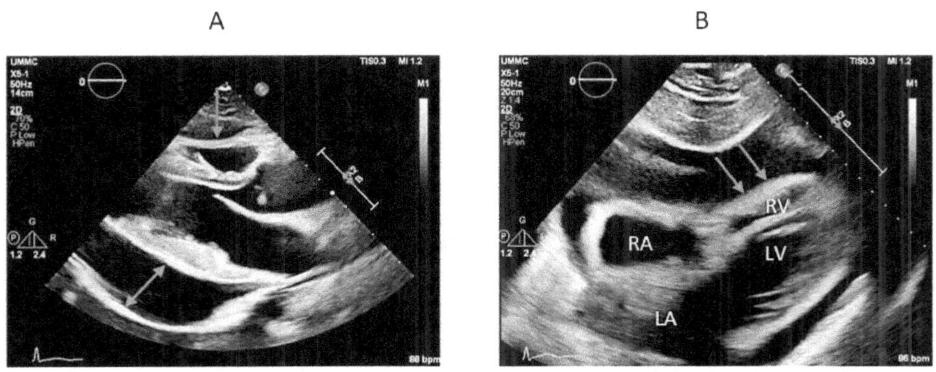

A. Urgent pericardiocentesis

B. Cardiac MRI

C. Inflammatory markers

D. Cardiac CT

711. 35-year-old male with resistant hypertension and progressive dyspnoea. The X-ray chest is shown below. Most likely diagnosis

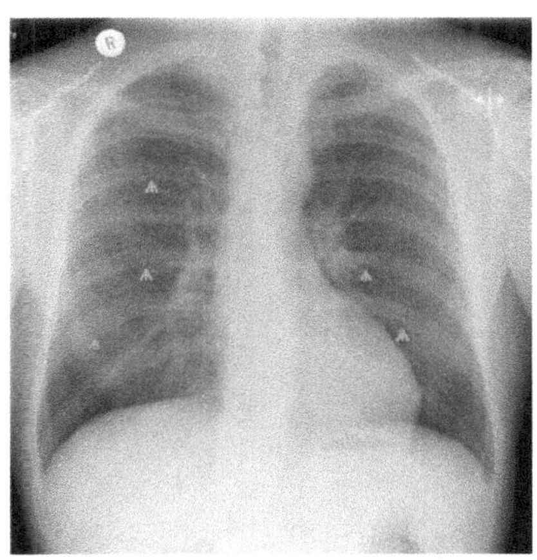

A. Aortic dissection

B. HFpEF

C. Coarctation aorta

D. Renal artery stenosis

712. Which of the following veins is commonly punctured while implanting a permanent pacemaker

A. Axillary vein

B. Superior venacava

C. Left brachial vein

D. Gastroepiploic vein

713. A 36-year-old woman presents with exertional dyspnea. RHC shows: mPAP: 42 mmHg, PCWP: 10 mmHg, CO: 4 L/min and PVR: 8 Wood units. What is the hemodynamic classification

A. Precapillary

B. Postcapillary

C. Mixed

D. Hyperdynamic PH

714. Correct statement regarding the procedure shown in the picture

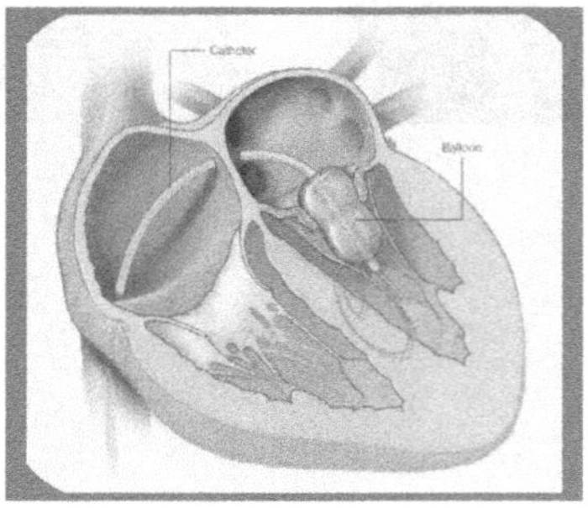

A. Commissural calcification is a contraindication

B. Left atrial thrombus is an indication for the procedure

C. Preferred ed in older individuals

D. A low Wilkins score indicates that the valve is not suitable for balloon valvotomy

715. The Gerbode defect is

A. LV to RA connection

B. RV to LA connection

C. Low velocity jet

D. Low gradient jet

716. False about Laplace law for cardiac wall tension

A. Wall tension is directly proportional to pressure

B. Wall tension is directly proportional to chamber dimension

C. Wall tension is inversely proportional to wall thickness

D. Wall tension is inversely proportional to chamber dimension

717. A 60-year-old male visited the echocardiography lab with a history of dizziness on exertion. Velocity across the aortic valve is 3 m/sec. What is the peak gradient across the aortic valve?

A. 36 mmHg

B. 64 mmHg

C. 60 mmHg

D. 9 mmHg

718. Which is an echocardiographic measure of right ventricular systolic function

A. TAPSE

B. E/a ratio

C. ESPVR

D. E′

719. The following echocardiographic M-mode pattern is seen in

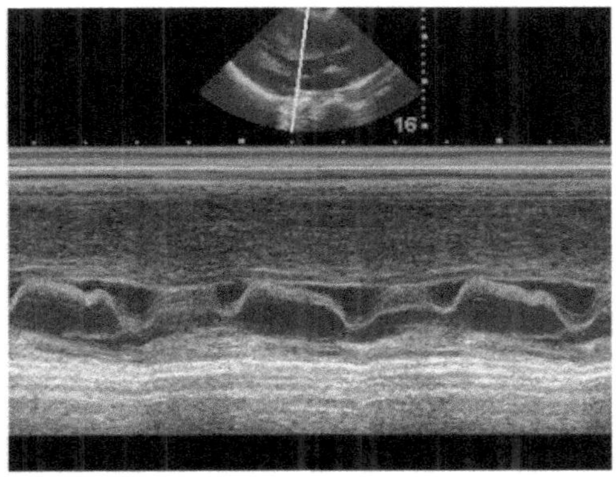

A. ARVC

B. Aortic stenosis

C. Amyloidosis

D. HOCM

720. Which of the following suggests ECG feature suggests posterior MI:

A. ST elevation in V1–V3

B. ST depression with tall R in V1–V3

C. ST elevation in II, III, aVF

D. T-wave inversion in V5–V6

721. AV dissociation with capture and fusion beats is diagnostic of:

A. SVT with aberrancy

B. Ventricular tachycardia

C. Junctional tachycardia

D. AF with pre-excitation

722. Electrical alternans with sinus tachycardia most often indicates:

A. Severe LV systolic dysfunction

B. Large pericardial effusion with tamponade

C. Supraventricular tachycardia

D. Digitalis toxicity

723. **Fragmented QRS** on surface ECG indicates:

A. Atrial conduction delay

B. Local myocardial scar or fibrosis

C. Reversible ischemia

D. Bundle branch block

724. **Epsilon wave** in V1–V3 is seen in:

A. Hypertrophic cardiomyopathy

B. ARVC

C. Brugada syndrome

D. Myocarditis

725. Ventricular tachycardia arising from the RVOT typically shows:

A. RBBB with inferior axis

B. LBBB with superior axis

C. LBBB with inferior axis

D. RBBB with superior axis

726. Differentiating VT from SVT with aberrancy: which of the following favours VT?

A. RS complex in all precordial leads

B. AV dissociation

C. QRS <140 ms

D. Initial R wave in V1

727. During cardiac catheterisation, a patient with dyspnea has: mPAP = 28 mmHg, PCWP = 18 mmHg and CO = 3.5 L/min. Pulmonary vascular resistance (PVR) =?

A. 1 Wood units

B. 3 WU

C. 4 WU

D. 6 WU

728. A 22-year-old male collapses during exercise. ECG shows coved-type ST elevation in V1–V3 with RBBB pattern. Which of the following gene mutations is most likely

A. SCN5A

B. KCNQ1

C. PKP2

D. LMNA

729. Hemodynamic hallmark of cardiac tamponade:

   A. Pulsus paradoxus and equalisation of diastolic pressures

   B. Square-root sign

   C. Kussmaul sign

   D. Elevated LVEDP

730. A 34-year-old woman presents with heart failure. MRI shows mid-myocardial late gadolinium enhancement in the basal septum. Endocardial biopsy revealed a non-caseating granuloma. Most likely diagnosis is

   A. Giant cell myocarditis

   B. Cardiac sarcoidosis

   C. Viral myocarditis

   D. Lymphocytic myocarditis

731. Cardiac resynchronisation therapy (CRT) is most beneficial in:

   A. QRS duration <120 ms

   B. LBBB morphology with QRS ≥150 ms

   C. RBBB with QRS ≥150 ms

   D. Atrial fibrillation with normal QRS

732. Which of the following causes of severe pulmonary hypertension shows a normal pulmonary capillary wedge pressure (PCWP)

   A. HFpEF

   B. Mitral stenosis

   C. Pulmonary veno-occlusive disease

   D. Left atrial myxoma

733. In severe acute AR, which sign is *least reliable*?

   A. Early diastolic murmur

   B. Wide pulse pressure

   C. Hyperdynamic apex beat

   D. Austin-Flint murmur

734. A 40-year-old with Marfan syndrome and an ascending aortic diameter of 5.2 cm. BP = 110/70 mmHg on β-blocker. The best management strategy is

   A. Continue medical therapy

   B. Add ACEI

   C. Schedule elective surgery

   D. Endovascular repair

735. Which condition shows *reverse splitting* of S_2?

A. Pulmonary hypertension

B. ASD

C. LBBB

D. RBBB

736. Which statement is *false* regarding sodium–glucose cotransporter-2 (SGLT2) inhibitors in HF?

A. Reduce CV death and HF hospitalisation

B. Useful in both diabetic and nondiabetic patients

C. Increase preload via osmotic diuresis

D. Contraindicated in eGFR < 20 mL/min/1.73 m^2

737. In cardiac amyloidosis, which ECG–echo combination is *characteristic*?

A. LVH on echo, high QRS voltage

B. Normal echo, low voltage

C. LVH on echo, low QRS voltage

D. Dilated LV, high voltage

738. In an acute STEMI, which reperfusion strategy has the *lowest mortality* when PCI is unavailable within 120 minutes?

A. Fibrinolysis alone

B. Rescue PCI after failed thrombolysis

C. Pharmacoinvasive approach (fibrinolysis → early PCI 3–24 h)

D. Transfer for delayed PCI > 24 h

739. During coronary angiography, a patient develops profound bradycardia and hypotension after RCA injection. Mechanism?

A. Coronary vasospasm

B. Bezold–Jarisch reflex

C. Contrast allergy

D. Coronary dissection

740. A 64-year-old with ischemic cardiomyopathy (LVEF 25%) on optimal GDMT is evaluated for device therapy. ECG shows QRS = 150 ms with LBBB morphology, NYHA III. Which device offers *maximum survival benefit*?

A. ICD alone

B. CRT-P

C. CRT-D

D. No device indicated

741. In restrictive cardiomyopathy, which of the following is *true*?

A. LV systolic dysfunction

B. Thickened myocardium

C. Marked biatrial enlargement

D. Small pericardial effusion

742. The *most specific marker* for myocardial necrosis is:

A. CK-MB

B. Myoglobin

C. Troponin I

D. LDH-1

743. A patient with a prosthetic mitral valve and persistent high-grade fever. Multiple blood cultures were negative. The most likely organism is:

A. Staphylococcus aureus

B. HACEK group

C. Coxiella burnetii

D. Enterococcus faecalis

744. Which of the following drug is *contraindicated* in hypertrophic obstructive cardiomyopathy (HOCM)?

A. Metoprolol

B. Dysopiramide

C. Nitroglycerin

D. Verapamil

745. In acute inferior wall MI with hypotension and clear lungs, the *next step* in management is:

A. Give IV furosemide

B. Start IV nitroglycerin

C. Give IV fluids bolus

D. Immediate β-blocker

746. A 58-year-old hypertensive man presents with sudden tearing chest pain radiating to the back. BP 180/100 mmHg, pulse 90/min. ECG is normal. What should be the next step

A. TEE

B. TTE

C. CT aortogram

D. Coronary angiogram

747. A 52-year-old male with a history of rest angina for the last 2 days presented with acute heart failure. Examination revealed a soft pansystolic murmur over the left parasternal area. The ECG obtained at presentation is shown below. What should be the management plan for this patient?

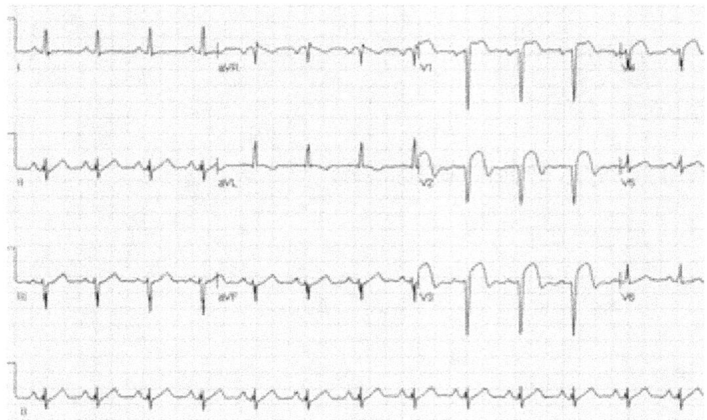

A. Thrombolysis

B. PCI

C. Surgery

D. Medical management only

748. False about Baxdrostat

A. Gyenaecomastia not common

B. Useful in resistant hypertension

C. Hyperkalemia is an adverse effect

D. Aldosterone receptor inhibitor

749. False statement regarding management of NSTEMI

A. Loading antiplatelet with aspirin 300mg

B. Early coronary revascularisation

C. Medical therapy is equally effective

D. CABG is preferred in complex triple-vessel disease

750. A 58-year-old man with a history of chronic smoking and diabetes has had effort angina for the last 6 months. Over the previous 2 days, he has had multiple episodes of rest angina. ECG showed ST depression in precordial leads. What should be the next step in the management

A. CT coronary angiogram

B. Invasive coronary angiogram

C. Stress ECG

D. Stress echocardiography

751. Duke score assessed during

   A. Stress ECG testing

   B. SPECT

   C. Cardiac MRI

   D. CT coronary calcium

752. False statement regarding stress testing in stable CAD

   A. Stress ECG has less diagnostic value

   B. Stress echo is most specific for obstructive CAD

   C. Stress testing is useful in patients with high pretest probability for CAD

   D. Prognosis depends upon the severity of ischemia

753. False statement regarding coronary stents

   A. Increased thrombosis with bioabsorbable scaffold

   B. Use of DES and BMS is equally common now

   C. Intracoronary imaging is useful in stent optimisation

   D. Rotablation is used for calcified coronary stenosis

754. A 42-year-old female with chronic heart failure and an LV ejection fraction of 30%. Which of the following statement is false about the management of this patient

   A. ARNI is preferred over ACE inhibitors

   B. AICD is more useful in non-ischemic than ischemic cardiomyopathy

   C. Digoxin improves quality of life

   D. Vericiguat in patients with worsening heart failure

755. First in man TAVI (transcatheter aortic valve implantation) was done by

   A. Andreas Gruentzig

   B. Alain Cribier

   C. Mason Sones

   D. Mirouski

756. Which investigation modality best differentiates restrictive cardiomyopathy and constrictive pericarditis

   A. Cardiac catheterisation

   B. Echocardiography

   C. Cardiac CT

   D. Transesophageal echocardiography

757. false statement regarding management of Heart failure with preserved EF (HFpEF)

A. NT-proBNP and BNP are useful in the diagnosis and monitoring of therapy

B. ARNI has shown a survival benefit

C. SGLT2 inhibitors reduce CV events

D. Diuretics are useful for decongestion irrespective of aetiology

758. A 24-year-old man had a syncopal attack while playing football. His father had a premature death at the age of 47 years. Evaluation revealed hypertrophic cardiomyopathy with an LV outflow gradient of 2o mmHg. What should be the management choice for this patient?

A. AICD with beta blocker

B. Beta blocker only

C. Assessment with cardiac MRI

D. Endocardial biopsy

759. A 62-year-old man presents with progressive dyspnoea and pedal swelling for the last 6 months. He also complains of a lack of sensation in both hands. Echocardiography revealed hypertrophied ventricles with restrictive filling. Most likely diagnosis is

A. Loefler endocarditis

B. Hypereosinophillic syndrome

C. ATTR amyloidosis

D. Fabry disease

760. Tuberculosis of the heart usually presents as

A. Fulminant myocarditis

B. Chronic pericarditis

C. Ventricular arrhythmia

D. Heart failure

761. Coronary artery calcium is best assessed by

A. Transesophageal echocardiography

B. Cardiac MRI

C. Non-contrast cardiac gated CT

D. Contrast-enhanced cardiac CT

762. False matching about cardiac MRI findings

A. LGE- Fat content

B. Midseptal LGE- Idiopathic DCMP

C. Patchy subendocardial LGE- ICMP

D. Diffuse subendocardial LGE- Amyloidosis

763. A 13-year-old boy was hospitalised with fever, joint pain and dyspnoea for one week. Examination revealed a pansystolic murmur over the precordium. Which of the following statement best describes the management of this condition

A. Lifelong penicillin prophylaxis

B. Steroid helpful for acute rheumatic carditis

C. Erythromycin is preferred over benzathine penicillin for secondary prophylaxis

D. The severity of carditis is not a predictor of chronic rheumatic heart disease

764. A 32-year-old primigravida, diagnosed with severe mitral stenosis in the first trimester of pregnancy. She is minimally symptomatic with dyspnoea and palpitation. Echocardiography revealed a non-calcific mitral valve and a valve area of 0.8 cm2. What should be the best management strategy for this patient?

A. Urgent mitral valve surgery

B. Balloon mitral valvotomy immediately

C. Balloon mitral valvotomy in the second trimester

D. Medical management only and surgery after childbirth

765. The most common cause of primary mitral regurgitation in Western countries is

A. Mitral valve prolapse

B. Ischemic MR

C. Iatrogenic

D. Post-CABG

766. A 37-year-old woman presents with progressive dyspnoea and mild pedal swelling for the last 1 year. Echocardiography revealed a dilated right ventricle and pulmonary artery systolic pressure of 80 mmHg. Contrast-enhanced CT chest revealed evidence of chronic pulmonary embolism involving bilateral proximal pulmonary artery branches. What is the best management option for this patient?

A. Bosentan

B. Selexipag

C. Pulmonary endarterectomy

D. Combination of ambrisentan and tadalafil

767. **A 32-year-old woman** presents with progressive dyspnea on exertion and fatigue over the past 6 months. She denies cough or wheeze. Examination reveals elevated JVP with prominent a-waves, a loud P_2, and a right ventricular heave. ECG shows right axis deviation and RV hypertrophy. Echocardiography confirms right atrial and right ventricular dilatation with an estimated pulmonary artery systolic pressure of 70 mmHg. Routine investigations, including V/Q scan and HRCT, are normal. What is the next best step in management

A. Right heart catheterisation and vasoreactivity testing

B. Empirical high-dose CCB

C. Empirical sildenafil

D. Coronary angiography

768. Sotatercept- an activin signalling inhibitor, useful in

A. Severe PAH

B. AL-amyloidosis

C. Fabry disease

D. ATTR-amyloidosis

769. False about cardioplegia during cardiac surgery

A. Systolic cardiac arrest

B. High potassium-containing solution used

C. Antegrade arrest uses the administration of cardioplegia fluid in the aortic root

D. Retrograde cardioplegia via the coronary sinus

770. False statement regarding surgical coronary revascularisation (CABG)

A. Preferred over PCI in diabetes with multivessel disease

B. Left internal mammary graft has the best long-term outcome

C. Venous graft has a similar outcome to arterial grafts

D. The radial artery can be used as an arterial graft

771. A 60-year-old male has been symptomatic for the last 4 months with progressive dyspnoea and pedal swelling. There are blackening around the eyes and lower backache. The strain imaging bull's-eye map is shown below. Most likely diagnosis is

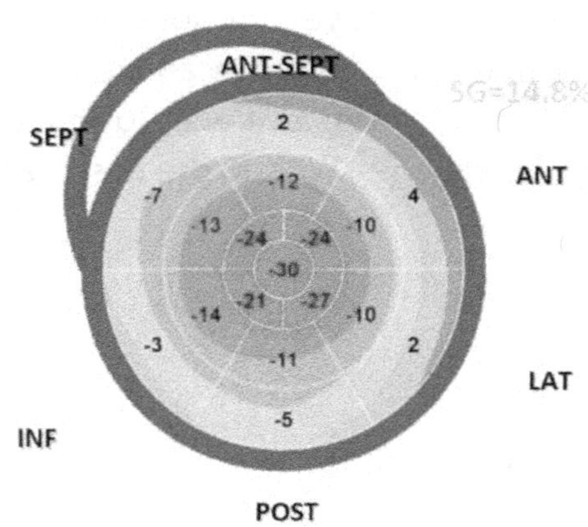

A. Cardiac sarcoidosis

B. Hypertrophic cardiomyopathy

C. Cardiac amyloidosis

D. Hemochromatosis

772. A 24-year-old male had an episode of syncope during sports. His mother had a sudden death at the age of 47 years without prior clinical history. Screening ECG of the patient shown below. What is the most appropriate therapy for this patient?

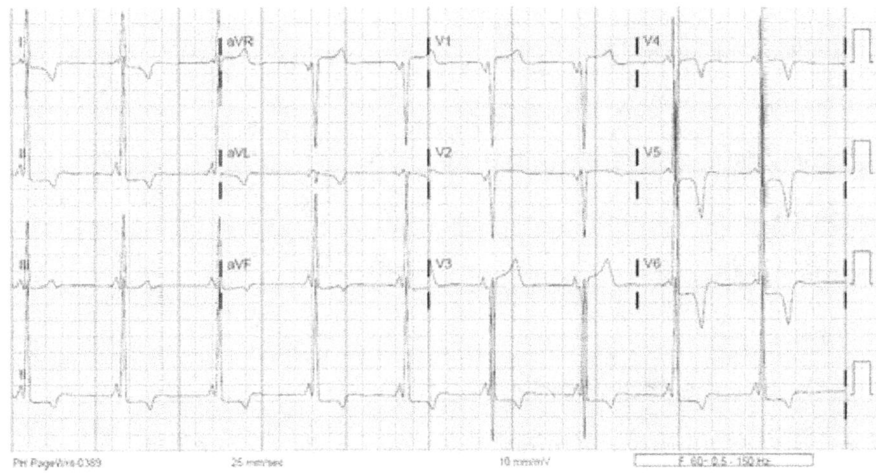

A. ICD implantation

B. Beta blocker

C. Dysopiramide

D. Genetic testing

773. The commonest mutation involved in sarcomeric HCM is

A. MYBPC3

B. TTN

C. MHC

D. MYH

774. Which of the following predicts the chances of sudden cardiac death in hypertrophic cardiomyopathy

A. Very high LV thickness

B. Family history of SCD

C. High LVOT gradient

D. Significant scar in cardiac MRI

775. Which of the following manifestations is most prevalent in acute rheumatic fever

A. Carditis

B. Polyarthritis

C. Chorea

D. Erythema marginatum

776. Preferred treatment option for symptomatic severe mitral stenosis in the 2nd trimester pregnancy

A. BMV (Balloon mitral valvotomy)

B. Surgical valvotomy

C. Mitral valve replacement surgery

D. Medical therapy only

777. Which is not a characteristic of juvenile mitral stenosis-

A. Thromboembolism more common

B. Left atrial enlargement is not common

C. More severe PAH

D. Symptom onset before the 2nd decade

778. A 34-year-old female with a history of progressive dyspnoea for the last 3 years and recent worsening symptoms. Echocardiography revealed severe mitral stenosis with non-calcific mitral leaflets (Valve area 0.8 cm2) and no regurgitation. Which of the following is the most appropriate management for this patient?

A. Medical therapy only

B. Balloon Mitral Valvotomy (BMV)

C. Mitral valve replacement

D. Transcatheter mitral valve replacement (TMVR)

779. Wilkin score, for the assessment of mitral valve before balloon mitral valvotomy, includes all of the following except-

A. Leaflet thickening

B. Leaflet calcification

C. Subvalvular involvement

D. Left atrial thrombus

780. Which of the following findings does not indicate severe mitral stenosis

A. Shortened S2-OS interval

B. Long duration murumur

C. Loud MDM

D. Mitral valve area less than 1 cm2

781. False statement regarding management of ventricular tachycardia

A. ICD is indicated if the LV ejection fraction is less than 30%

B. Amiodarone is indicated in heart failure patients with ventricular tachycardia

C. Catheter ablation is not effective in idiopathic VT

D. Flecainide is contraindicated in CAD patients

782. Causes of bidirectional VT all except

A. Organophosphate poisoning

B. CPVT

C. Aconite toxicity

D. Digoxin toxicity

783. Which of the following antiarrhythmic drugs is contraindicated in a patient with coronary artery disease and heart failure

A. amiodarone

B. lidocaine

C. flecainide

D. sotalol

784. Which of the following statement is false regarding the management of a large atrial septal defect (ASD)

A. Device closure in defects more than 40mm

B. Device closure indicated in the ostium secundum ASD

C. ASD closure is indicated when there is RV volume overload

D. Severe obstructive PAH is a contraindication for shunt closure

785. A 9-month-old infant with a history of recurrent respiratory tract infection and a loud pansystolic murmur visits for a second opinion. Echocardiography revealed a large perimembranous VSD with a dilated left ventricle. Which is the best management option for this patient

A. Surgical closure

B. Device closure

C. Medical stabilisation only

D. Cardiac catheterization

786. Which is not an ECG feature of Tetralogy of Fallot

A. Left axis deviation

B. Right ventricular hypertrophy

C. Sudden transition of R to S in v2/v3

D. Sinus rhythm

787. X-ray chest of a 3-year-old baby with central cyanosis(Spo2- 87%) and a loud systolic murmur at the pulmonary area is shown below. Which of the following statement is false regarding the management of this condition

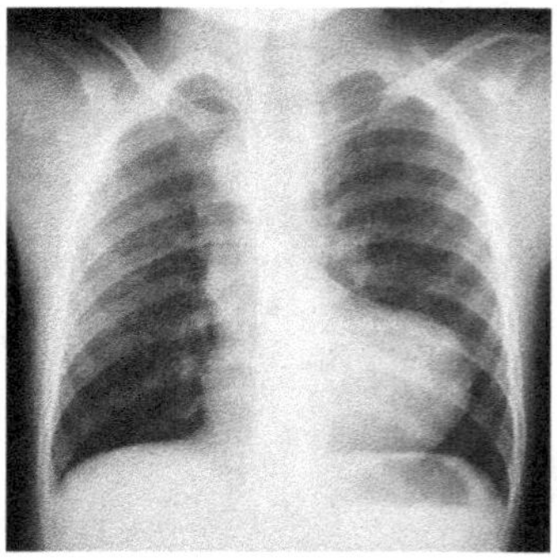

A. Surgical repair is not indicated at this age

B. The BT shunt is indicated in refractory cyanotic spells

C. Beta blockers are useful in spells

D. Severe pulmonary regurgitation if a transannular patch is used for pulmonary stenosis

788. False statement regarding cyanotic congenital heart disease

A. Ebstein anomaly- apical displacement of the mitral leaflet

B. Ventricular inversion on L-TGA

C. Large VSD in tetralogy of Fallot

D. Infracardiac TAPVC is usually obstructive

789. According to the CSI clinical practice guideline, what is the target LDL level recommended in a patient with diabetes and a recent episode of acute coronary syndrome?

A. Less than 100 mg/dl

B. Less than 70 mg/dl

C. Less than 55 mg/dl

D. Less than 40 mg/dl

790. Which of the following lipid-lowering drug is safe in pregnancy

A. Simvastatin

B. Evolocumab

C. Rosuvastatin

D. Bile acid sequestrants

791. Which of the following lipid-lowering drugs causes hyperuricemia/gout

    A. Bempedoic acid

    B. Simvastatin

    C. Gemfibrozil

    D. Incliseran

792. False statement regarding sitostorelemia

    A. ABC transporter mutation

    B. Episodic hemolysis

    C. Rapid response to high-intensity statin

    D. Avoidance of dietary plant sterol-containing food

793. Which of the following drugs acts independent of LDL receptor activity and is recommended in Familial hypercholesterolemia

    A. Evinacumab

    B. Evolocumab

    C. Alirocumab

    D. incliseran

794. Which of the following drug has the maximal LDL-lowering effect

    A. Evolocumab

    B. Rosuvastatin

    C. Bempedoic acid

    D. Ezetimibe

795. False statement regarding Lipoprotein a(Lpa)

    A. Thrombogenic property

    B. Statin lowers Lp(a) level

    C. Pelacarsen newer therapy

    D. Genetically determined risk factor for ASCVD

796. Pulsus paradoxus is seen in

    A. Severe COPD

    B. Tamponade

    C. Constrictive pericarditis

    D. All of the above

797. The most specific clinical sign of severe aortic regurgitation

A. Hill sign

B. Corrigans pulse

C. Increased pulse pressure

D. De musset sign

798. Reverse pulsus paradoxus is seen in

A. HOCM

B. Tamponade

C. Constrictive pericarditis

D. Severe AR

799. False statement regarding hang-out interval

A. Longer for the pulmonary valve than the aortic valve

B. Depends on vascular resistance

C. Responsible for the physiological splitting of the first heart sound (S1)

D. Shortened in pulmonary hypertension

800. The wrong match is

A. Corrigan's pulse- Severe AR

B. Kussmaul's sign- constrictive pericarditis

C. Pulsus paradoxus- cardiac tamponade

D. Fixed split-second heart sound- large VSD

Answer Key Level II

401. B (Ref summary-14)

402. A (Ref summary-16)

403. D, Orthodromic AVRT conducts through the AV node and the normal conduction system, leading to a narrow complex tachycardia (Ref summary-19)

404. C. Both are short RP tachycardia (Ref summary-19)

Both are short RP tachycardia

405. B. JVP elevated in both conditions (Ref summary-12)

406. D (Ref summary-21)

407. A (Ref summary-21)

408. A. AF is common in short QT syndrome (Ref summary-21)

409. B. Phase 2 reentry underlies arrhythmogenesis (Ref summary-21,44)

410. A. Epicardiac RVOT focus may be targeted for ablation in Brugada (Ref summary-21)

411. B (Ref summary-21)

412. B (Ref summary-20)

413. D. Autosomal dominant common (Ref summary-21)

414. B (Ref summary-21)

415. B (Ref summary-19)

416. A. Pulmonary stenosis is predominantly congenital.

417. A (Ref summary-25)

418. A. Balloon dilation is the treatment of choice in critical PS or AS in a neonate

419. B (Ref summary-35)

420. B (Ref summary-26)

421. C. increased filling pressure and dilated LA are hallmarks of diastolic dysfunction. (Ref summary-26)

422. A (Ref summary-32)

423. A (Ref summary-10)

424. D. SGLT2 inhibitors have shown a favourable outcome in HFrEF and HFpEF even in patients without diabetes (Ref summary-8)

425. D. Cardiac MRI is crucial for the diagnosis of cardiac amyloidosis (Ref summary-28)

426. B. Coronary calcium score is useful in low/borderline risk score (Ref summary-44)

427. C (Ref summary-39)

428. A. Elevated in both HFpEF and HFpEF (Ref summary-8)

429. D (Ref summary-2)

430. D (Ref summary-2)
431. D. Short systolic murmur in acute MR
432. A. Flecainide contraindicated in the presence of CAD/structural heart disease (Ref summary-20)
433. C (Ref summary-43)
434. C (Ref summary-34)
435. A (Ref summary-34)
436. D (Ref summary-34)
437. A (Ref summary-34)
438. A. Right arm BP elevated due to Coanda effect (Ref summary-44)
439. B (Ref summary-8)
440. A. Bicuspid aortic valve is very common with coarctation.
441. A (Ref summary-16)
442. C (Ref summary-40)
443. D. High negative predictive value/ruling out value (Ref summary-44)
444. B (Ref summary-7)
445. A (Ref summary-24)
446. A. Increased availability of Na in distal tubules leads to exchange of K and H ions, resulting in hypokalemia and alkalosis.
447. C (Ref summary-25)
448. B (Ref summary-25)
449. D (Ref summary-10)
450. A (Ref summary-10)
451. A (Ref summary-44)
452. A. AV block and bradycardia are common in IWMI with RCA occlusion. (Ref summary-44)
453. B. ECG suggestive of preexcited AF and evidence of preexcitation in baseline ECG. Catheter ablation is strongly indicated to prevent recurrence. (Ref summary-19)
454. B. Epsilon waves and T inversion in precordial leads are characteristic of ARVC (Ref summary-21)
455. A.ECG suggestive of Brugada syndrome, and Quinidine is the drug of choice (Ref summary-21)
456. B (Ref summary-21)
457. A. Evidence of preexcitation/ WPW pattern suggests likely episodes of AVRT (Ref summary-19)
458. A. Coarse AF in mitral stenosis with a dilated left atrium mimics atrial flutter.
459. B. Procainamide is the drug of choice in patients with stable preexcited AF (Ref summary-19)

460. B (Ref summary-34)

461. D. ECG suggestive of regularised AF (AF with complete heart block and regular junctional escape), seen in digoxin toxicity (Ref summary-8)

462. C. ECG suggestive of Wenckebach phenomena, and the usual site of block is AV node (Ref summary-30)

463. A. (Ref summary-41)

464. B. RBBB after a long-short cycle in AF is known as Ashman's phenomenon. Secondary to the longer refractory period of the right bundle.

465. (Ref summary-)

466. A. Warfarin dose up to 5 mg is considered safe in pregnancy (Ref summary-39)

467. A. Cine wave pattern suggestive of hyperkalemia, and Calcium gluconate is the initial drug for cardiac membrane stabilisation.

468. C. Wide QRS slow rhythm with AV dissociation indicate AIVR. Common after reperfusion in MI.

469. B. convex upward ST elevation with PR depression suggestive of acute pericarditis

470. B. Sinus pause in a Holter study suggestive of sick sinus syndrome and a permanent pacemaker indicated (Ref summary-30)

471. A (Ref summary-28)

472. A (Ref summary-28)

473. D (Ref summary-28)

474. B (Ref summary-28)

475. B (Ref summary-3)

476. D (Ref summary-3)

477. A (Ref summary-3)

478. D (Ref summary-21)

479. A (Ref summary-7)

480. C (Ref summary-22)

481. B (Ref summary-19)

482. A (Ref summary-22)

483. B (Ref summary-22)

484. C (Ref summary-22)

485. A (Ref summary-10)

486. B (Ref summary-38)

487. A (Ref summary-38)

488. A (Ref summary-7)

489. A (Ref summary-7)
490. D (Ref summary-44)
491. A (Ref summary-31)
492. D (Ref summary-32)
493. C (Ref summary-32)
494. C. Mipomersan is an antisense oligonucleotide that inhibits apoB production. (Ref summary-32)
495. B (Ref summary-44)
496. D (Ref summary-31)
497. B. AMBITION Trial- Combination of tadalafil and ambrisentan is superior to monotherapy (Ref summary-31)
498. A (Ref summary-31)
499. B. NOAC contraindicated in patients with prosthetic heart valves (Ref summary-18)
500. D (Ref summary-18)
501. D (Ref summary-37)
502. A (Ref summary-16)
503. A (Ref summary-36)
504. B (Ref summary-36)
505. A. Exercise ECG has the least diagnostic value in predicting obstructive CAD amongst all diagnostic tests. (Ref summary-2)
506. B (Ref summary-2)
507. B (Ref summary-8)
508. A. DELIVER, EMPORER PRESERVED trial (Ref summary-9)
509. D (Ref summary-25)
510. B (Ref summary-32)
511. A. Pulsus alternans is seen in LV failure, and electrical alternans in cardiac tamponade. (Ref summary-40)
512. A (Ref summary-)
513. (Ref summary-)
514. A (Ref summary-31)
515. D. CS fistula involves a left-to-right shunt without causing paradoxical embolism.
516. D (Ref summary-40)
517. B (Ref summary-22)
518. A

519. B (Ref summary-39)
520. D. (Ref summary-23)
521. B. Irreversible PAH usually sets in by 2 years of age. (Ref summary-23,24)
522. B (Ref summary-14)
523. A (Ref summary-13)
524. D (Ref summary-25)
525. A (Ref summary-14)
526. A (Ref summary-33)
527. B
528. A (Ref summary-31)
529. A. Chicken wing LAA is the least thrombogenic morphology.
530. A (Ref summary-1)
531. B (Ref summary-21)
532. (Ref summary-)
533. (Ref summary-)
534. D
535. A. Glucagon activates adenylate cyclase, increasing cAMP production, increasing heart rate and contractility independent of beta receptor activity.
536. B. Refer Framingham Heart Study
537. C (Ref summary-8)
538. A. Primary prevention trials with aspirin in diabetes have shown mixed results. (Ref summary-44)
539. A
540. D (Ref summary-19)
541. D. (Ref summary-8)
542. C.
543. (Ref summary-)
544. C (Ref summary-2)
545. C. Phenylephrine is a vasoconstrictor, increases systemic vascular resistance and is used in the management of spells (Ref summary-25)
546. D
547. D (Ref summary-29)
548. B

549. C. ALCAPA (Anomalous origin of left coronary artery from pulmonary artery). Ischemic ECG changes are common. Usually present with heart failure in early childhood.

550. D (Ref summary-25)

551. B. Aorto-mitral continuity is seen in normally related great arteries. D-TGA involves pulmonary-mitral continuity (Ref summary-25)

552. A. 99-67/99-83 = 2. Pulmonary vein saturation is presumed to be 99%. (Ref summary-7)

553. A (Ref summary-25)

554. A (Ref summary-25)

555. D. Hypokalemia due to aldosterone excess (Ref summary-29)

556. A. SERCA activity is reduced with decreased contractility

557. A. Equally seen in male and female (Ref summary-13)

558. C. Safety data of NOAC in pregnancy is not there as of now (Ref summary-39)

559. A (Ref summary-38)

560. A. Asymptomatic mild to moderate PS is usually followed conservatively and does not need surgery.

561. A (Ref summary-44)

562. A. No graft used in arterial switch in TGA where PA and aorta are exchanged surgically (Ref summary-25)

563. D. Regadaneson is a selective agonist with fewer side effects (Ref summary-2)

564. A (Ref summary-2)

565. A (Ref summary-1)

566. C. Load-independent measures of ventricular contractility- ESPVR, Tei index, dp/dt and strain rate.

567. C (Ref summary-36)

568. C (Ref summary-26)

569. A (Ref summary-40)

570. A (Ref summary-7)

571. C. Gerbode defect is usually a high velocity jet, usually >4 m/sec (Ref summary-23)

572. C (Ref summary-10)

573. D. Isometric exercise is associated with an increase in diastolic BP due to sustained muscle contraction.

574. A. An increase in pulse pressure after PVC indicates AS. Decrease in pulse pressure suggests HOCM (Ref summary-7)

575. B

576. B

577. A (Ref summary-25)

578. A. Rsr with r<0.5 indicates RBBB, not RVH.
579. A. VT during exercise/ sympathetic activity (Ref summary-21)
580. A (Ref summary-21)
581. C (Ref summary-37)
582. D (Ref summary-29)
583. C (Ref summary-5)
584. A. Lung uptake suggests increased hold of radiotracers in the lung, indirectly indicating left ventricular dysfunction and raised LVEDP (Ref summary-28)
585. A. 100-120 compression per minute as per ACLS guideline
586. D. Murmur in the left 2nd intercostal space indicates increased flow across the pulmonary valve. Increased flow is associated with MS/MR due to increased left-to-right shunt. Eisenmanger leads to decreased pulmonary flow and a decrease in the flow murmur.
587. C (Ref summary-1)
588. C (Ref summary-26)
589. A (Ref summary-5)
590. B (Ref summary-44)
591. B. Hypertensive heart disease usually leads to diastolic heart failure (HFpEF) without cardiomegaly.
592. A. EPS and catheter ablation indicated.
593. A
594. A (Ref summary-39)
595. D (Ref summary-4)
596. D. TOTAL trial- Manual aspiration thrombectomy during primary angioplasty does not have a mortality benefit and increases stroke risk (Ref summary-4)
597. A. Trial comparing Warfarin Vs Rivaroxaban in rheumatic AF, stopped early due to increased events in the rivaroxaban arm.
598. A (Ref summary-38)
599. A (Ref summary-19)
600. C (Ref summary-11)
601. B (Ref summary-32)
602. B (Ref summary-32)
603. C. Endocarditis risk is similar between mechanical and bioprosthetic valves (Ref summary-18)
604. D (Ref summary-36)
605. D. ECG of severe LVH suggestive of HCM. Cardiac MRI should be done next to further characterise and assess LGE (Ref summary-10)

606. A. SBP usually decreases with IABP and increases MAP and DBP (Ref summary-41)
607. D (Ref summary-25)
608. A (Ref summary-41)
609. D. P2 is usually soft in Ebstein anomaly (Ref summary-25)
610. D. Anticoagulation is not indicated after valve repair. (Ref summary-18)
611. D (Ref summary-43)
612. B. Complete necrosis by 12 to 24 hours.
613. A. Refer to the STITCH and STITCHES trials
614. B. Increased A-a gradient suggests V/Q mismatch, and decreased gradient suggests hypoventilation
615. D. All are features of high-output heart failure.
616. D. Presence of ASD decompresses LA pressure in mitral stenosis.
617. B (Ref summary-40)
618. B (Ref summary-24)
619. A (Ref summary-28)
620. C (Ref summary-5)
621. A. Situs inversus dextrocardia is usually not associated with congenital heart disease.
622. D. PA pressure is high at birth and does not allow a severe shunt in a large VSD. VSD usually become symptomatic over days as PA pressure falls.
623. B (Ref summary-8)
624. A (Ref summary-8)
625. A (Ref summary-8)
626. D
627. D. No antiarrhythmic drug has shown mortality benefit in ventricular tachycardia.
628. C. Cavotricuspid isthmus is the common source of atrial flutter. (Ref summary-19)
629. B (Ref summary-21)
630. B (Ref summary-4)
631. B. (Ref summary-35)
632. A
633. C (Ref summary-21)
634. B. Congenital AS/Bicuspid aortic valve/HLHS has the highest paternal inheritance.
635. C. Antiarrhythmic drugs have not shown survival benefit after MI.
636. B. Common in young females.

637. B (Ref summary-2)
638. D. (Ref summary-44)
639. C. Thiazide causes hypercalcemia
640. A (Ref summary-25)
641. C. PAPVC draining to IVC. (Ref summary-23)
642. D. Short early diastolic murmur is seen in acute AR due to raised LVEDP in a non-dilated ventricle. (Ref summary-40)
643. C (Ref summary-40)
644. D (Ref summary-8)
645. A (Ref summary-44)
646. B (Ref summary-44)
647. D
648. B (Ref summary-21)
649. A (Ref summary-20)
650. A
651. C (Ref summary-36)
652. A. Absent spleen leads to Howell-Jolly bodies in RBC. Right isomerism causes asplenia
653. A (Ref summary-30)
654. A (Ref summary-29)
655. A (Ref summary- 38, ALLHAT trial)
656. A (Ref summary-21)
657. A. Aldosterone synthase inhibitor (Ref summary-29)
658. A. Aldosterone synthase inhibitor for resistant hypertension (Ref summary-29)
659. A (Ref summary-14)
660. D (Ref summary-14)
661. B (Ref summary-14)
662. A (Ref summary-14)
663. B (Ref summary-14)
664. B, LVEDP is usually normal in MS (Ref summary-14)
665. A (Ref summary-14)
666. A (Ref summary-14)
667. B (Ref summary-15)

668. A (Ref summary-15)

669. A (Ref summary-20)

670. B (Ref summary-7)

671. C (Ref summary-9)

672. A. recurrent DVT of the left leg due to mechanical compression of the left iliac vein by the right iliac artery.

673. D (Ref summary-44)

674. D (Ref summary-44)

675. A. DIGIT-HF trial (Ref summary-8)

676. B. ODISSY-HCM trial- no clinical benefit in non-obstructive HCM (Ref summary-10)

677. A (Ref summary-4)

678. B. Cardiomegaly is uncommon in Eisenmenger syndrome (Ref summary-24)

679. A (Ref summary-24)

680. D (Ref summary-33)

681. D. STRONG-HF trial (Ref summary-8)

682. B. AIVR is a marker of reperfusion.

683. A. Phase 4 potential in the SA nodal cell is responsible for automaticity (Ref summary-43)

684. A. AIVR has all the features of VT except rate.

685. A. LCX from the right coronary sinus is the commonest coronary anomaly

686. A (Ref summary-43)

687. B (Ref summary-8)

688. A (Ref summary-34)

689. A. (Ref summary-43)

690. C. (Ref summary-34)

691. (Ref summary-)

692. B. Antiplatelet is enough for the bioprosthetic valve in TAVI (Ref summary-16)

693. A. (Ref summary-30)

694. D (Ref summary-16)

695. A (Ref summary-16)

696. D. Pulsus alternans is seen in severe heart failure (Ref summary-40)

697. A. Severe AR and ASD, where pulsus paradoxus is absent despite tamponade (Ref summary-40)

698. A (Ref summary-1)

699. B (Ref summary-4)

700. D (Ref summary-15)

701. A. Low voltage complex with electrical alternans is expected in massive pericardial effusion.

702. B. Success rate is more than 90% in PSVT.

703. C (Ref summary-43)

704. C (Ref summary-20)

705. B. CXR suggestive of mitral stenosis. Echocardiography should be the next step to confirm the diagnosis. (Ref summary-14)

706. A

707. C. The left recurrent laryngeal nerve is likely to be affected by PDA device closure

708. A. Large VSD should be closed before the age of 1 year to prevent the development of irreversible vascular changes (Ref summary-23)

709. A (Ref summary-23)

710. A. Echofree space around myocardium and RV collapse suggests pericardial tamponade (Ref summary-26)

711. C. Clinical details and rib notching in CXR suggest coarctation of the aorta (Ref summary-44)

712. A (Ref summary-42)

713. B. Normal PCWP with elevated PVRI suggests precapillary PH (Ref summary-7)

714. A. Picture of BMV procedure (Ref summary-14)

715. A. LV to RA connection with high velocity jet (Ref summary-23)

716. D. $T = P\, r/2t$, P- pressure, r- radius, t-wall thickness

717. A. Peak gradient = 4 V2 (Ref summary-26)

718. A (Ref summary-26)

719. D. LVH with SAM is characteristic of HOCM (Ref summary-10)

720. B (Ref summary-45)

721. B (Ref summary-20)

722. B

723. B

724. B (Ref summary-21)

725. C (Ref summary-20)

726. B (Ref summary-20)

727. B. $PVR = [28 - 18]/3.5 = 2.85 \approx 3$ WU (Ref summary-7)

728. A (Ref summary-21)

729. A

730. B (Ref summary-11)

731. B (Ref summary-8)

732. C. PCWP is elevated in left heart pathology

733. B. Wide pulse pressure may not be there in acute severe AR (Ref summary-17)

734. C. High risk of dissection once the aortic diameter is over 5 cm

735. C. (Ref summary-40)

736. C. Decrease preload by diuresis mechanism (Ref summary-8)

737. C. LVH on echo, but ECG voltages are low due to damping of voltage by amyloid infiltration. (Ref summary-11)

738. C (Ref summary-4)

739. C. Increased vagal activity due to stimulation of ventricular mechanoreceptors. Common in inferior wall MI

740. C. LBBB with a wide QRS would benefit from CRT, and LVEF less than 35% is a candidate for AICD. CRTD is ideal for this patient.

741. C. Normal ventricular thickness, diastolic dysfunction and marker biatrial enlargement are characteristic of RCMP (Ref summary-12)

742. C

743. C. Bartonella, Brucella, Coxiella, Legionella, and Tropheryma do not grow in routine culture media, causing IE (Ref summary-37)

744. C. Nitrates reduce preload and afterload, increasing LVOT obstruction, and should be avoided in HOCM (Ref summary-10)

745. C. IV fluids in this situation, as RV is preload-dependent. Nitroglycerin should be avoided as it reduces preload.

746. C. Clinical details suggestive of aortic dissection.

747. C. Pansystolic murmur in the setting of STEMI suggests ventricular septal rupture, for which surgical closure in required.

748. D. Baxdrostat is a newer aldosterone synthesis inhibitor (Ref summary-29)

749. C. Revascularisation with PCI/CABG has a mortality benefit in ACS (Ref summary-3)

750. B (Ref summary-1)

751. A (Ref summary-2)

752. C (Ref summary-2)

753. B (Ref summary-5)

754. B. DANISH trial showed better survival benefit of AICD in ischemic cardiomyopathy (Ref summary-8)

755. B (Ref summary-6)

756. A (Ref summary-12)

757. B (Ref summary-9)

758. A. Syncope is an indication for AICD in HCM. Beta blocker for symptomatic relief of LVOT obstruction. (Ref summary-10)

759. B. RCMP with sensory neuropathy points towards ATTR amyloidosis (Ref summary-11)

760. B. Chronic pericarditis with effusion is the commonest affection of TB in the heart.

761. C (Ref summary-27)

762. A. LGE indicates fibrosis in the myocardium (Ref summary-27)

763. B (Ref summary-13)

764. C (Ref summary-14)

765. A (Ref summary-15)

766. C. Clinical details consistent with CTEPH (Ref summary-31)

767. A. Right heart catheterisation to confirm PAH and vasoreactivity testing to predict the effect of CCB (Ref summary-31)

768. A. STELLAR, HYPERION Trial (Ref summary-31)

769. A. Diastolic arrest using a high concentration of potassium-containing solution (Ref summary-44)

770. C. Venous grafts occlude faster than arterial grafts (Ref summary-44)

771. C. Cherry on the top pattern is characteristic of cardiac amyloidosis (Ref summary-11)

772. A. ECG suggestive of HCM and clinical history indicative of high risk for SCD (Ref summary-10)

773. A (Ref summary-10)

774. C (Ref summary-10)

775. A (Ref summary-13)

776. A (Ref summary-14)

777. A (Ref summary-14)

778. B (Ref summary-14)

779. D (Ref summary-14)

780. C (Ref summary-14)

781. C (Ref summary-20)

782. A (Ref summary-20)

783. C (Ref summary-20)

784. A. Device closure is possible in defects up to 40mm (Ref summary-23)

785. A (Ref summary-23)

786. A. Right axis deviation and RVH are seen in TOF. (Ref summary-25)

787. A. X-ray and clinical details of TOF. Surgery is indicated in childhood irrespective of age. (Ref summary-25)

788. A (Ref summary-25)

789. C (Ref summary-32)

790. D (Ref summary-32)

791. A (Ref summary-32)

792. C. No response to statin (Ref summary-32)

793. A (Ref summary-32)

794. A (Ref summary-32)

795. B. (Ref summary-32)

796. D. (Ref summary-40)

797. A. (Ref summary-17)

798. A. (Ref summary-40)

799. C. Physiological splitting of S2 (Ref summary-40)

800. D. Fixed split S2 seen in large ASD (Ref summary-40)

www.ingramcontent.com/pod-product-compliance
Lightning Source LLC
LaVergne TN
LVHW060022210926
848481LV00013B/3767
* 9 7 9 8 9 0 3 9 2 9 3 6 8 *